T0198201

Advances in Radiotherapy

Editor

TERENCE M. WILLIAMS

SURGICAL ONCOLOGY CLINICS OF NORTH AMERICA

www.surgonc.theclinics.com

Consulting Editor
TIMOTHY M. PAWLIK

July 2023 • Volume 32 • Number 3

ELSEVIER

1600 John F. Kennedy Boulevard • Suite 1800 • Philadelphia, Pennsylvania, 19103-2899

http://www.theclinics.com

SURGICAL ONCOLOGY CLINICS OF NORTH AMERICA Volume 32, Number 3
July 2023 ISSN 1055-3207, ISBN-13: 978-0-443-18213-6

Editor: John Vassallo (j.vassallo@elsevier.com)
Developmental Editor: Malvika Shah

Surgical Oncology Clinics of North America (ISSN 1055-3207) is published quarterly by Elsevier Inc., 360 Park Avenue South, New York, NY 10010-1710. Months of publication are January, April, July, and October. Business and Editorial Offices: 1600 John F. Kennedy Blvd., Ste. 1800, Philadelphia, PA 19103-2899. Customer Service Office: 3251 Riverport Lane, Maryland Heights, MO 63043. Periodicals postage paid at New York, NY and additional mailing offices. Subscription prices are $335.00 per year (US individuals), $651.00 (US institutions) $100.00 (US student/resident), $374.00 (Canadian individuals), $823.00 (Canadian institutions), $100.00 (Canadian student/resident), $484.00 (foreign individuals), $823.00 (foreign institutions), and $205.00 (foreign student/resident). Foreign air speed delivery is included in all *Clinics* subscription prices. All prices are subject to change without notice. **POSTMASTER**: Send address changes to *Surgical Oncology Clinics of North America,* Elsevier Health Science Division, Subscription Customer Service, 3251 Riverport Lane, Maryland Heights, MO 63043. **Customer Service: 1-800-654-2452 (US and Canada). 314-447-8871 (outside US and Canada). Fax: 314-447-8029. E-mail: journalscustomerservice-usa@elsevier.com (for print support); journalsonline support-usa@elsevier.com (for online support).**

Reprints. For copies of 100 or more, of articles in this publication, please contact the Commercial Reprints Department, Elsevier Inc., 360 Park Avenue South, New York, New York 10010-1710. Tel. 212-633-3874; Fax: 212-633-3820; E-mail: reprints@elsevier.com.

Surgical Oncology Clinics of North America is covered in *MEDLINE/PubMed (Index Medicus) and EMBASE/ Excerpta Medica, Current Contents/Clinical Medicine, and ISI/BIOMED.*

Contributors

CONSULTING EDITOR

TIMOTHY M. PAWLIK, MD, MPH, PhD, FACS, FRACS (Hon.)
Professor and Chair, Department of Surgery; The Urban Meyer III and Shelley Meyer Chair
for Cancer Research; Professor of Surgery, Oncology, and Health Services Management
and Policy; Surgeon in Chief; The Ohio State University, Wexner Medical Center,
Columbus, Ohio

EDITOR

TERENCE M. WILLIAMS, MD, PhD
Professor and Chair, Department of Radiation Oncology, City of Hope National Medical
Center, Duarte, California

AUTHORS

ARYA AMINI, MD
Associate Professor, Department of Radiation Oncology, City of Hope National Medical
Center, Duarte, California

JOSE G. BAZAN, MD, MS
Associate Professor, Department of Radiation Oncology, The Ohio State University
Wexner Medical Center, The Arthur G. James Cancer Hospital and Solove Research
Institute, The Ohio State University Comprehensive Cancer Center, Columbus, Ohio

SASHA J. BEYER, MD, PhD
Department of Radiation Oncology, The Ohio State University Wexner Medical Center,
Columbus, Ohio

DUKAGJIN M. BLAKAJ, MD, PhD
Department of Radiation Oncology, The Ohio State University Wexner Medical Center,
Columbus, Ohio

MICHAEL D. CHUONG, MD
Department of Radiation Oncology, Miami Cancer Institute, Miami, Florida

JOSHUA CINICOLA, PharmD, RPh
Ernest Mario School of Pharmacy, Rutgers University, Piscataway, New Jersey

KYLE C. CUNEO, MD
Associate Professor, Department of Radiation Oncology, University of Michigan, Ann
Arbor, Michigan

SAVITA DANDAPANI, MD, PhD
Associate Professor, Department of Radiation Oncology, City of Hope National Medical
Center, Duarte, California

MATTHEW P. DEEK, MD
Department of Radiation Oncology, Rutgers Cancer Institute of New Jersey, Rutgers Robert Wood Johnson School of Medicine, Rutgers University, New Brunswick, New Jersey

NICHOLAS EUSTACE, MD, PhD
Resident Physician, Department of Radiation Oncology, City of Hope National Medical Center, Duarte, California

SHERA FEINSTEIN, MD
Department of Radiation Oncology, University of California, Davis Medical Center, Sacramento, California

SUJANA GOTTUMUKKALA, MD
Department of Radiation Oncology, University of Texas Southwestern, Dallas, Texas

CLAIRE HAO, BS
Clinical Research Associate, Department of Radiation Oncology, City of Hope National Medical Center, Duarte, California

DANIEL J. HERR, MD, PhD
Department of Radiation Oncology, University of Michigan, Ann Arbor, Michigan

JARED HUNT
Department of Radiation Oncology, University of California, Davis Medical Center, Sacramento, California

DANIEL E. HYER, PhD
Department of Radiation Oncology, University of Iowa, Iowa City, Iowa

SALMA K. JABBOUR, MD, FASTRO
Department of Radiation Oncology, Rutgers Cancer Institute of New Jersey, Rutgers Robert Wood Johnson School of Medicine, Rutgers University, New Brunswick, New Jersey

ARI KASSARDJIAN, MD
Department of Radiation Oncology, City of Hope National Medical Center, Duarte, California

SOO KYOUNG KIM, MD
Department of Radiation Oncology, University of California, Davis Medical Center, Sacramento, California

AMAR U. KISHAN, MD
Department of Radiation Oncology, University of California, Los Angeles, Los Angeles, California

COLTON LADBURY, MD
Resident Physician, Department of Radiation Oncology, City of Hope National Medical Center, Duarte, California

ALEXANDER LIN, MD
Department of Radiation Oncology, Perelman School of Medicine, University of Pennsylvania, Philadelphia, Pennsylvania

TIMOTHY LIN, MD, MBA
Department of Radiation Oncology, Department of Molecular Radiation Sciences, Johns Hopkins School of Medicine, Baltimore, Maryland

SWATI MAMIDANNA, MD
Department of Radiation Oncology, Rutgers Cancer Institute of New Jersey, Rutgers Robert Wood Johnson School of Medicine, Rutgers University, New Brunswick, New Jersey

JENNIFER K. MATSUI, PhD
College of Medicine, The Ohio State University, Columbus, Ohio

ALIAH MCCALLA, BS
College of Medicine, Central Michigan University, Mount Pleasant, Michigan

ERIC D. MILLER, MD, PhD
Department of Radiation Oncology, The Ohio State University, Comprehensive Cancer Center, Columbus, Ohio

ARTA M. MONJAZEB, MD, PhD
Professor of Radiation Oncology, Department of Radiation Oncology, University of California, Davis Medical Center, Sacramento, California

AMOL NARANG, MD
Department of Radiation Oncology, Department of Molecular Radiation Sciences, Johns Hopkins School of Medicine, Baltimore, Maryland

RUSSELL F. PALM, MD
Department of Radiation Oncology, Moffitt Cancer Center, Tampa, Florida

JOSHUA D. PALMER, MD
Department of Radiation Oncology, The Ohio State University Wexner Medical Center, Columbus, Ohio

HALEY K. PERLOW, MD
Department of Radiation Oncology, The Ohio State University Wexner Medical Center, Columbus, Ohio

RAJU R. RAVAL, MD, DPhil
Department of Radiation Oncology, The Ohio State University Wexner Medical Center, Columbus, Ohio

ALEX R. RITTER, MD
Department of Radiation Oncology, The Ohio State University Comprehensive Cancer Center, Department of Radiation Oncology, Arthur G. James Cancer Hospital and Richard J. Solove Research Institute, Columbus, Ohio

SAMER SALAMEKH, MD
Cancer Specialists of North Florida, Jacksonville, Florida

NINA N. SANFORD, MD
Department of Radiation Oncology, University of Texas Southwestern, Dallas, Texas

KRISTEN SPENCER, DO, MPH
New York Langone Perlmutter Cancer Center, New York, New York

ANDREW TAM, MD
Department of Radiation Oncology, City of Hope National Medical Center, Duarte, California

EVAN M. THOMAS, MD, PhD
Department of Radiation Oncology, The Ohio State University Wexner Medical Center, Columbus, Ohio

MICHAEL C. TJONG, MD, MPH
Department of Radiation Oncology, Dana-Farber Cancer Institute, Boston, Massachusetts

JACOB TROTTER, MD
Department of Radiation Oncology, Perelman School of Medicine, University of Pennsylvania, Philadelphia, Pennsylvania

RITURAJ UPADHYAY, MD
Department of Radiation Oncology, The Ohio State University Wexner Medical Center, Columbus, Ohio

CHARLES X. WANG, MD, PhD
Department of Radiation Oncology, University of California, Davis Medical Center, Sacramento, California

HOWARD WEST, MD
Department of Medical Oncology, City of Hope National Medical Center, Duarte, California

TERENCE M. WILLIAMS, MD, PhD
Professor and Chair, Department of Radiation Oncology, City of Hope National Medical Center, Duarte, California

JEFFREY WONG, MD
Professor, Department of Radiation Oncology, City of Hope National Medical Center, Duarte, California

NIKHIL YEGYA-RAMAN, MD
Department of Radiation Oncology, University of Pennsylvania, Philadelphia, Pennsylvania

Contents

Studies suggest select patients from across the pancreatic adenocarcinoma (PDAC) disease spectrum may benefit from adding radiation therapy
(RT) to multi-modality care. In resectable PDAC, there is an evolving role
for neoadjuvant RT with adjuvant RT reserved for patients with increased
recurrence risk. In borderline resectable PDAC, neoadjuvant chemoradiation likely improves R0 resection rates and in unresectable PDAC, definitive RT may prolong survival for some patients. Recent developments in
RT delivery are promising but additional studies are needed to determine
the benefit of these technologies and to optimize the role of RT in multimodality care.

During the past 30 years, several advances have been made allowing for
safer and more effective treatment of patients with liver cancer. This report
reviews recent advances in radiation therapy for primary liver cancers
including hepatocellular carcinoma and intrahepatic cholangiocarcinoma.
First, studies focusing on liver stereotactic body radiation therapy (SBRT)
are reviewed focusing on lessons learned and knowledge gained from
early pioneering trials. Then, new technologies to enhance SBRT treatments are explored including adaptive therapy and MRI-guided and
biology-guided radiation therapy. Finally, treatment with Y-90 transarterial
radioembolization is reviewed with a focus on novel approaches focused
on personalized therapy.

Esophageal cancer is the eighth most common cancer worldwide and is
the sixth most common cause of cancer-related mortality. The paradigm
has shifted to include a multimodality approach with surgery, chemotherapy, targeted therapy (including immunotherapy), and radiation therapy. Advances in radiotherapy through techniques such as intensity
modulated radiotherapy and proton beam therapy have allowed for the

more dose homogeneity and improved organ sparing. In addition, recent studies of targeted therapies and predictive approaches in patients with locally advanced disease provide clinicians with new approaches to modify multimodality treatment to improve clinical outcomes.

The current preferred standard of care management for patients with locally advanced rectal cancer is total neoadjuvant therapy, in which all chemotherapy and radiotherapy is delivered before surgery. Within this approach, developed in response to persistently high distant failure rates despite excellent local control with preoperative chemoradiotherapy, there remains questions regarding the optimal radiotherapy regimen (short course vs long course) and sequencing of chemotherapy (induction vs consolidation).

The development of large-field intensity-modulated radiation therapy (IMRT) has enabled the implementation of total marrow irradiation (TMI), total marrow and lymphoid irradiation (TMLI), and IMRT total body irradiation (TBI). IMRT TBI limits doses to organs at risk, primarily the lungs and in some cases the kidneys and lenses, which may mitigate complications. TMI/TMLI allows for dose escalation above TBI radiation therapy doses to malignant sites while still sparing organs at risk. Although still sparingly used, these techniques have established feasibility and demonstrated promise in reducing the adverse effects of TBI while maintaining and potentially improving survival outcomes.

Oligoprogressive disease (OPD) is an emerging concept that describes patients who have progression of disease in a limited number of metastatic sites while on systemic therapy. Growing evidence has suggested the integration of local ablative therapy with systemic agents in patients with OPD further improves survival. In oligoprogressive non-small cell lung cancer, stereotactic body radiotherapy may have an important role in the effective local control of selective progressing metastases, which may translate to better patient outcomes. This review explores the treatment paradigm of this subset of patients and provides an update on the current existing literature on this topic.

SURGICAL ONCOLOGY
CLINICS OF NORTH AMERICA

SERIES OF RELATED INTEREST

Advances in Surgery
https://www.advancessurgery.com
Surgical Clinics of North America
https://www.surgical.theclinics.com
Thoracic Surgery Clinics
https://www.thoracic.theclinics.com

Foreword

Advances in Radiotherapy

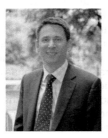

Timothy M. Pawlik, MD, MPH,
PhD, FACS, FRACS (Hon.)
Consulting Editor

This issue of the *Surgical Oncology Clinics of North America* focuses on Advances in Radiotherapy. In 1896, Wilhelm Conrad Roentgen, a German physics professor, presented a lecture on a new kind of "X ray" and in 1901 received the first Nobel Prize awarded in physics for this work.[1] Around this same time, Maria Sklodowska-Curie discovered radium as a source of radiation and subsequently reported on the physiologic effects of radium rays.[2] The earliest radiation treatments involved skin conditions, like eczema and lupus, although radiotherapy was described in the treatment of a patient with gastric cancer as early as the nineteenth century.[3] Following these early applications, a generation of technological innovations has ushered in multiple breakthroughs that has established radiation therapy as a cornerstone of cancer treatment. In fact, data from the US Surveillance, Epidemiology, and End Results suggest that radiation is commonly used in the treatment of a wide array of primary malignancies, ranging from 30% to 75% depending on the type and anatomic location of the tumor. In addition, for patients in need of palliative interventions, more than one-half of patients with cancer will receive some type of radiotherapy during at least one point in their care.[4] In turn, it is critical that providers who care for patients with cancer be up-to-date about the latest advances, applications, and data related to radiation therapy. To that end, this current issue of *Surgical Oncology Clinics of North America* is a timely and practical resource that provides an important update on the topic. We are fortunate to have Terence Williams, MD, PhD as our Guest Editor. Dr Williams is Professor and Chair, Department of Radiation Oncology, City of Hope National Medical Center, Duarte, California. Dr Williams received his MD and PhD from Albert Einstein College of Medicine in New York and completed his residency in radiation oncology and internship in internal medicine at University of Michigan Medical Center. Before joining City of Hope, he held several leadership roles at The James Cancer Hospital and Comprehensive Cancer Center at The Ohio State University. He has a National

Surg Oncol Clin N Am 32 (2023) xiii–xiv
https://doi.org/10.1016/j.soc.2023.03.006
1055-3207/23/© 2023 Published by Elsevier Inc.

surgonc.theclinics.com

Institutes of Health–funded research laboratory, which focuses on stereotactic body radiation therapy, experimental therapeutics, radiogenomics, DNA repair, radiobiology, nutrient scavenging, and theranostics. Dr Williams has received much funding and numerous awards from the National Cancer Institute, National Institutes of Health, American Society of Radiation Oncology, American Society of Clinical Oncology, American Cancer Society, and the Radiologic Society of North America. He also serves as a permanent member of the National Institutes of Health Radiation Therapeutics and Biology study section, as vice-chair of American Society for Radiation Oncology biology scientific programs, and serves on numerous committees for NRG Oncology and Alliance for Clinical Trials in Oncology. Dr Williams specializes in treating patients with thoracic and gastrointestinal cancers, with an emphasis on non–small cell lung, pancreatic, and hepatobiliary malignancies.

The issue covers a number of important topics, including advances in radiotherapy for a wide range of cancers, including pancreas, liver, lung, and breast, among others. In addition, other important topics, such as the role of intraoperative radiation therapy, proton radiotherapy, as well as MRI-linear accelerator technology, are covered. Furthermore, biology-guided radiotherapy and radioimmunomodulation are also discussed.

I want to thank Dr Williams for identifying such a great group of coauthors to contribute to this issue of *Surgical Oncology Clinics of North America*. The authors have done a fantastic job delineating the current important clinical topics related to radiation therapy. This issue of *Surgical Oncology Clinics of North America* will assist all who care for patients with cancer, helping providers understand the important advances and current role of radiotherapy in oncologic care. Once again, thank you to Dr Williams and all the contributing authors.

Timothy M. Pawlik, MD, MPH, PhD,
FACS, FRACS (Hon.)
Department of Surgery
The Ohio State University
Wexner Medical Center
395 West 12th Avenue, Suite 670
Columbus, OH 43210, USA

E-mail address:
tim.pawlik@osumc.edu

REFERENCES

1. Rontgen WC. Uber eine neue Art von Strahlen. Vorläufige Mitteilung. In: Sitzungsberichtë der physikalisch-medicinischen Gesellschaft zu Würzburg, Sitzung. 1985;30:132–141.
2. Becquerel AH, Curie P. Action physiologique des rayons de radium. Compt Rend Acad Sci 1901;132:1289–91.
3. Hodges PC. The life and times of Émil H. Grubbé. Chicago: University of Chicago Press; 1964. p. xi, 135.
4. Connell PP, Hellman S. Advances in radiotherapy and implications for the next century: a historical perspective. Cancer Res 2009;69(2):383–92.

Preface

Advances in Radiotherapy

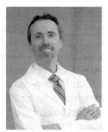

Terence M. Williams, MD, PhD
Editor

Radiation Oncology is a cornerstone of cancer therapy, partnering with Surgery and Medical/Hematology Oncology to enhance outcomes for patients with cancer. In the past few decades, advances in technology have largely driven the administration of more personalized radiation therapy (RT). The advent of intensity-modulated radiation therapy (IMRT), stereotactic body radiotherapy (SBRT/stereotactic ablative radiotherapy [SABR]), and stereotactic radiosurgery (SRS) allowed radiation oncologists to better "carve" radiation dose around critical normal structures, allowing sparing of normal tissues and/or opening up opportunities for radiation dose intensification. In the coming decades, the future of Radiation Oncology remains bright with continued advances in intraoperative radiation (IORT), brachytherapy, particle therapy (protons, carbon), magnetic resonance–guided radiotherapy (MRgRT), PET-guided radiotherapy using biology-guided radiotherapy (BgRT), and radioimmunomodulation (using radiation to harness the immune system). In this Issue, we convey the state-of-the-art with leading Radiation Oncology experts in gastrointestinal (GI), hematologic, thoracic, breast, central nervous system, head and neck malignancies, and advanced technologies.

First, Sanford and colleagues review the controversial role of RT in various stages of pancreatic cancer and highlight new efforts at dose escalation, palliation through celiac plexus radiosurgery, and use of RT for oligometastatic disease. Cuneo and colleagues cover the development of SBRT in primary liver cancer discussing the challenges of treating an organ that is often diseased to start with. They discuss the use of Y90 dosimetry, combination Y90 and SBRT, novel MRI technologies, BgRT, ionizing radiation acoustic imaging, and how to determine and mitigate liver toxicity from radiation using biomarkers and adaptive split course techniques. Jabbour and colleagues provide a timely summary of the role of targeted therapy in combination with RT for esophagogastric cancer, including HER2, EGFR, VEGF, and immunotherapy, but also on the role of radiation and radiation dose in the preoperative and

Surg Oncol Clin N Am 32 (2023) xv–xvi
https://doi.org/10.1016/j.soc.2023.03.005
1055-3207/23/© 2023 Published by Elsevier Inc.

definitive settings, the role of proton RT, and novel methods to measure treatment response (eg, functional MRI, ctDNA). In rectal cancer, Narang and colleagues summarize the development of the total neoadjuvant therapy paradigm, short-course versus long-course RT, timing of surgery, and the burgeoning concept of nonoperative management.

Outside of GI malignancies, Amini and colleagues explore the use of RT in lung cancer as an ablative therapy beyond oligometastatic disease for patients with oligoprogressive disease and summarize the nascent literature on the use of surgery and needle ablation in order to better define the roles of these other local ablative therapies. In breast cancer, Bazan and colleagues provide a comprehensive review of how RT has changed in the last two decades going from 2D to 3D to IMRT, as well as hypofractionation/ultra-hypofractionation, IORT, and accelerated partial breast radiation. The summary also covers where the field stands on omitting radiotherapy for certain patient subsets, the use of prone radiation and protons to spare heart toxicity, and the use of RT in the metastatic setting. In the area of brain metastasis, Palmer and team update readers on how to optimize patient selection for whole brain RT, SRS, fractionated SRS, and preoperative SRS through clinical factors, including advanced imaging methods, with the goal to maximize tumor control and minimize toxicity (eg, radionecrosis). Outside of solid tumors, Dandapani and colleagues relate cutting-edge radiation technology in the field of hematologic malignancies, specifically, the use of total marrow/lymphoid irradiation through the advent of IMRT for hematopoietic stem cell transplant to minimize debilitating side effects of total body irradiation, as well as novel concepts of boosting areas of active bone marrow with radiation.

Toward the tail end of this Issue, you will find exceptional summaries of novel RT technologies provided for proton and FLASH RT (using head and neck [H&N] as an example by Lin and team), IORT (Miller and colleagues), MRgRT (by Chuong and colleagues), and BgRT (Ladbury/Williams and colleagues). Last, a section by Monjazeb and team summarizing the available data on how RT may be able to prime and activate the immune system to generate systemic responses to RT through alteration of the tumor microenvironment, and activation of adaptive/innate immunity, rounds out our journey on modern radiotherapy. Taken together, the future of Radiation Oncology is very promising with continued advances in imaging and physics technology, but also with the influx of biology that is long overdue, enabling radiation oncologists to further personalize the treatment of patients with cancer.

Terence M. Williams, MD, PhD
Professor and Chair
Department of Radiation Oncology
City of Hope National Medical Center
1500 East Duarte Road
Duarte, CA 91010, USA

E-mail address:
terwilliams@coh.org

Current State and Future Directions of Radiation Therapy for Pancreas Adenocarcinoma

Sujana Gottumukkala, MD[a], Samer Salamekh, MD[b],
Nina N. Sanford, MD[a],*

KEYWORDS

- Pancreatic ductal adenocarcinoma • Radiation therapy • Tumors • Pancreas cancer
- SBRT

KEY POINTS

- In resectable PDAC, neoadjuvant radiation is institution dependent with adjuvant radiation used for patients with close/positive margins, lymphovascular invasion, or multiple lymph nodes.
- The role of neoadjuvant chemoradiation in borderline resectable PDAC is contested but the ongoing PREOPANC-3 and PANDAS-PRODIGE 44 trials are expected to provide clarification.
- Advanced delivery techniques such as SAbR or SMART allow for escalation of the biologically effective dose with favorable toxicity profiles.

INTRODUCTION

The prognosis of pancreatic ductal adenocarcinoma (PDAC) remains poor, with only 11% surviving more than 5 years after diagnosis.[1] Given such low survival rates coupled with increasing incidence of PDAC, the overall burden of PDAC is sharply rising. By 2040, PDAC is expected to become the second most common cause of cancer mortality.[2,3] Complete surgical resection, although associated with better survival, is necessary but insufficient for cure.[4,5] However, only a minority of patients, approximately 15% to 20%, present with resectable disease at diagnosis.[6] Nevertheless, even after a successful resection, the majority of patients will develop recurrent disease. Although the majority of these patients present with metastatic PDAC, many will also have tumors that progress locally; some studies have reported a local failure

[a] Department of Radiation Oncology, University of Texas Southwestern, 2280 Inwood Road, Dallas, TX 75390-9303, USA; [b] Cancer Specialists of North Florida, Jacksonville, FL, USA
* Corresponding author.
E-mail address: Nina.Sanford@UTSouthwestern.edu

Surg Oncol Clin N Am 32 (2023) 399–414
https://doi.org/10.1016/j.soc.2023.02.001
1055-3207/23/© 2023 Elsevier Inc. All rights reserved.

surgonc.theclinics.com

rate as high as 50% post-operatively including a proportion who have local only recurrence up until the time of death. Given these statistics, the potential for radiation therapy (RT) to optimize locoregional control in PDAC is appealing; however, given conflicting data including several negative randomized controlled trials, the role of RT in PDAC is not clearly defined and practices vary significantly across institutions.

What are the potential benefits of improved locoregional control with RT in PDAC? In the pre-operative setting, RT can be used to improve the rate of R0 resection; in the post-operative setting to sterilize any microscopic residual disease; and in the inoperable setting to maximize local control and for symptomatic palliation. How do these measures translate to the clinically-relevant endpoints for patients living longer (overall survival [OS]) or better (quality of life)? Most large, randomized trials of RT in PDAC have used OS as a primary endpoint and have been negative. In contrast, single-arm and/or single-institution studies have reported favorable outcomes with the use of RT across the PDAC disease spectrum, suggesting that select patients do benefit from the addition of RT to multi-modality care. Improvements in systemic therapy for PDAC have demonstrated the need for intensive chemotherapy and early control of micrometastatic disease even in cases where tumors appear radiographically favorable (early stage). The improved systemic control with chemotherapy has also, in our opinion, amplified the potential benefit of local therapy including RT. In addition, recent technological developments in radiation delivery, such as stereotactic ablative radiation therapy (SAbR), MRI-linear accelerators (MR-LINAC), and adaptive RT, have enabled more safe delivery of higher doses of radiation. In this review, we will discuss the evolving role of RT in PDAC with a focus on recent trials and future directions.

RESECTABLE PANCREATIC DUCTAL ADENOCARCINOMA

Resectable PDAC includes tumors where upfront R0 resection appears achievable due to no or minimal contact with surrounding vasculature and luminal structures. Current National Comprehensive Cancer Network (NCCN) guidelines recommend adjuvant chemotherapy for resectable PDAC with consideration of neoadjuvant therapy in select patients with high-risk features (very high CA 19–9, large tumors, excessive weight loss, and extreme pain).[7] Many centers routinely treat nearly all patients with resectable PDAC with upfront chemotherapy with the goal of early control of micrometastatic disease and to "allow" poor biology tumors to manifest such that patients can avoid a Whipple procedure with subsequent early distant progression. Despite this trend for neoadjuvant therapy across all gastrointestinal cancer types, there remains an equipoise between the two strategies. The ongoing Alliance trial, A021806 (NCT04340141), randomizes patients to surgery with adjuvant chemotherapy versus peri-operative chemotherapy. Pending successful recruitment and follow-up, this study is anticipated to provide level 1 evidence regarding the optimal chemotherapy sequencing for resectable disease. Notably, neither arm in this cooperative group trial includes RT.

Nevertheless, RT does have a role in patients whose tumors are initially deemed resectable, although the indications and practices vary from center to center. Historically, RT was initially studied in the post-operative setting for resectable tumors. One positive RT study with many caveats, GITSG 91-73,[8] was followed by several negative trials: EORTC 40891,[9,10] ESPAC-1,[11,12] among others. Furthermore, a meta-analysis with patient-level data was published in 2005 of six trials and reported that adjuvant chemotherapy provided a 25% reduction in death, whereas chemoradiation did not provide a benefit in the overall cohort.[13]

Modern RT cooperative group studies for resectable pancreatic cancer have also been performed in the adjuvant setting. RTOG 9704 reported on 451 patients with resectable PDAC. After resection, patients were randomized to either 3 weeks of 5-FU followed by chemoradiation (CRT) (50.4 Gy in 28 fractions with 5-FU) and additional 3 months of standalone 5-FU or 3 weeks of gemcitabine followed by CRT and additional 3 months of gemcitabine. There was no survival difference in the two arms of the trial.[14] Although the radiation protocol was the same in both arms, the trial provided important information regarding predictors of outcomes. Secondary analysis of the trial revealed that patients who received RT per protocol had improved survival compared with those who did not (median survival 20.9 months compared with 17.5 months), without a difference in toxicity.[15] Additional analysis revealed patients without nodal involvement and those with a post-operative CA 19-9 <180U/mL had improved survival (higher CA 19–9 associated with larger tumors).[16] The study was used as a basis for the randomized NRG/RTOG 0848 trial which was designed to answer two questions: whether adding erlotinib to gemcitabine in the post-operative setting improves survival and whether RT improved survival in the adjuvant setting. Patients with PDAC who underwent resection and had post-resection serum CA 19-9 <180U/mL were randomized to either 6 months of gemcitabine or 6 months of gemcitabine with erlotinib. After assessing for disease progression and completing systemic therapy, patients underwent a second randomization to receive chemotherapy or CRT (50.4 Gy in 28 fractions with capecitabine or 5-FU). The addition of erlotinib did not improve survival in these patients. The results of the radiotherapy randomization have not yet been presented.

Given the above, clearly not all patients with resected PDAC benefit from the addition of adjuvant radiotherapy because the most common sites of progression are distant (ie, outside of the radiation field). Studies have attempted to define subsets of patients for whom adjuvant radiotherapy may improve outcomes. In practice, adjuvant RT is generally reserved for patients with pathologic risk factors for local recurrence or residual disease, such as an R1 resection, close margins, lymphovascular invasion, or high nodal positivity rate. These patients will generally complete adjuvant chemotherapy first, undergo restaging scans, and then adjuvant radiotherapy presuming no metastatic disease progression. It can also be argued, however, that reserving RT for salvage local therapy is a reasonable option, given that (1) some of these patients may ultimately develop metastatic progression first, and (2) being able to visualize gross disease on scans will aid in designing a better RT plan with higher dose to tumor and lower dose to surrounding organs.

Given the trend toward neoadjuvant therapy including RT across gastrointestinal cancers, is there a role for RT in the neoadjuvant setting for resectable PDAC? Currently, pre-operative RT is omitted for resectable disease as, by definition, clear margins are generally believed to be achievable upfront and as such, the risks of RT are believed to outweigh any potential benefits. One reason for this hesitancy is that delivery of a 6-week course of CRT in the pre-operative setting would delay surgery and subsequent adjuvant systemic therapy. Shorter courses of neoadjuvant CRT may provide benefit to patients without the delay of long-course CRT. A phase I/II trial from Massachusetts General Hospital investigated the use of a short course of neoadjuvant chemoradiation with protons (5 fractions of 5 Gy-equivalents) and capecitabine followed by early surgery and adjuvant gemcitabine. The study reported favorable rates of toxicity (4.1% grade 3 toxicity and no grade 4/5 toxicity) and no treatment-related delays to surgery.[17] A smaller phase I study from the University of Wisconsin escalated the dose of neoadjuvant chemoradiation to 35 Gy in 5 fractions to the tumor and 25 Gy in 5 to elective nodal volume, with concurrent capecitabine. No acute grade 3 or higher toxicity was seen and all patients who underwent surgery had R0 resection. Currently, the use of neoadjuvant RT in resectable PDAC is largely institution dependent, with its use primarily at institutions where most, if not almost all patients, receive RT at some point in their treatment path for non-metastatic PDAC.

BORDERLINE RESECTABLE DISEASE

PDAC is generally considered borderline resectable if resection is technically feasible, but would result in an R1 resection. Historically, management of borderline resectable PDAC has been heterogenous due to the wide range of cancers that fall within this category and variation in how different centers/clinicians define borderline resectable. This definition has been further complicated after the advent of neoadjuvant therapy that may be able to improve resectability in up to one-third of patients who were initially believed to be locally advanced/unresectable.[18] Per NCCN guidelines, the current treatment paradigm consists of neoadjuvant therapy followed by restaging and consideration of surgery for patients without disease progression.[7] There remains discrepancy on the specific type of neoadjuvant regimen and also where RT should be included.

Numerous studies have demonstrated that neoadjuvant therapy improves pathologic outcomes including R0 resection rates, nodal positivity, and even results in a pathologic complete response for a small proportion of patients. However, the debate remains whether the addition of RT in the neoadjuvant setting can translate to a survival benefit. In a retrospective series of 160 patients with borderline resectable PDAC, one of the earliest studies defining this group, who received neoadjuvant treatment with chemotherapy, CRT (50.4 Gy in 28 fractions or 30 Gy in 10 fractions), or both, Katz and colleagues reported high R0 resection rates and favorable survival for patients able to complete neoadjuvant treatment and subsequent surgery.[19] Of the initial 160 patients, 125 patients (78%) were able to complete neoadjuvant therapy and restaging with 66 patients (41%) ultimately undergoing surgery. Of those patients who underwent surgery, 94% achieved R0 resection with a partial pathologic response noted in 56% of patients. Median survival was significantly higher for patients who were able to undergo resection compared with those who were unable to receive surgery (40 months vs 13 months). However, this was a retrospective series, thus, the survival benefit could have been driven by selection biases rather than neoadjuvant therapy. Several recently published studies including borderline resectable PDAC may shed further light on the role of RT.

The preoperative chemoradiotherapy for resectable or borderline resectable pancreatic cancer (PREOPANC) study randomized 246 patients with resectable or borderline resectable PDAC to immediate surgery followed by adjuvant gemcitabine versus neoadjuvant CRT with gemcitabine followed by surgery and adjuvant chemotherapy. Patients who underwent neoadjuvant CRT had higher R0 resection rates (71% vs 40%) and improved median disease-free survival and locoregional failure-free interval.[20] At median follow-up of 27 months, there was no difference in median OS between arms for the overall cohort. However, a pre-planned subgroup analysis of patients with borderline resectable disease demonstrated a median OS benefit with pre-operative CRT (17.6 months vs 13.2 months). The long-term results of the study were recently published.[21] With median follow-up of 59 months, the OS was better in the neoadjuvant chemoradiotherapy group than in the upfront surgery group (hazard ratio, 0.73; 95% CI, 0.56–0.96; $P = .025$). Although the difference in median survival was only 1.4 months (15.7 months vs 14.3 months), the 5-year OS rate was 20.5% (95% CI, 14.2–29.8) with neoadjuvant chemoradiotherapy and 6.5% (95% CI, 3.1–13.7) with upfront surgery.

The effect of neoadjuvant chemoradiotherapy was consistent across the prespecified subgroups, including resectable and borderline resectable pancreatic cancer, with the latter group seeming to derive the most benefit (HR 0.67, 95% CI 0.45–0.99). One interpretation of this finding is that neoadjuvant treatment provides a potential long-term survival benefit for those patients who do not develop metastatic disease in the first few years after surgery. A key limitation of the PREOPANC trial is the use of gemcitabine rather than more modern chemotherapy regimens such as FOLFIRINOX or gemcitabine/nab-paclitaxel, which are the current standard of care in the neoadjuvant setting. The PREOPANC-2 trial seeks to address this limitation by randomizing patients to either eight cycles of neoadjuvant FOLFIRINOX followed by surgery versus three cycles of neoadjuvant gemcitabine with a hypofractionated course of radiation during the second cycle (36 Gy in 15 fractions) followed by surgery and four cycles of adjuvant gemcitabine.[22] A potential limitation of this study, however, is that the arm receiving hypofractionated RT is not treated with FOLFIRINOX. In a phase II/III Korean study randomizing 58 patients to neoadjuvant gemcitabine-based CRT followed by surgery versus upfront surgery followed by adjuvant CRT, interim analysis demonstrated higher R0 resection rates with neoadjuvant CRT (51.8% vs 26.1%) as well as improved 1-year OS, 2-year OS, and median survival.[23]

The Alliance A021501 trial randomized 126 patients with borderline resectable PDAC to either eight cycles of neoadjuvant mFOLFIRINOX followed by resection and four cycles of adjuvant mFOLFOX or four cycles of neoadjuvant mFOLFIRINOX, RT (33–40 Gy in 5 fractions, or 25 Gy in 5 fractions), resection, and four cycles of adjuvant mFOLFOX.[24] The primary endpoint of the trial was 18-month OS, which was higher with neoadjuvant chemotherapy alone than neoadjuvant chemotherapy with RT (66.4% vs 47.3%) even among patients who underwent pancreatectomy (93.1% vs 78.9%). Although the trial was not meant to be a comparison between the two treatment arms, rather two separate comparisons against historical controls, many have interpreted the trial as evidence that radiation is ineffective, or worse, harmful, in patients with borderline resectable pancreatic cancer. Notable limitations of the study were that although randomized, patients in the RT arm had higher baseline CA19-9 (median 171 U/mL compared with 248 U/mL), possibly signifying more aggressive disease, and also had more frequent dose delays and reductions in chemotherapy. Furthermore, fewer patients in the RT arm underwent surgery (51% compared with 58%) and even fewer underwent pancreatectomy (35% compared with 48%). From the report, there is no clear rationale of why the addition of radiation could lead to worse OS, which we surmise is most likely related to imbalance of underlying characteristics and differences in pancreatectomy. A secondary analysis of RT quality assurance is currently being performed.

A single-institution phase II clinical trial was performed with 48 borderline resectable patients. The patients received eight cycles of FOLFIRINOX followed by either short-course radiation for those who were resectable based on restaging imaging (25 GyE in 5 or 30 Gy in 10 photons) or long-course chemoradiation for those with persistent vascular involvement (50.4 Gy in 28 with Capecitabine or 5-FU).[25] Sixty seven percent of the patients were able to undergo resection and an R0 resection rate of 97% was achieved. The 2-year OS was 56% for the overall cohort and 72% for patients who underwent resection. The discordant results between the Alliance phase III trial and the single-institution phase II are likely multifactorial and may include heterogeneity in treatment when enrolled in cooperative setting compared with single-institution expertise/bias. In addition, patients in the phase II study received eight cycles of FOLFIRINOX, which is the same number of cycles patients in the control arm of the Alliance study received, whereas the RT arm in the Alliance study received only seven cycles.

However, the difference in findings is likely too large to be explained by a single cycle of chemotherapy. The ongoing PREOPANC-2 as described above (EudraCT: 2017–002036–17) is comparing outcomes of neoadjuvant FOLFIRINOX to gemcitabine and CRT (36 Gy in 15 fractions)[22] whereas PANDAS-PRODIGE 44 (NCT02676349) is investigating the addition of CRT (50.4 Gy in 28 with capecitabine) to FOLFIRINOX. The results of these and other trials will provide additional clarification on the role of neoadjuvant RT in borderline resectable PDAC.

LOCALLY ADVANCED DISEASE

Locally advanced PDAC generally refers to a disease which is unresectable due to the involvement of critical vasculature or adjacent organs, however, there is heterogeneity in the definition. Some clinicians restrict the definition of locally advanced to patients who will "never" undergo surgery, whereas others include patients who could become resectable/borderline resectable with some degree of downstaging. The heterogeneity in defining locally advanced by treatment facility, individual providers and in study inclusion criteria has made creation of guidelines more difficult. Nevertheless, management of patients with locally advanced PDAC consists of starting with systemic therapy with subsequent RT considered in patients with good performance status and without systemic progression after chemotherapy.[7] In this setting, RT can be used pre-operatively or definitively.

There is no level 1 data to support the routine use of conventional RT for locally advanced PDAC. In the LAP07 trial, investigators used a two-step randomization process to investigate the effect of gemcitabine versus erlotinib and CRT versus chemotherapy on survival.[26] In the first randomization, patients were randomized to four cycles of gemcitabine versus gemcitabine and erlotinib. Patients without disease progression after 4 months underwent a second randomization to long-course CRT with capecitabine versus 2 more months of their initial chemotherapy. There was no difference in survival with the addition of erlotinib. Patients who received CRT had significantly decreased local progression compared with those who received additional chemotherapy (32% vs 46%); however, there was no difference in survival. Formal RT quality assurance of the trial suggests that only 32% of patients in the CRT arm were treated per protocol, which may have diminished the impact of CRT.

The results of the CONKO-007 trial were recently presented at American Society of Clinical Oncology (ASCO) in 2022.[27] This was a randomized trial of 180 patients with locally advanced PDAC who received induction chemotherapy and then were randomized to receive chemoradiation or not. Despite being a trial in locally advanced PDAC, the primary endpoint was R0 resection rate, again highlighting the discrepancy in characterization of locally advanced disease. There was no difference in R0 resection rate or median OS between arms. However, for patients who did undergo surgery (122 total), the arm receiving chemoradiation had higher rates of pathologic complete response (18% vs 2%, $P = 0.004$), R0 resection (69% vs 50%, $P = 0.04$) and negative circumferential margin (47% vs 25%, $P = 0.01$). Furthermore, although there was no difference in median OS, the 5-year OS was doubled (9.6% vs 4.3%) in patients receiving neoadjuvant chemoRT. Among the subgroup undergoing surgery and receiving FOLFIRINOX, the 5-year OS was an impressive 26.9% with the addition of chemoRT, versus 13% with induction chemotherapy alone. As in PREOPANC, RT appears to prolong the survival tail for a "favorable" subgroup of patients with locally advanced disease–those able to undergo surgery and receive FOLFIRINOX. Further research is needed to better define this subset a priori to better tailor therapies including the addition of RT.

Stereotactic Ablative Radiation Therapy

SAbR, also known as stereotactic body radiotherapy (SBRT), provides a method for dose escalation while protecting organs at risk (OARS) and can be used in the neoadjuvant, adjuvant, or definitive setting. The success of SAbR is predicated on highly precise patient and tumor immobilization and tumor visualization permitting delivery of high doses to small, well-defined targets, over few treatments. Immobilization using SBRT, motion monitoring, and image-guided RT provides a process for reducing treatment margins and subsequent dose delivered to OARS. This not only improves the tolerability of treatment but provides an opportunity to escalate the biologically effective dose (BED) with the goal of completely eradicating the tumor and improving local control.

Koong and colleagues reported one of the earliest studies of SAbR in PDAC in a phase I dose escalation with 15 patients who were treated from 15 to 25 Gy at a single fraction with no acute dose-limiting toxicity.[28] Metallic fiducial markers were placed and were tracked by orthogonal x-ray during treatment, which was performed with breath hold to minimize target motion during the respiratory cycle. Most centers performing SAbR for PDAC utilize a similar technique today; however, the radiation is delivered in approximately 5 fractions to provide some averaging/repair of dose received by OARs, while still delivering a condensed course of treatment. The change from 1 fraction to 5 fractions was based upon subsequent studies showing higher rates of late toxicity with single fraction SAbR, thus the BED of 1 fraction SAbR was converted to an equivalent in 5 fractions. For example, Pollom and colleagues retrospectively analyzed 167 patients who received a biologically equivalent dose of either 25 Gy in 1 fraction or 33 Gy in 5 fractions using the universal survival curve[29] and found that there was no difference in control rates or survival between the groups. However, there was higher grade $\geq$ 2 gastrointestinal (GI) toxicity in patients who received a single fraction compared with 5 fractions.[30] Therefore, 33 Gy in 5 fractions became a frequently used SAbR dose.

Several retrospective[31–34] and prospective single-arm studies[30] have been performed demonstrating low toxicity and excellent local control (LC) with SAbR in locally advanced PDAC. The results of these studies and multi-institutional analyses have suggested that patients receiving higher BED may have improved survival; however, the conclusions are limited by selection bias in that patients who are able to receive a higher dose of SAbR may have more favorable tumors. The pooled analysis in unresectable locally advanced pancreatic cancer (PAULA-1) study analyzed 54 PDAC patients treated with SAbR between 2013 and 2018 and found that both LC and OS were better in patients receiving $\geq$ 48 Gy BED 10.[35] Currently, many institutions aim to treat to a BED of ~100 or greater, such as via 50 Gy in 5 fractions or 67.5 Gy in 15 fractions, although prospective data on the role of dose escalation are lacking at this time. A sample SAbR plan of a patient treated to 50 Gy in 5 fractions is shown in **Fig. 1**. There are several ongoing randomized studies investigating the role of SAbR in PDAC such as the AGITG MASTERPLAN (ACTRN12619000409178).[36]

Radiation Volume Definition

The RT target volume remains a topic of debate, again with widely variable practices across institutions. As described above, RT in PDAC was initially studied in the postoperative setting using conventionally fractionated radiation therapy treatment including primary tumor as well as the regional lymph nodes. Initially, these landmarks were based upon bony anatomy, this transitioned to vascular anatomy such as in RTOG 0848, where a contouring atlas was provided and has become a standard

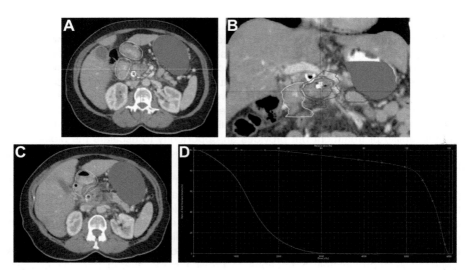

Fig. 1. A 54-year-old woman with locally advanced pancreatic cancer. She was treated with FOLFORINOX x 8 cycles and then proceeded to SAbR on a clinical trial to a dose of 50 Gy in 5 fractions. The target volume is shown (panels *A* and *B*). The gross tumor volume is outlined in pink and the clinical target volume in red. Please note the adjacent vasculature including the SMA and SMV at the level of the tumor is included in the clinical target volume, but no further elective nodal irradiation. The OARS include the duodenum, stomach, and jejunum also outlined in the panels. A plan was created (panel *C*) with maximum dose approximately 120% of the prescription dose and with carving of dose around the duodenum (*yellow line*), where the target volume was intentionally underdosed. A composite organ at risk was created including the duodenum, jejunum, and small bowel (*pink line*) and this was kept to a maximum of 33 Gy for less than 0.5 cc (panel *D*). Given the proximity to mucosal structures, 83% of the planning target volume received the prescription dose of 50 Gy (*red line*). The patient completed SAbR without toxicity. SMA, Superior mesenteric artery; SMV, Superior mesenteric vein.

reference in designing pancreatic radiation fields today.[37] In this atlas, comprehensive target volumes included the post-operative tumor bed, anastomoses, and regional nodal volume. In contrast, when SAbR was introduced, target volumes included the tumor alone with an isotropic margin. This was in part due to concerns of gastrointestinal toxicity with treatment of mucosal structures to high dose per fraction. Currently, The American Society for Radiation Oncology (ASTRO), European Society for Radiotherapy and Oncology (ESTRO), and the Australasian Gastrointestinal Trials Group/Trans-Tasman Radiation Oncology Group (AGITG/TROG) recommend against treating elective nodal radiation when using SAbR in locally advanced PDAC due to lack of evidence of benefit.[38–40]

However, a significant proportion of PDAC has perineural and/or lymphovascular involvement, with surgical series suggesting occult metastasis rates as high as 80%.[41] As such, there is increased concern that treating only the tumor with SAbR doses may be associated with increased risk of regional recurrence, especially around the celiac and superior mesenteric vasculature.[42,43] These areas are also high-risk locations for surgical complications, common sites of positive margins, and can be more difficult to treat with salvage therapy. As such, some centers have adopted an elective target coverage in SAbR at an intermediate dose level, such as 25 Gy in 5 fractions. Retrospective studies have demonstrated improved progression free survival

(PFS) with this approach.[42] A recent retrospective analysis, with propensity score matching, compared outcomes of patients treated at a single institution with either SAbR to the tumor (33–40 Gy in 5 fractions) or SAbR to the tumor and 25 Gy in 5 fractions elective nodal radiation.[44] The 2-year locoregional recurrence was lower with elective nodal radiation (22.6% compared with 44.6%) which came at the expense of higher acute grade 1/grade 2 GI toxicity (60% compared with 20%). OS was similar in the two cohorts. However, given the mounting level of evidence supporting coverage of elective areas along with demonstrated low toxicity rates, there has been a trend to also treat areas of high risk adjacent to the tumor including vessels and nodal volumes, albeit to a lower dose than the gross tumor. The specific volume to treat has been a subject of debate, with some clinicians advocating for extensive elective nodal coverage whereas others treating the tumor with adjacent vasculature given higher rates of recurrence found around the celiac and superior mesenteric artery. Although there are unlikely to be future randomized trials focused on radiation target volume definition in particular, having defined volumes in prospective studies will allow for systematic analysis of different target volume strategies.

MRI-LINEAR ACCELERATORS

An MR-LINAC combines the high-energy beam output from a linear accelerator with MRI-guided radiation delivery. There are two commercially available systems: a 0.35 T MRIdian from ViewRay (Oakwood Village, Ohio, USA) and 1.5 T Unity from Elekta (Stockholm, Sweden). These machines offer several advantages compared with traditional linear accelerators with image guidance. Pancreatic tumors are difficult to visualize on CT without using contrast; however, the tumors are more readily visualized using MRI. Both commercial systems allow for MRI while radiation treatment is being delivered, resulting in true intra-fraction motion monitoring. This is particularly important for visualizing the stomach, duodenum, and jejunum where radiotherapy hotspots may result in significant toxicity.[45] Imaging during radiation treatment has demonstrated significant variability and unpredictability in the motion of both the tumor as well as the nearby organs at risk (OARs).[46] Furthermore, since MR image is obtained for image alignment at every fraction, MR-LINAC allows for daily adaptation to both the tumor as well as OARS (ie, creation of a new radiotherapy plan with each fraction).

There have been several retrospective reports on utilizing MR-LINAC for the treatment of PDAC. Most of these reports are of patients treated with the ViewRay machine because it has been Food and Drug Administration (FDA) approved longer (initially with a Cobalt-60 radiation source and later with a linear accelerator radiation source). One of the first studies on utilizing MR-LINAC for stereotactic MR-guided adaptive RT, termed SMART, for the treatment of PDAC was reported by Bohoudi and colleagues, who treated 10 tumors to 40 Gy in 5 fractions.[47] Shortly thereafter, Henke and colleagues reported on a series of five PDAC patients treated to 50 Gy in 5 fractions.[48] There have been several larger retrospective studies demonstrating good efficacy with favorable GI toxicity profiles.[49–51] One of these studies divided patients by treatment BED and reported higher OS in patients who received >70 Gy BED 10 (49% vs 30%).[49] This is a rapidly evolving area that is driven by continued technological progress and significant opportunities for improvement remain.[52] In a recent multi-institutional review of 148 PDAC patients treated on the MRIdian using SMART (57% locally advanced, 29% borderline resectable, 14% medically inoperable), 23% of patients underwent pancreaticoduodenectomy, and survival (median OS 26 months) was significantly higher than the historic controls.[53] Grade 3 acute toxicity was 4.1% and late toxicity 12.8%, with no grade 4 toxicity. Most patients received induction chemotherapy and 50 Gy in 5 fractions. A prospective phase II trial for SMART-based treatment on MRIdian (NCT03621644) and a prospective registry for those treated on Unity (MOMENTUM NCT04075305) are currently underway, with a plan for presentation of SMART results in the fall of 2022. A phase III randomized trial assessing the addition of MR-guided RT to chemotherapy in locally advanced pancreatic cancer will soon be enrolling.

PALLIATION

Patients with pancreatic cancer may have poor quality of life (QOL) due to tumor progression resulting in jaundice, obstruction, weight loss, and/or pain. Unfortunately, approximately 80% of patients with advanced PDAC will experience severe pain before death, which is often due to the primary tumor.[54] Specifically, the pancreas is near the celiac plexus; compression at this location can result in intense pain that is often difficult to adequately manage. These patients often have poor prognoses, thus, delivering a condensed course of RT to palliate pain while minimizing treatment burden which may be a prudent strategy to improve QOL. In one of the largest single-institution studies, 61 patients with celiac axis pain related to their PDAC received 8 Gy x 1, 8 Gy x 2, 8 Gy x 3, with at least 66% of patients achieving pain relief.[55] Most other studies utilizing 1 to 6 fractions also demonstrated improvement in pain after RT.[56] A recent single-arm prospective clinical trial (NCT02356406) assessed treatment with single fraction RT to 25Gy encompassing the entire retroperitoneal celiac plexus.[57] Among 18 patients treated, 16 (84%) reported decreased pain 3 weeks after treatment and 4 patients had complete eradication of pain. The authors concluded that celiac plexus radiosurgery appeared effective in pain relief. A phase II multicenter trial using this regimen is currently accruing. However, one study of 22 patients who received 45 Gy in 3 fractions via SAbR demonstrated overall deterioration, increased nausea, and greater pain after RT.[58] Notably, this study used one of the highest doses and was one of the early studies utilizing SAbR, which may have led to poorer outcomes. Importantly, however, it demonstrates the need to carefully select patients and design safe treatment plans, particularly when the intent of therapy is palliative. The PAINPANC is a prospective single-arm trial currently underway that treats patients with PDAC-related celiac axis pain to 27 Gy in 3 fractions (NL4896, NTR5143).

OLIGOMETASTATIC DISEASE

The concept of oligometastasis was first introduced in 1995 as a state of limited systemic metastasis that may be amenable to local treatments that result in cure.[59] This has been shown for several metastatic GI malignancies with liver and lung metastasis such as colorectal cancer.[59] Although PDAC frequently metastasizes to liver and lung, given high rates of early disseminated progression, it has not been clear that such a state exists for a meaningful proportion of patients with metastatic PDAC.

There are case reports of long-term survivors of PDAC with metastectomy; the clinical course in these patients is often of slow progression with recurrences several years after initial resection.[60] In total, most large retrospective series report few long-term survivors after metastasectomy.[61] This suggests that a small proportion of PDAC with limited metastasis may have favorable biology that portends a more indolent course more amendable to aggressive local therapy. Genomic studies in PDAC suggest that there are metastatic clones in the primary tumor many years before dissemination and that dissemination to distant organs precedes the development of the first clinical site of metastasis by several years.[62]

Advances in biomarkers may better stratify patient's metastatic potential and advances in systemic therapy may slow the growth of metastatic clones such that local therapy may provide a meaningful benefit, whether in OS or time off systemic therapy. Several factors have been identified that portend a better prognosis in limited metastatic disease including fewer number of liver metastasis, low CA 19-9, and presence of lung metastasis compared with liver metastasis.[61,63] Additional therapy appears to improve survival in those with limited metastatic disease; however, studies are limited by selection bias and there remain limited survivors beyond 5 years.[63]

SAbR provides an appealing treatment option that balances local control and QOL compared with surgical metastasectomy. SAbR can be selectively used in patients on chemotherapy to maximize time off systemic therapy, often resulting in improvement in QOL, while minimizing disease progression. The use of SAbR has been shown to improve survival for other diseases and may be beneficial for patients with limited metastatic disease. There are at least two randomized trials examining the role of SAbR in oligometastatic PDAC (NCT04975516, OligoRARE NCT04498767).

Our institution recently published a retrospective series on the use of SAbR for oligometastatic PDAC.[64] This report included 41 patients with oligometastatic PDAC, defined as 1 to 5 metastases without progression for at least 5 months. Of these patients, 20 received SAbR and 21 did not. Out of the 20 SAbR-treated patients, 17 (85%) had 6 or more months of time off chemotherapy, compared with 7 patients (33.3%) among the chemotherapy-treated group. Median polyprogression-free survival was 40 and 14 months (HR = 0.2; 95% CI, 0.07–0.54; P =.0009), and OS was 42 and 18 months (HR = 0.21; 95% CI, 0.08–0.53; P =.0003), for SAbR and chemotherapy-treated cohorts, respectively. The results from this study are hypothesis generating given selection biases with retrospective data. However, they suggest that an oligometastatic subset does exist in PDAC that may benefit from local therapy, and further efforts are needed to better define this population and optimize their treatment.

SUMMARY

Improvements in prognosis for patients diagnosed with PDAC have largely been attributed to better surgery and advancements in multiagent systemic therapy. Most trials have demonstrated that RT improves locoregional control, but this often has not translated into a survival benefit. The majority of studies have unfortunately not included rigorous measuring of QOL metrics. However as systemic therapy continues to decrease rates of distant metastasis/recurrence in PDAC, improvements in locoregional control may become more important with greater likelihood of improving survival and QOL. Although some patients benefit from RT, currently it is difficult to know in whom and when RT should be utilized. Recent developments in RT delivery with SAbR as well as MR-LINAC technology can better optimize the therapeutic ratio of RT by providing higher doses of radiation in a more conformal manner that minimizes toxicity. Preliminary studies are highly encouraging but additional randomized studies are necessary to determine the benefit of these new technologies and to optimize the sequencing/timing of RT in relation to systemic therapy and surgery.

CLINICS CARE POINTS

- Current guidelines recommend against elective nodal irradiation with SAbR but given concern for regional recurrence when treating the tumor alone, some centers have adopted the practice of treating an elective volume to an intermediate dose level such as 25 Gy in 5 fractions.

CONFLICTS OF INTEREST

None.

DISCLOSSURE

The Authors have nothing to disclose.

REFERENCES

1. Siegel RL, Miller KD, Jemal A. Cancer statistics, 2020. CA Cancer J Clin 2020; 70(1):7–30.
2. Rahib L, Wehner MR, Matrisian LM, et al. Estimated projection of US cancer incidence and death to 2040. JAMA Netw Open 2021;4(4):e214708.
3. Iacobuzio-Donahue CA, Fu B, Yachida S, et al. DPC4 gene status of the primary carcinoma correlates with patterns of failure in patients with pancreatic cancer. J Clin Oncol 2009;27(11):1806–13.
4. Ducreux M, Cuhna AS, Caramella C, et al. Cancer of the pancreas: ESMO clinical practice guidelines for diagnosis, treatment and follow-up. Ann Oncol 2015; 26(Suppl 5):v56–68.
5. Tempero MA, Malafa MP, Al-Hawary M, et al. Pancreatic adenocarcinoma, Version 2.2021, NCCN clinical practice guidelines in oncology. J Natl Compr Cancer Netw 2021;19(4):439–57.
6. Geer RJ, Brennan MF. Prognostic indicators for survival after resection of pancreatic adenocarcinoma. Am J Surg 1993;165(1):68–72.
7. NCCN. Pancreatic adenocarcinoma (Version 2.2021), Available at: https://www.nccn.org/professionals/physician_gls/pdf/pancreatic.pdf, 2021. Accessed September 1, 2022.
8. Kalser MH, Ellenberg SS. Pancreatic cancer. Adjuvant combined radiation and chemotherapy following curative resection. Arch Surg 1985;120(8):899–903.
9. Klinkenbijl JH, Jeekel J, Sahmoud T, et al. Adjuvant radiotherapy and 5-fluorouracil after curative resection of cancer of the pancreas and periampullary region: phase III trial of the EORTC gastrointestinal tract cancer cooperative group. Ann Surg 1999;230(6):776–82 [discussion: 782-774].
10. Smeenk HG, van Eijck CH, Hop WC, et al. Long-term survival and metastatic pattern of pancreatic and periampullary cancer after adjuvant chemoradiation or observation: long-term results of EORTC trial 40891. Ann Surg 2007;246(5): 734–40.
11. Neoptolemos JP, Dunn JA, Stocken DD, et al. Adjuvant chemoradiotherapy and chemotherapy in resectable pancreatic cancer: a randomised controlled trial. Lancet 2001;358(9293):1576–85.
12. Neoptolemos JP, Stocken DD, Friess H, et al. A randomized trial of chemoradiotherapy and chemotherapy after resection of pancreatic cancer. N Engl J Med 2004;350(12):1200–10.
13. Stocken DD, Buchler MW, Dervenis C, et al. Meta-analysis of randomised adjuvant therapy trials for pancreatic cancer. Br J Cancer 2005;92(8):1372–81.
14. Regine WF, Winter KA, Abrams R, et al. Fluorouracil-based chemoradiation with either gemcitabine or fluorouracil chemotherapy after resection of pancreatic adenocarcinoma: 5-year analysis of the US Intergroup/RTOG 9704 phase III trial. Ann Surg Oncol 2011;18(5):1319–26.
15. Abrams RA, Winter KA, Regine WF, et al. Failure to adhere to protocol specified radiation therapy guidelines was associated with decreased survival in RTOG

9704–a phase III trial of adjuvant chemotherapy and chemoradiotherapy for patients with resected adenocarcinoma of the pancreas. Int J Radiat Oncol Biol Phys 2012;82(2):809–16.

16. Berger AC, Garcia M, Hoffman JP, et al. Postresection CA 19-9 Predicts overall survival in patients with pancreatic cancer treated with adjuvant chemoradiation: a prospective validation by RTOG 9704. J Clin Oncol 2008;26(36):5918–22.

17. Hong TS, Ryan DP, Borger DR, et al. A phase 1/2 and biomarker study of preoperative short course chemoradiation with proton beam therapy and capecitabine followed by early surgery for resectable pancreatic ductal adenocarcinoma. Int J Radiat Oncol Biol Phys 2014;89(4):830–8.

18. Gillen S, Schuster T, Meyer Z, Buschenfelde C, et al. Preoperative/neoadjuvant therapy in pancreatic cancer: a systematic review and meta-analysis of response and resection percentages. PLoS Med 2010;7(4):e1000267.

19. Katz MH, Pisters PW, Evans DB, et al. Borderline resectable pancreatic cancer: the importance of this emerging stage of disease. J Am Coll Surg 2008;206(5): 833–46 [discussion: 846-838].

20. Versteijne E, Suker M, Groothuis K, et al. Preoperative chemoradiotherapy versus immediate surgery for resectable and borderline resectable pancreatic cancer: results of the dutch randomized phase III PREOPANC trial. J Clin Oncol 2020; 38(16):1763–73.

21. Versteijne E, van Dam JL, Suker M, et al. Neoadjuvant chemoradiotherapy versus upfront surgery for resectable and borderline resectable pancreatic cancer: long-term results of the dutch randomized PREOPANC trial. J Clin Oncol 2022;40(11): 1220–30.

22. Janssen QP, van Dam JL, Bonsing BA, et al. Total neoadjuvant FOLFIRINOX versus neoadjuvant gemcitabine-based chemoradiotherapy and adjuvant gemcitabine for resectable and borderline resectable pancreatic cancer (PREOPANC-2 trial): study protocol for a nationwide multicenter randomized controlled trial. BMC Cancer 2021;21(1):300.

23. Jang JY, Han Y, Lee H, et al. Oncological benefits of neoadjuvant chemoradiation with gemcitabine versus upfront surgery in patients with borderline resectable pancreatic cancer: a prospective, randomized, open-label, multicenter phase 2/3 trial. Ann Surg 2018;268(2):215–22.

24. Katz MHG, Shi Q, Meyers JP, et al. Alliance A021501: preoperative mFOLFIRINOX or mFOLFIRINOX plus hypofractionated radiation therapy (RT) for borderline resectable (BR) adenocarcinoma of the pancreas. J Clin Oncol 2021; 39(3_suppl):377.

25. Murphy JE, Wo JY, Ryan DP, et al. Total neoadjuvant therapy with FOLFIRINOX followed by individualized chemoradiotherapy for borderline resectable pancreatic adenocarcinoma: a phase 2 clinical trial. JAMA Oncol 2018;4(7):963–9.

26. Hammel P, Huguet F, van Laethem JL, et al. Effect of chemoradiotherapy vs chemotherapy on survival in patients with locally advanced pancreatic cancer controlled after 4 months of gemcitabine with or without erlotinib: the LAP07 randomized clinical trial. JAMA 2016;315(17):1844–53.

27. Fietkau R, Ghadimi M, Grützmann R, et al. Randomized phase III trial of induction chemotherapy followed by chemoradiotherapy or chemotherapy alone for nonresectable locally advanced pancreatic cancer: First results of the CONKO-007 trial. J Clin Oncol 2022;40(16_suppl):4008.

28. Koong AC, Le QT, Ho A, et al. Phase I study of stereotactic radiosurgery in patients with locally advanced pancreatic cancer. Int J Radiat Oncol Biol Phys 2004;58(4):1017–21.

29. Park C, Papiez L, Zhang S, et al. Universal survival curve and single fraction equivalent dose: useful tools in understanding potency of ablative radiotherapy. Int J Radiat Oncol Biol Phys 2008;70(3):847–52.
30. Pollom EL, Alagappan M, von Eyben R, et al. Single- versus multifraction stereotactic body radiation therapy for pancreatic adenocarcinoma: outcomes and toxicity. Int J Radiat Oncol Biol Phys 2014;90(4):918–25.
31. Song YC, Yuan ZY, Li FT, et al. Analysis of clinical efficacy of CyberKnife (R) treatment for locally advanced pancreatic cancer. OncoTargets Ther 2015;8.
32. Ryan JF, Rosati LM, Groot VP, et al. Stereotactic body radiation therapy for palliative management of pancreatic adenocarcinoma in elderly and medically inoperable patients. Oncotarget 2018;9(23):16427–36.
33. Mellon EA, Hoffe SE, Springett GM, et al. Long-term outcomes of induction chemotherapy and neoadjuvant stereotactic body radiotherapy for borderline resectable and locally advanced pancreatic adenocarcinoma. Acta Oncol 2015;54(7):979–85.
34. Jung J, Yoon SM, Park JH, et al. Stereotactic body radiation therapy for locally advanced pancreatic cancer. PLoS One 2019;14(4):e0214970.
35. Arcelli A, Guido A, Buwenge M, et al. Higher biologically effective dose predicts survival in SBRT of pancreatic cancer: a multicentric analysis (PAULA-1). Anticancer Res 2020;40(1):465–72.
36. Oar A, Lee M, Le H, et al. AGITG MASTERPLAN: a randomised phase II study of modified FOLFIRINOX alone or in combination with stereotactic body radiotherapy for patients with high-risk and locally advanced pancreatic cancer. BMC Cancer 2021;21(1).
37. Wang RC, Goepfert H, Barber AE, et al. Unknown primary squamous cell carcinoma metastatic to the neck. Arch Otolaryngol Head Neck Surg 1990;116(12):1388–93.
38. Brunner TB, Haustermans K, Huguet F, et al. ESTRO ACROP guidelines for target volume definition in pancreatic cancer. Radiother Oncol 2021;154:60–9.
39. Oar A, Lee M, Le H, et al. Australasian gastrointestinal trials group (AGITG) and trans-tasman radiation oncology group (TROG) guidelines for pancreatic stereotactic body radiation therapy (SBRT). Pract Radiat Oncol 2020;10(3):e136–46.
40. Palta M, Godfrey D, Goodman KA, et al. Radiation therapy for pancreatic cancer: executive summary of an ASTRO clinical practice guideline. Pract Radiat Oncol 2019;9(5):322–32.
41. Brunner TB, Merkel S, Grabenbauer GG, et al. Definition of elective lymphatic target volume in ductal carcinoma of the pancreatic head based on histopathologic analysis. Int J Radiat Oncol Biol Phys 2005;62(4):1021–9.
42. Kharofa J, Mierzwa M, Olowokure O, et al. Pattern of marginal local failure in a phase II trial of neoadjuvant chemotherapy and stereotactic body radiation therapy for resectable and borderline resectable pancreas cancer. Am J Clin Oncol 2019;42(3):247–52.
43. Zhu X, Ju X, Cao Y, et al. Patterns of local failure after stereotactic body radiation therapy and sequential chemotherapy as initial treatment for pancreatic cancer: implications of target volume design. Int J Radiat Oncol Biol Phys 2019;104(1):101–10.
44. Miller JA, Toesca DAS, Baclay JRM, et al. Pancreatic stereotactic body radiation therapy with or without hypofractionated elective nodal irradiation. Int J Radiat Oncol Biol Phys 2021;112(1):131–42.
45. Elhammali A, Patel M, Weinberg B, et al. Late gastrointestinal tissue effects after hypofractionated radiation therapy of the pancreas. Radiat Oncol 2015;10:186.

46. Heerkens HD, van Vulpen M, van den Berg CA, et al. MRI-based tumor motion characterization and gating schemes for radiation therapy of pancreatic cancer. Radiother Oncol 2014;111(2):252–7.
47. Bohoudi O, Bruynzeel AME, Senan S, et al. Fast and robust online adaptive planning in stereotactic MR-guided adaptive radiation therapy (SMART) for pancreatic cancer. Radiother Oncol 2017;125(3):439–44.
48. Henke L, Kashani R, Robinson C, et al. Phase I trial of stereotactic MR-guided online adaptive radiation therapy (SMART) for the treatment of oligometastatic or unresectable primary malignancies of the abdomen. Radiother Oncol 2018; 126(3):519–26.
49. Rudra S, Jiang N, Rosenberg SA, et al. Using adaptive magnetic resonance image-guided radiation therapy for treatment of inoperable pancreatic cancer. Cancer Med 2019;8(5):2123–32.
50. Chuong MD, Bryant J, Mittauer KE, et al. Ablative 5-fraction stereotactic magnetic resonance-guided radiation therapy with on-table adaptive replanning and elective nodal irradiation for inoperable pancreas cancer. Pract Radiat Oncol 2021; 11(2):134–47.
51. Hassanzadeh C, Rudra S, Bommireddy A, et al. Ablative five-fraction stereotactic body radiation therapy for inoperable pancreatic cancer using online MR-guided adaptation. Adv Radiat Oncol 2021;6(1):100506.
52. Hall WA, Small C, Paulson E, et al. Magnetic resonance guided radiation therapy for pancreatic adenocarcinoma, advantages, challenges, current approaches, and future directions. Front Oncol 2021;11:628155.
53. Chuong MD, Kirsch C, Herrera R, et al. Long-term multi-institutional outcomes of 5-fraction ablative stereotactic mr-guided adaptive radiation therapy (SMART) for inoperable pancreas cancer with median prescribed biologically effective dose of 100 Gy10</sub>. Int J Radiat Oncol Biol Phys 2021;111(3):S147–8.
54. Perone JA, Riall TS, Olino K. Palliative care for pancreatic and periampullary cancer. Surg Clin North Am 2016;96(6):1415–30.
55. Ebrahimi G, Rasch CRN, van Tienhoven G. Pain relief after a short course of palliative radiotherapy in pancreatic cancer, the Academic Medical Center (AMC) experience. Acta Oncol 2018;57(5):697–700.
56. Buwenge M, Macchia G, Arcelli A, et al. Stereotactic radiotherapy of pancreatic cancer: a systematic review on pain relief. J Pain Res 2018;11:2169–78.
57. Hammer L, Hausner D, Ben-Ayun M, et al. Single-fraction celiac plexus radiosurgery: a preliminary proof-of-concept phase 2 clinical trial. Int J Radiat Oncol Biol Phys 2022;113(3):588–93.
58. Hoyer M, Roed H, Sengelov L, et al. Phase-II study on stereotactic radiotherapy of locally advanced pancreatic carcinoma. Radiother Oncol 2005;76(1):48–53.
59. Weichselbaum RR, Hellman S. Oligometastases revisited. Nat Rev Clin Oncol 2011;8(6):378–82.
60. Hagiwara K, Harimoto N, Araki K, et al. Long-term survival of two patients with pancreatic cancer after resection of liver and lung oligometastases: a case report. Surg Case Rep 2020;6(1):309.
61. Saedon M, Maroulis I, Brooks A, et al. Metastasectomy of pancreatic and periampullary adenocarcinoma to solid organ: The current evidence. J BUON 2018; 23(6):1648–54.
62. Yachida S, Jones S, Bozic I, et al. Distant metastasis occurs late during the genetic evolution of pancreatic cancer. Nature 2010;467(7319):1114–7.

63. Yamanaka M, Hayashi M, Yamada S, et al. A possible definition of oligometastasis in pancreatic cancer and associated survival outcomes. Anticancer Res 2021; 41(8):3933–40.

64. Elamir AM, Karalis JD, Sanford NN, et al. Ablative radiation therapy in oligometastatic pancreatic cancer to delay polyprogression, limit chemotherapy, and improve outcomes. Int J Radiat Oncol Biol Phys 2022;114(4):792–802.

Advances in Radiation Therapy for Primary Liver Cancer

Kyle C. Cuneo, MD*, Daniel J. Herr, MD, PhD

KEYWORDS

- Stereotactic body radiation therapy • Adaptive radiation therapy
- Y-90 radioembolization • Y-90 segmentectomy • Hepatocellular carcinoma

KEY POINTS

- Liver stereotactic body radiation therapy (SBRT) is a safe and effective treatment of patients with hepatocellular carcinoma.
- Recent advances in SBRT include MR-guided and biology-guided radiotherapy.
- Adaptive radiation is an exciting new option for patients at higher risk for toxicity.
- Personalized Y-90 radioembolization has the potential to improve outcomes in patients.

INTRODUCTION

Management of patients with primary liver cancer including hepatocellular carcinoma and cholangiocarcinoma is challenging because of underlying liver disease, associated comorbidities, and the sensitivity of the liver to locoregional therapies. Ideally, treatment decisions should be made with input from a multidisciplinary team including surgery, hepatology, medical oncology, radiology, radiation oncology, and pathology. Radiation therapy in the form of stereotactic body radiation therapy (SBRT) or Yttrium-90 transarterial radioembolization (TARE) is an effective tool in the management of patients with primary liver cancer. Several recent advances in the field have made these treatments safer and more effective leading to increased utilization. Here, we discuss recent advances in radiation therapy for the management of primary liver cancers including hepatocellular carcinoma and intrahepatic cholangiocarcinoma.

Stereotactic Body Radiation Therapy

SBRT involves the delivery of relatively high doses of radiation over a small number of fractions (1–6) typically using advanced treatment planning techniques and image guidance. The first reports of using SBRT in the liver to treat cancer are from the

Department of Radiation Oncology, University of Michigan, 1500 E Medical Center Dr, Ann Arbor, MI 48109, USA
* Corresponding author.
E-mail address: kcuneo@umich.edu

Surg Oncol Clin N Am 32 (2023) 415–432
https://doi.org/10.1016/j.soc.2023.02.002
1055-3207/23/© 2023 Elsevier Inc. All rights reserved.

surgonc.theclinics.com

mid-1990s.[1,2] During the past 3 decades the ability to precisely delivery radiation and our understanding of normal tissue and tumor radiation dose response have improved considerably.

SBRT is most commonly delivered using a linear accelerator-based treatment system with daily image guidance and respiratory motion management; however, several other treatment platforms exist. Patients undergo initial simulation scans with contrast-enhanced computed tomography (CT) and, in many cases, MRI, which are fused with the planning CT scan for improved target delineation (**Fig. 1**). At the time of simulation, strategies for respiratory motion are determined. These include various breath hold techniques that have been previously reviewed[3,4] or 4-dimensional CT scans, which allow for visualization of tumor motion for planning purposes.[5] Often radiopaque markers called fiducials are placed percutaneously around the tumor to assist with daily alignment.[6,7] More recently, newer technologies (reviewed below and in accompanying articles in this issue) including magnetic resonance imaging (MRI) and positron emission tomography (PET) guidance have been incorporated into linear accelerators to facilitate daily set up and motion tracking of tumors during treatment. These advances have allowed for tighter treatment planning margins and improved accuracy and precision in the delivery of radiation therapy to a patient.

Several prospective clinical trials have demonstrated that liver SBRT is a safe and effective treatment option for patients with liver cancer. The group from Princess Margaret Hospital published several of the early prospective studies using SBRT for patients with liver cancer. These studies showed promising local control rates near 90% but had relatively high rates of liver decompensation.[8,9] These early studies identified the importance of baseline liver function on the risk of toxicity from liver radiation, mainly that patients with Child Pugh class B liver function are at a high risk of liver decompensation. During the following 2 decades, improvements in technology and our understanding of factors associated with toxicity from SBRT have led to lower rates of toxicity with improved control rates. Most modern series demonstrate control rates between 90% and 95% with the risk of liver decompensation being less than 10% in appropriately selected patients (**Table 1**).

SBRT can be used as an alternative to microwave and radiofrequency ablation to target 1 to 3 or more tumors in the liver in a single course. SBRT is commonly used

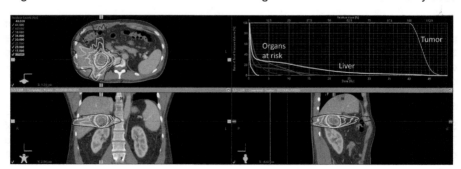

Fig. 1. Treatment planning images from Eclipse (Varian) for a patient receiving liver SBRT. Shown are axial, coronal, and sagittal planes with the targeted tumor and isodose lines. Each isodose line represents a specific dose distribution within the patient. The upper right panel shows a dose value histogram (DVH), which provides a graphical representation of the dose per volume for the tumor and adjacent organs. In this plan, the whole tumor receives a high dose of radiation (>40 Gy in 3 fractions), whereas OARs receive much lower doses. The radiation plan is created using treatment planning software to meet preset dose constraints and target goals.

Table 1
Select prospective studies of liver stereotactic body radiation therapy

Study	Phase	N	Dose	Outcomes	Liver Toxicity
Bujold et al,[8] 2013	I/II	CPA 102	24–54 Gy/6 fx	LC 1y 87% OS 1y 55%	29%
Culleton et al,[9] 2014	II	CPB 29	30 Gy/6 fx	Median OS 7.9 mo	63%
Lasley et al,[10] 2015	I/II	CPA 38 CPB 21	CPA 48 Gy/3 fx CPB 40 Gy/5 fx	CPA LC 2y 91% CPB LC 2y 82%	CPA 11% CPB 38%
Weiner et al,[11] 2016	I/II	CPA 23 CPB 3	55 Gy/5 fx	LC 1y 91%	35%
Feng et al,[12] 2018	II	CPA 69 CPB 21	23–60 Gy/3–5 fx Adaptive	LC 2y 95%	7%
Durand-Labrunie et al,[13] 2020	II	CPA 37 CPB 5	45 Gy/3 fx	LC 18 mo 98%	10%
Yoon et al,[14] 2020	II	CPA 50 (<5 cm)	45 Gy/3 fx	LC 5y 97%	4%

over ablation for larger tumors (>3 cm) given the improved local control rates in these situations.[15] Additionally, SBRT is useful to treat tumors not amenable to ablation due to location (eg, liver dome or deep central tumors) or proximity to major blood vessels (heat sink effect). The decision of which treatment modality to pursue for a patient is best determined in a multidisciplinary tumor board setting and depends on the resources and expertise available at an institution. Most large centers, which have ablation and SBRT available currently view these treatments as being interchangeable for small tumors given similar rates of local control and toxicity.[15–17] Advantages of ablation over SBRT include fewer visits for the patient, less cost in most circumstances, and the ability to biopsy the tumor at the same time. Advantages of SBRT include its noninvasive nature and ability to treat tumors not amenable to ablation.

Delivering high doses of radiation to the liver can be challenging due to the radiosensitivity of adjacent organs at risk, mainly the liver, bowel, and stomach.[18,19] The liver is quite sensitive to radiation therapy,[10,20,21] however, this organ has a considerable amount of reserve, so as long as a specific volume healthy liver is kept to a safe dose (approximately 700 cc), the risk of liver injury is relatively low. Adjacent bowel and stomach are also very sensitive to radiation, and unlike the liver, these organs are limited by the maximum dose they can receive given their serial functional subunit organization.[22,23] Further complicating these matters are the daily positional changes and respiratory associated motion that occurs in stomach, bowel, and other organs, which can add uncertainty into the true dose these organs receive. Fortunately, new technologies have allowed us to address many of these issues allowing for safer and more effective treatments.

Although SBRT is a safe and effective treatment of patients with small tumors and good liver function,[15] most of the large studies demonstrating safety and efficacy of treatment have enrolled predominantly patients with Child Pugh A (CP-A) disease.[8,24] Treatment of patients with compromised liver function remains a challenge, with greater rates of functional hepatic decline following SBRT in these patients.[9,10,25] For example, a recent prospective analysis of 29 patients with Child-Pugh B and C disease undergoing SBRT for HCC to a mean dose of 34 Gy in 6 fractions demonstrated a 34% rate of Child-Pugh score increase of 2 or more points within a month of treatment.[9] Another recent large retrospective study of 146 patients undergoing SBRT to 50 Gy in 5 fractions or hypofractionated RT to 45 Gy in 18 fractions demonstrated similar findings. Of the 51 patients with Child Pugh (CP) B8 or worse disease included in this analysis, 35% experienced a 2-point or greater worsening of CP score within 6 months of treatment.[25] Methods to optimize the therapeutic ratio for these patients have been promising in terms of achieving acceptable local control and minimizing risk of liver injury. In this review, we discuss recent advances in radiation therapy for patients with liver cancer.

Charged Particle Therapy

Most radiation therapy treatments are administered using high energy x-rays or electrons. Several other forms of radiation exist, many of which have superior physical properties to standard x-ray photons, including proton therapy and carbon ion therapy. Protons have a fixed range in tissue meaning the deposition of their energy is over a limited volume resulting in their characteristic Bragg Peak. Theoretically, the lack of exit dose can allow for lower radiation dose to dose-limiting adjacent organs at risk. However, protons are still subject to the limitations seen with standard x-ray treatments in the liver, including poor tumor delineation on set up imaging, organ motion, and deformation. Carbon ion therapy has the advantages of protons in terms of limiting exit dose in addition to superior radiation biology properties over traditional x-rays and protons. The major barrier to these treatments being more available is their extremely high cost and the high level of physics support and expertise to perform these therapies safely. Recently, more cost-effective proton units have been developed allowing for expanded access to these treatments for patients. Carbon ions facilities remain very limited and costly.

Earlier studies using particle therapy for liver cancers have shown promising results (**Table 2**). Bush and colleagues performed a 76 patient prospective trial in patients with liver cancer treated with proton therapy. On this study, 54 patients had Child Pugh class B disease and no grade 3+ toxicity liver was reported.[26] Hong and colleagues reported on a 44 patient trial with protons with 9 patients with Child Pugh class B disease showing a 2-year control rates of 95% and only 4% grade 3+ liver toxicity in the cohort.[27] Additionally, Kasuya and colleagues performed a large prospective study in 127 patients with liver cancer treated with carbon ion therapy. This study had excellent local control rates of 95% at 1 year and 90% at 5 years with only 5% liver toxicity.[28] Prospective studies comparing particle therapy to x-ray-based SBRT are greatly needed to determine the value of these modalities.

Adaptive Radiation Therapy

Adaptative radiation therapy is an emerging concept, which uses information obtained before and during treatment to modify and optimize therapy. Adaptation can be incorporated into multiple parts of the treatment course. During the treatment itself, information can be obtained from advanced imaging and treatment planning techniques to adjust the radiation plan based off tumor and organ at risk positional changes. This ability to adapt during treatment has been driven by improvements in on board imaging technology including MRI-guided and PET-guided linear accelerators, which are discussed below. Additionally, adaptation can be performed in between fractions in a treatment course using imaging and predictive biomarkers of response and toxicity to modify the prescription dose and dose distribution, as described below.

Magnetic Resonance Imaging-Guided Therapy

A major challenge in treating patients with liver cancer with SBRT is the limited ability to visualize the tumor and normal tissue at the time of treatment delivery due to the limited soft tissue delineation capabilities of standard on board imaging modalities such as cone beam CT. CT-based image guidance systems typically use surrogates such as the edges of normal liver, patient exterior anatomy, or fiducial markers to align and deliver treatment. Several factors can lead to inconsistencies with these approaches including irregular breathing patients, liver deformation (from ascites for example), and normal organ motion. To overcome these issues, MRI-guided treatment systems have been developed with 2 recently approved for clinical use by the Food and Drug Administration. The major advantage of MR-linac systems is the ability for real-time visualization of the tumor and surrounding organs.[30]

Different approaches using an MR-linac to treat liver cancer have been developed. A commonly used technique is online adaptation.[30,31] Online adaptation involves real-time assessment of the target and organs at risk followed by radiation plan adaptation while the patient is on the treatment table. Given the poor soft tissue delineation with standard cone beam CT imaging, this process is only feasible at this time using an MRI-guided linac system.[32,33]

Several studies have examined the potential feasibility, safety, and efficacy of MR-guided radiation therapy for liver cancer. Rosenberg and colleagues treated 26 patients with HCC and metastatic cancer using an MRI-linac. This study showed a long-term local control rate of 80% with 2 grade 3+ toxicities.[34] Feldman and

Table 2
Prospective studies of liver particle therapy

Study	Phase	N	Dose	Outcomes	Toxicity
Bush et al,[26] 2011 Proton	II	22 HCC CPA 36 HCC CPB 18 HCC CBC	63 GyE/15 fx	LC 80% 3y PFS 60%	0% liver 7% Grade 2 gastrointestinal
Hong et al,[27] 2016 Proton	II	44 HCC 37 ICC 2 HCC/ICC	67.5 GyE/15 fx (median 58 GyE)	LC 94.8% HCC LC 94.1% ICC	4.8% G3 toxicity 3.6% liver
Fukumitsu et al,[29] 2009 Proton	II	51 HCC	66 GyE/10 fx	3y LC 94.5%	16% CP decline
Kasuya et al,[28] 2017 Carbon	I/II	129 HCC	MTD 52.8 GyE/4 fx	1y LC 94.7% 3y LC 91.4%	5% CP increase at 6 mo

colleagues reported on 29 patients with 31 lesions treated with an MR-linac.[35] This study showed no grade 3 toxicity with local control greater than 90%. Additionally, Henke and colleagues performed a study using stereotactic MR-guided adaptive radiation therapy. Their study had no grade 3 toxicity events with a 1-year local control rate of 89%[36] (**Table 3**). Multiple studies using these technologies are ongoing.

Although, MR-guided radiation therapy clearly demonstrates the improved ability to delineate the tumor and normal tissues over conventional approaches, the technology has limitations. First off, the equipment needed to perform this treatment is considerably more expensive than traditional linac-based SBRT systems. Additionally, although dosimetric studies suggest these techniques can lower dose to normal tissues and allow for tighter treatment planning margins on the target tumor, the benefit over traditional SBRT approaches has not been demonstrated in an appropriately powered randomized prospective study. Finally, these treatments are more time and resource dependent. All these reasons have limited the use of MR adaptive therapy to mainly academic research centers at this time.

Biology-Guided Radiotherapy

Biology-guided radiotherapy (Bg-RT) is an exciting new technology that incorporates PET/CT imaging with radiation therapy in one system. PET allows for real-time visualization of biological processes. In addition to the commonly used tracer fluorodeoxyglucose (FDG), many other tracers exist, which target varying biological processes within the tumor and tissue. The systems being developed are currently focusing on using the radiotracer signal to monitor and track the tumor in real time during treatment delivery. In this sense, the tumor can act as its own fiducial marker.

There is currently one approved Bg-RT treatment system in the United States. The RefleXion X1 system (RefleXion Medical, Inc, Hayward, CA) recently received U.S. Food and Drug Administration (FDA) clearance for an investigational new device exemption clinical trial.[37] There are a handful of these units installed at academic centers in the United States and we are awaiting clinical data from the first patients treated with this technology.

Currently, Bg-RT is in the early steps of development with a focus mainly on tumor tracking during therapy. Several other applications of Bg-RT potentially exist. Liver tumors can be quite heterogenous in terms of their biology and microenvironment. Radiosensitivity depends on several factors that can vary substantially within an individual tumor including the amount of oxygen present, which is required for free radical production resulting in DNA damage. Using novel tracers, such as hypoxia markers, may allow for boosting select regions of a tumor deemed to be radioresistant through the oxygen effect.[38,39] Additionally, other functional imaging modalities such as functional MRI could be used to dose large heterogenous tumors based off regions of radiosensitivity. This technique potentially could allow for lower doses to portions of the tumor adjacent to organs at risk (OARs) in addition to increased doses to regions of the tumor thought to be more radioresistant.

Ionizing Radiation Acoustic Imaging

A major limitation in current radiation treatment approaches is the inability to detect where and how much radiation is delivered to a target. Currently, these parameters are estimated based off imaging and computer calculations obtained before delivery. Although, MR and PET-guided systems potentially improve our ability to localized and target the tumor, neither of these systems tells us what dose is actually delivered to the target. Understanding this information has the potential to optimize the delivery of

Table 3
MR-guided radiation therapy studies

Study	Phase	N	Dose	Outcomes	Liver Toxicity
Henke et al,[36] 2018	I	20 (10 liver)	50 Gy/5 fx Adaptive	6 mo PFS 89%; 66% of fractions had improved PTV coverage	0%
Feldman et al,[35] 2019	Retrospective	29	45–50 Gy/5 fx Not adaptive	LC 1 y 97%	0%
Rosenberg et al,[34] 2019	Retrospective	26	50 Gy/5 fx Not adaptive	FFLP 80% all pts FFLP 100% HCC	0% Grade 4+
Luterstein et al,[76] 2020	Retrospective	17 (cholangio)	40 Gy/5 fx Adaptive	LC 1 y 86%	0%
Boldrini et al,[77] 2021	Retrospective	10	50–55 Gy/5 fx	LC 90%	10%

radiation to patients. One system currently being developed is ionizing radiation acoustic imaging (iRAI).[40–43]

iRAI is a novel medical imaging modality that allows for real-time determination of the radiation dose being delivered. This technology uses the thermoacoustic effect[40] where acoustical waves are generated from the small transient temperature increase in irradiated tissue resulting in thermal expansion. Currently, this technology is limited to preclinical systems[40,44–46] and ongoing early phase clinical studies. Preclinical studies have demonstrated the potential of iRAI for monitoring in real time the alignment of the target and radiation beam in conventional and ultra-high dose rate systems such as FLASH.[42,43] By removing the uncertainties in dose delivery to the target and organs at risks, smaller treatment margins could be used and theoretically higher doses could be delivered in situations where mobile organs at risk (bowel, stomach, colon) are adjacent to the target.

Adaptive Split Course Radiation

One novel concept that has recently been proposed to reduce toxicity related to treatment in patients at higher risk of liver decompensation is adaptive radiation treatment in a split course. This treatment paradigm uses a 1-month treatment break following the first 3 fractions of SBRT, with reassessment of hepatic function before proceeding with the final 2 fractions. In 2017, Feng and colleagues prospectively assessed this concept in a single arm phase II trial, which enrolled 90 patients.[12] In this study, hepatic function was directly assessed at baseline by evaluating indocyanine green retention at 15 minutes (ICGR15). Patients then received 3 fractions of a planned 5 fraction SBRT course, followed by a 4-week treatment break to allow for reassessment of subclinical liver function change. After this break, ICGR15 was reevaluated before proceeding with the final 2 fractions with dose adaptation utilizing statistical modeling to predict the posttreatment ICGR15 based on baseline and midtreatment ICGR15, dose delivered in the first 3 fractions, and planned dose for the final 2 fractions. If midtreatment ICGR15 was less than 44%, no further treatment was given. In total, 69% of patients completed all 5 planned fractions. Using this approach, only 7% of patients experienced at 2+-point decline in CP score within 6 months, with a local control rate of 99% at 1 year and 95% at 2 years.

Subsequently, the same group analyzed 178 patients receiving either conventional or adaptive SBRT in 3 or 5 fractions with the goal of comparing local control and treatment-related toxicity between these 2 groups. This analysis demonstrated equivalent local control, with a 1-year local control rate of 98% for patients treated with a 1-month break and 93% for patients treated without a break. Inverse probability of treatment weighting controlling for the number of earlier liver-directed therapies, mean liver dose, and receipt of a treatment break demonstrated a decreased risk of treatment-related toxicity in patients receiving a midtreatment break.[47]

Although the aforementioned studies demonstrate similar efficacy and improved toxicity with adaptive SBRT, they only evaluated a limited number of patients with Child Pugh B or worse liver disease. These patients are at greater risk of hepatic decompensation following treatment and, therefore, are more likely to benefit from toxicity reduction with adaptive treatment. The use of adaptive SBRT to mitigate treatment-related toxicity in this population was retrospectively assessed in 2 recent studies. One analysis of prospectively collected data for 80 patients treated on clinical trials at a single institution revealed a 22.5% rate of CP score decline of 2 points or more at 6 months with local control rates of 93% and 86% at 1 and 2 years, respectively.[48] Another retrospective single-institution study of 37 patients receiving SBRT for HCC included 9 patients with CP $\geq$ B8 disease, who were treated with split course

SBRT with a planned total dose of 50 Gy in 5 fractions. Although this study did not report change in CP scores, only 1 out of 9 patients with CP $\geq$ B8 disease experienced a grade 3+ treatment-related toxicity.[49] Given the reduced rates of treatment-related toxicity associated with adaptive SBRT, this approach has the promise to expand treatment to patients with worse liver function, who historically have prohibitively high rates of treatment-related toxicity with standard SBRT.

One possible limitation to the widespread adaptation of the split-course adaptive approach is the reliance on ICGR15 for baseline hepatic function assessment, which is more time consuming and specialized than standard laboratory tests. This has prompted investigation into other measures of hepatic function that are more convenient and less invasive to the patient. A recent study assessing baseline and midtreatment ICGR15 and albumin-bilirubin (ALBI) scores for 151 patients undergoing adaptive SBRT for hepatocellular carcinoma revealed that ALBI-centric predictive models performed similarly to indocyanine green (ICG)-centric models on multivariate analyses predicting treatment-related toxicity.[50] Given that ALBI can be conveniently calculated from standard laboratory tests that are routinely performed in patients with hepatocellular carcinoma, this approach offers great promise as a routine measure of hepatic function that can be leveraged for midtreatment adaptation of SBRT.

Biomarker-Guided Therapy

Currently liver function is mainly classified using either Child Pugh or ALBI scoring systems. Both of these methods are dependent on serum values of albumin and bilirubin, with Child Pugh score adding international normalized ratio (INR) and partially subjective clinical factors. The classification systems have been associated with overall survival; however, their use in guiding radiation therapy and patient selection may not be optimal. Understanding the biological processes behind radiation liver injury and tumor response would be helpful for patient selection and dose modification.

In addition to the standard markers listed above, cytokines and other proteins have been correlated with outcomes and toxicity. Earlier studies have identified several biomarkers associated with liver function and treatment-related toxicity including hepatocyte growth factor (HGF), CD40 L, transforming growth factor-beta (TGFβ), and tumor necrosis factor-alpha (TNFα).[51–54]

TNFα in particular has been linked to acute and chronic liver injury in several studies[55–57] in addition to its well-defined role in multiple inflammatory conditions.[58–60] Several drugs exist, which target these pathways and are in clinical use for multiple inflammatory conditions. A limitation of TNFα in clinical use is its short half-life (20–70 minutes); however, one of the major receptors of TNFα, TNFR1, has been shown to be a stable marker of inflammation.[58,59] In 2 recently published studies, pretreatment TNFR1 levels were shown to be predictive of radiation-associated liver injury after liver SBRT and Y90 treatment.[60–62] Currently, concepts to target the TNF axis using off-label FDA-approved therapies such as anti-TNF drugs and steroids are being explored.

Another serum marker of interest is HGF. HGF is the major ligand for the kinase cMET. As the name infers, HGF plays an important role in liver regeneration after injury and in organ development. Multiple groups have identified HGF as a potential predictive and prognostic biomarker for toxicity and outcome following liver SBRT.[53,54] Additionally, drugs which target the HGF-MET axis and recombinant HGF proteins are being developed for potential clinical use.

Improved understanding of the mechanisms behind radiation-induced liver injury has the potential to improve outcomes in patients undergoing liver radiation. Using biomarkers in the pretreatment setting to help select patients and select dose may provide for improved patient selection over Child Pugh and ALBI scores. Additionally, targeting these pathways has the potential to mitigate toxicity and improve the therapeutic ratio in patients.

Yttrium-90 Radioembolization

TARE is another form of radiation therapy available for patients. Unlike external beam radiation, TARE involves injecting Y-90 embedded in glass beads (Theraspheres) or resin (SIR-Spheres) into the hepatic artery and its branches. This therapy is possible due to the dual blood supply to the liver. Earlier studies have shown that tumors receive most of their blood supply from the arterial system, whereas the healthy liver receives most of its blood supply from the portal venous system.[63,64]

Y-90 is a pure beta emitter with a half-life of 64.2 hours and average tissue penetrance is 2.4 mm, making it an excellent source for therapeutic treatments. A standard Y-90 TARE treatment involves an initial mapping session using technetium-99m macroaggregated albumin as a surrogate for Y-90 dose distribution. The mapping session determines the estimated dose that would be delivered to the lungs, maps the vasculature to check for perfusion to organs at risk, and provides the volume of liver to be targeted for dose vial ordering. Patients typically undergo treatment 2 weeks after the mapping session. Major advantages of Y-90 include no requirement for hospitalization, relatively few visits for the patient, and the ability to cover multiple tumors in one setting. Disadvantages include the need for 2 or more invasive procedures, rare but potentially severe complications such as liver, bowel, stomach, and lung injury, and the fact it is largely limited to patients with relatively good underlying liver function (Child Pugh A). Historically, Y-90 treatment has been administered to an entire lobe of the liver via direct injection into the left or right hepatic artery. This method has been shown to be effective and safe leading to full FDA approval.

Radiation Segmentectomy

A major issue with lobar Y-90 dosing is that the total dose delivered to the tumor is limited by normal liver tolerance and heterogeneity between and within the arterially perfused targets. Recent studies have demonstrated that lobar treatments can underdose target tumors, and tumors receiving lower doses are at a higher risk of failure.[65] More recently, segmental treatment strategies have been developed, which allow for considerably higher doses to be delivered to smaller volumes. Studies using radiation segmentectomy Y-90 TARE have shown encouraging response rates around 80% and low risks of toxicities[66-71] (**Table 4**). However, prospective studies evaluating the use of segmentectomy specifically comparing it to other modalities are lacking.

Dosimetry-Guided Treatment

Given the uncertainty of the actual dose delivered and the dependence of dose on response, several groups have developed methods to determine if a tumor receiving Y-90 is adequately dosed. One method to estimate the dose delivered to the tumor uses the 99mTc-macroaggregated albumin (MAA) SPECT/CT scan obtained at mapping to predict what dose each tumor will receive.[65,72] Predicted dose delivered to the target using this method has been correlated with clinical response.[65] The DOSISPHERE-01 study used MAA SPECT/CT-based planning to assure delivery of high doses to the target tumor. This study suggested there was a survival benefit for patients treated to a threshold dose of greater than 205 Gy over conventional dosing based off the perfused liver volume.[73]

Another method is to use PET to measure the dose delivered posttreatment.[74,75] Secondary radioisotope decay from Y-90 emits positron signals that can be directly measured using standard PET scanners. This information can be used to accurately

Table 4
Select retrospective studies of Y-90 segmentectomy

Study	Phase	N	Dose	Outcomes	Liver Toxicity
Salem et al,[66] 2021	Retrospective	162	Median 410 Gy	ORR 88%	19.1% G3 any
Lewandowski et al,[67] 2018	Retrospective	70	Not reported >190 Gy	CR 59% 5y LC 72%	5.7% G3 liver
Vouche et al,[68] 2014	Retrospective	104	Median 242 Gy	CR 47% PR 39%	9.6% bilirubin elevation
Riaz et al,[69] 2011	Retrospective	84	Median 521 Gy	RR 81%	9% liver toxicity
Biederman et al,[70] 2018	Retrospective	55	Not reported	CR 81%	5.5% G3+ liver
Padia et al,[71] 2017	Retrospective	101	Not reported >200 Gy	RR 84%	9.9% biochemical toxicity

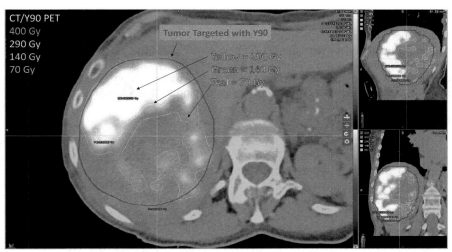

Fig. 2. Posttreatment Y-90 PET imaging. This image was acquired shortly after Y-90 administration to the right lobe of the liver. Using advanced software, the PET signal from Y-90 decay is converted into isodose lines and overlayed on a planning or diagnostic CT scan. This image demonstrates the heterogeneity of dose distribution in a large tumor treated with Y-90. A portion of the tumor received less than 140 Gy and 70 Gy, which is associated with an increased risk of local failure. Targeting the underdosed regions with an external beam radiation boost was planned for this patient as part of a clinical trial (NCT04518748).

determine the true dose delivered to the tumor and has several advantages over SPECT imaging including higher spatial resolution and improved ability to quantify absolute dose delivered[75] (**Fig. 2**).

A novel approach, which is currently being tested in a clinical trial (NCT04518748), is to use external beam radiation therapy to boost underdosed lesions following Y-90 administration. This approach has the potential to offer ablative local regional therapy to patients with multiple tumors treated with Y-90 where one or more tumors are not adequately dosed with the initial infusion.

SUMMARY

The development of novel radiation treatment techniques for patients with liver cancer represents a major advancement in oncology. The ability to personalize and adapt therapy has the potential to maximize the therapeutic ratio in patients, especially those with poor baseline liver function. Given the potential costs of these new technologies, testing in a clinical trial setting would be vital to demonstrate safety and efficacy over standard approaches.

CLINICS CARE POINTS

- Stereotactic body radiation therapy (SBRT) is a safe and effective treatment option for hepatocellular carcinoma.
- Emerging techinques to personalize treatment include MR-guided, biology-guided and split-course adaptive SBRT.
- Recent refinements in the delivery of Y-90 radioembolization may improve outcomes.

DECLARATION OF INTERESTS

K.C. Cuneo has a patent pending related to iRAI: U.S. Application No. 17/600,564, National Phase of International Application No. PCT/US20/32,385, Title: Combined Radiation Acoustics and Ultrasound for Radiotherapy Guidance and Cancer. K.C. Cuneo is also the principal investigator on a clinical trial involving Y-90 and SBRT combination therapy and iRAI and receives NIH funding for these projects.

REFERENCES

1. Blomgren H, Lax I, Näslund I, et al. Stereotactic high dose fraction radiation therapy of extracranial tumors using an accelerator. Clinical experience of the first thirty-one patients. Acta Oncol 1995;34(6):861–70.
2. Lax I, Blomgren H, Larson D, et al. Extracranial stereotactic radiosurgery of localized targets. J Radiosurg 1998;1:135–48.
3. Soni PD, Palta M. Stereotactic Body Radiation Therapy for Hepatocellular Carcinoma: Current State and Future Opportunities. Dig Dis Sci 2019;64(4):1008–15.
4. Boda-Heggemann J, Knopf AC, Simeonova-Chergou A, et al. Deep Inspiration Breath Hold-Based Radiation Therapy: A Clinical Review. Int J Radiat Oncol Biol Phys 2016;94(3):478–92.
5. Giraud P, Morvan E, Claude L, et al. Respiratory gating techniques for optimization of lung cancer radiotherapy. J Thorac Oncol 2011;6(12):2058–68.
6. Ezzell GA, Galvin JM, Low D, et al. Guidance document on delivery, treatment planning, and clinical implementation of IMRT: report of the IMRT Subcommittee of the AAPM Radiation Therapy Committee. Med Phys 2003;30(8):2089–115.
7. Xing L, Thorndyke B, Schreibmann E, et al. Overview of image-guided radiation therapy. Med Dosim 2006;31(2):91–112.
8. Bujold A, Massey CA, Kim JJ, et al. Sequential phase I and II trials of stereotactic body radiotherapy for locally advanced hepatocellular carcinoma. J Clin Oncol 2013;31(13):1631–9.
9. Culleton S, Jiang H, Haddad CR, et al. Outcomes following definitive stereotactic body radiotherapy for patients with Child-Pugh B or C hepatocellular carcinoma. Radiother Oncol 2014;111(3):412–7.
10. Lasley FD, Mannina EM, Johnson CS, et al. Treatment variables related to liver toxicity in patients with hepatocellular carcinoma, Child-Pugh class A and B enrolled in a phase 1-2 trial of stereotactic body radiation therapy. Pract Radiat Oncol 2015;5(5):e443–9.
11. Weiner AA, Olsen J, Ma D, et al. Stereotactic body radiotherapy for primary hepatic malignancies - Report of a phase I/II institutional study. Radiother Oncol 2016;121(1):79–85.
12. Feng M, Suresh K, Schipper MJ, et al. Individualized Adaptive Stereotactic Body Radiotherapy for Liver Tumors in Patients at High Risk for Liver Damage: A Phase 2 Clinical Trial. JAMA Oncol 2018;4(1):40–7.
13. Durand-Labrunie J, Baumann AS, Ayav A, et al. Curative Irradiation Treatment of Hepatocellular Carcinoma: A Multicenter Phase 2 Trial. Int J Radiat Oncol Biol Phys 2020;107(1):116–25.
14. Yoon SM, Kim SY, Lim YS, et al. Stereotactic body radiation therapy for small (≤5 cm) hepatocellular carcinoma not amenable to curative treatment: Results of a single-arm, phase II clinical trial. Clin Mol Hepatol 2020;26(4):506–15.
15. Wahl DR, Stenmark MH, Tao Y, et al. Outcomes After Stereotactic Body Radiotherapy or Radiofrequency Ablation for Hepatocellular Carcinoma. J Clin Oncol 2016;34(5):452–9.

16. Lee J, Shin IS, Yoon WS, et al. Comparisons between radiofrequency ablation and stereotactic body radiotherapy for liver malignancies: Meta-analyses and a systematic review. Radiother Oncol 2020;145:63–70.
17. Cacciola A, Parisi S, Tamburella C, et al. Stereotactic body radiation therapy and radiofrequency ablation for the treatment of liver metastases: How and when? Rep Pract Oncol Radiother 2020;25(3):299–306.
18. Eriguchi T, Takeda A, Sanuki N, et al. Acceptable toxicity after stereotactic body radiation therapy for liver tumors adjacent to the central biliary system. Int J Radiat Oncol Biol Phys 2013;85(4):1006–11.
19. Barney BM, Olivier KR, Macdonald OK, et al. Clinical outcomes and dosimetric considerations using stereotactic body radiotherapy for abdominopelvic tumors. Am J Clin Oncol 2012;35(6):537–42.
20. Velec M, Haddad CR, Craig T, et al. Predictors of Liver Toxicity Following Stereotactic Body Radiation Therapy for Hepatocellular Carcinoma. Int J Radiat Oncol Biol Phys 2017;97(5):939–46.
21. Pan CC, Kavanagh BD, Dawson LA, et al. Radiation-associated liver injury. Int J Radiat Oncol Biol Phys 2010;76(3 Suppl):S94–100.
22. Kavanagh BD, Pan CC, Dawson LA, et al. Radiation dose-volume effects in the stomach and small bowel. Int J Radiat Oncol Biol Phys 2010;76(3 Suppl):S101–7.
23. Miften M, Vinogradskiy Y, Moiseenko V, et al. Radiation Dose-Volume Effects for Liver SBRT. Int J Radiat Oncol Biol Phys 2021;110(1):196–205.
24. Tse RV, Hawkins M, Lockwood G, et al. Phase I study of individualized stereotactic body radiotherapy for hepatocellular carcinoma and intrahepatic cholangiocarcinoma. J Clin Oncol 2008;26(4):657–64.
25. Nabavizadeh N, Waller JG, Fain R, et al. Safety and Efficacy of Accelerated Hypofractionation and Stereotactic Body Radiation Therapy for Hepatocellular Carcinoma Patients With Varying Degrees of Hepatic Impairment. Int J Radiat Oncol Biol Phys 2018;100(3):577–85.
26. Bush DA, Kayali Z, Grove R, et al. The safety and efficacy of high-dose proton beam radiotherapy for hepatocellular carcinoma: a phase 2 prospective trial. Cancer 2011;117(13):3053–9.
27. Hong TS, Wo JY, Yeap BY, et al. Multi-Institutional Phase II Study of High-Dose Hypofractionated Proton Beam Therapy in Patients With Localized, Unresectable Hepatocellular Carcinoma and Intrahepatic Cholangiocarcinoma. J Clin Oncol 2016;34(5):460–8.
28. Kasuya G, Kato H, Yasuda S, et al. Progressive hypofractionated carbon-ion radiotherapy for hepatocellular carcinoma: Combined analyses of 2 prospective trials. Cancer 2017;123(20):3955–65.
29. Fukumitsu N, Sugahara S, Nakayama H, et al. A prospective study of hypofractionated proton beam therapy for patients with hepatocellular carcinoma. Int J Radiat Oncol Biol Phys 2009;74(3):831–6.
30. Witt JS, Rosenberg SA, Bassetti MF. MRI-guided adaptive radiotherapy for liver tumours: visualising the future. Lancet Oncol 2020;21(2):e74–82.
31. Bohoudi O, Bruynzeel AME, Senan S, et al. Fast and robust online adaptive planning in stereotactic MR-guided adaptive radiation therapy (SMART) for pancreatic cancer. Radiother Oncol 2017;125(3):439–44.
32. Green OL, Henke LE, Hugo GD. Practical Clinical Workflows for Online and Offline Adaptive Radiation Therapy. Semin Radiat Oncol 2019;29(3):219–27.
33. Mittauer K, Paliwal B, Hill P, et al. A New Era of Image Guidance with Magnetic Resonance-guided Radiation Therapy for Abdominal and Thoracic Malignancies. Cureus 2018;10(4):e2422.

34. Rosenberg SA, Henke LE, Shaverdian N, et al. A Multi-Institutional Experience of MR-Guided Liver Stereotactic Body Radiation Therapy. Adv Radiat Oncol 2019; 4(1):142–9.

35. Feldman AM, Modh A, Glide-Hurst C, et al. Real-time Magnetic Resonance-guided Liver Stereotactic Body Radiation Therapy: An Institutional Report Using a Magnetic Resonance-Linac System. Cureus 2019;11(9):e5774.

36. Henke LE, Olsen JR, Contreras JA, et al. Stereotactic MR-Guided Online Adaptive Radiation Therapy (SMART) for Ultracentral Thorax Malignancies: Results of a Phase 1 Trial. Adv Radiat Oncol 2019;4(1):201–9.

37. Oderinde OM, Shirvani SM, Olcott PD, et al. The technical design and concept of a PET/CT linac for biology-guided radiotherapy. Clin Transl Radiat Oncol 2021;29: 106–12.

38. Wouters BG, Brown JM. Cells at intermediate oxygen levels can be more important than the "hypoxic fraction" in determining tumor response to fractionated radiotherapy. Radiat Res 1997;147(5):541–50.

39. Stewart RD, Li XA. BGRT: biologically guided radiation therapy-the future is fast approaching. Med Phys 2007;34(10):3739–51.

40. Xiang L, Tang S, Ahmad M, et al. High Resolution X-ray-Induced Acoustic Tomography. Sci Rep 2016;6:26118.

41. Lei H, Zhang W, Oraiqat I, et al. Toward in vivo dosimetry in external beam radiotherapy using x-ray acoustic computed tomography: A soft-tissue phantom study validation. Med Phys 2018. https://doi.org/10.1002/mp.13070.

42. Oraiqat I, Zhang W, Litzenberg D, et al. An ionizing radiation acoustic imaging (iRAI) technique for real-time dosimetric measurements for FLASH radiotherapy. Med Phys 2020;47(10):5090–101.

43. Ba Sunbul NH, Zhang W, Oraiqat I, et al. A simulation study of ionizing radiation acoustic imaging (iRAI) as a real-time dosimetric technique for ultra-high dose rate radiotherapy (UHDR-RT). Med Phys 2021;48(10):6137–51.

44. Hickling S, Leger P, El Naqa I. On the Detectability of Acoustic Waves Induced Following Irradiation by a Radiotherapy Linear Accelerator. IEEE Trans Ultrason Ferroelectr Freq Control 2016;63(5):683–90.

45. Hickling S, Lei H, Hobson M, et al. Experimental evaluation of x-ray acoustic computed tomography for radiotherapy dosimetry applications. Med Phys 2017;44(2):608–17.

46. Hickling S, Xiang L, Jones KC, et al. Ionizing radiation-induced acoustics for radiotherapy and diagnostic radiology applications. Med Phys 2018;45(7): e707–21.

47. Jackson WC, Suresh K, Maurino C, et al. A mid-treatment break and reassessment maintains tumor control and reduces toxicity in patients with hepatocellular carcinoma treated with stereotactic body radiation therapy. Radiother Oncol 2019;141:101–7.

48. Jackson WC, Tang M, Maurino C, et al. Individualized Adaptive Radiation Therapy Allows for Safe Treatment of Hepatocellular Carcinoma in Patients With Child-Turcotte-Pugh B Liver Disease. Int J Radiat Oncol Biol Phys 2021;109(1): 212–9.

49. Baumann BC, Wei J, Plastaras JP, et al. Stereotactic Body Radiation Therapy (SBRT) for Hepatocellular Carcinoma: High Rates of Local Control With Low Toxicity. Am J Clin Oncol 2018;41(11):1118–24.

50. Jackson WC, Hartman HE, Gharzai LA, et al. The Potential for Midtreatment Albumin-Bilirubin (ALBI) Score to Individualize Liver Stereotactic Body Radiation Therapy. Int J Radiat Oncol Biol Phys 2021;111(1):127–34.

51. Anscher MS, Crocker IR, Jirtle RL. Transforming growth factor-beta 1 expression in irradiated liver. Radiat Res 1990;122(1):77–85.
52. Anscher MS, Peters WP, Reisenbichler H, et al. Transforming growth factor beta as a predictor of liver and lung fibrosis after autologous bone marrow transplantation for advanced breast cancer. N Engl J Med 1993;328(22):1592–8.
53. Hong TS, Grassberger C, Yeap BY, et al. Pretreatment plasma HGF as potential biomarker for susceptibility to radiation-induced liver dysfunction after radiotherapy. NPJ Precis Oncol 2018;2:22.
54. Cuneo KC, Devasia T, Sun Y, et al. Serum Levels of Hepatocyte Growth Factor and CD40 Ligand Predict Radiation-Induced Liver Injury. Transl Oncol 2019; 12(7):889–94.
55. Küsters S, Tiegs G, Alexopoulou L, et al. In vivo evidence for a functional role of both tumor necrosis factor (TNF) receptors and transmembrane TNF in experimental hepatitis. Eur J Immunol 1997;27(11):2870–5.
56. Heyninck K, Wullaert A, Beyaert R. Nuclear factor-kappa B plays a central role in tumour necrosis factor-mediated liver disease. Biochem Pharmacol 2003;66(8): 1409–15.
57. Yang YM, Seki E. TNFα in liver fibrosis. Curr Pathobiol Rep 2015;3(4):253–61.
58. Cope AP, Aderka D, Doherty M, et al. Increased levels of soluble tumor necrosis factor receptors in the sera and synovial fluid of patients with rheumatic diseases. Arthritis Rheum 1992;35(10):1160–9.
59. Aderka D, Wysenbeek A, Engelmann H, et al. Correlation between serum levels of soluble tumor necrosis factor receptor and disease activity in systemic lupus erythematosus. Arthritis Rheum 1993;36(8):1111–20.
60. Khoury SJ, Orav EJ, Guttmann CR, et al. Changes in serum levels of ICAM and TNF-R correlate with disease activity in multiple sclerosis. Neurology 1999;53(4): 758–64.
61. Cousins MM, Devasia TP, Maurino CM, et al. Pretreatment Levels of Soluble Tumor Necrosis Factor Receptor 1 and Hepatocyte Growth Factor Predict Toxicity and Overall Survival After. J Nucl Med 2022;63(6):882–9.
62. Cousins MM, Morris E, Maurino C, et al. TNFR1 and the TNFα axis as a targetable mediator of liver injury from stereotactic body radiation therapy. Transl Oncol 2021;14(1):100950.
63. Bierman HR, Byron RL, Kelley KH, et al. Studies on the blood supply of tumors in man. III. Vascular patterns of the liver by hepatic arteriography in vivo. J Natl Cancer Inst 1951;12(1):107–31.
64. Breedis C, Young G. The blood supply of neoplasms in the liver. Am J Pathol 1954;30(5):969–77.
65. Garin E, Lenoir L, Rolland Y, et al. Dosimetry based on 99mTc-macroaggregated albumin SPECT/CT accurately predicts tumor response and survival in hepatocellular carcinoma patients treated with 90Y-loaded glass microspheres: preliminary results. J Nucl Med 2012;53(2):255–63.
66. Salem R, Johnson GE, Kim E, et al. Yttrium-90 Radioembolization for the Treatment of Solitary, Unresectable HCC: The LEGACY Study. Hepatology 2021; 74(5):2342–52.
67. Lewandowski RJ, Gabr A, Abouchaleh N, et al. Radiation Segmentectomy: Potential Curative Therapy for Early Hepatocellular Carcinoma. Radiology 2018; 287(3):1050–8.
68. Vouche M, Habib A, Ward TJ, et al. Unresectable solitary hepatocellular carcinoma not amenable to radiofrequency ablation: multicenter radiology-pathology

correlation and survival of radiation segmentectomy. Hepatology 2014;60(1): 192–201.

69. Riaz A, Gates VL, Atassi B, et al. Radiation segmentectomy: a novel approach to increase safety and efficacy of radioembolization. Int J Radiat Oncol Biol Phys 2011;79(1):163–71.
70. Biederman DM, Titano JJ, Korff RA, et al. Radiation Segmentectomy versus Selective Chemoembolization in the Treatment of Early-Stage Hepatocellular Carcinoma. J Vasc Interv Radiol 2018;29(1):30–7.e2.
71. Padia SA, Johnson GE, Horton KJ, et al. Segmental Yttrium-90 Radioembolization versus Segmental Chemoembolization for Localized Hepatocellular Carcinoma: Results of a Single-Center, Retrospective, Propensity Score-Matched Study. J Vasc Interv Radiol 2017;28(6):777–85.e1.
72. Dewaraja YK, Chun SY, Srinivasa RN, et al. Improved quantitative. Med Phys 2017;44(12):6364–76.
73. Garin E, Tselikas L, Guiu B, et al. Personalised versus standard dosimetry approach of selective internal radiation therapy in patients with locally advanced hepatocellular carcinoma (DOSISPHERE-01): a randomised, multicentre, open-label phase 2 trial. Lancet Gastroenterol Hepatol 2021;6(1):17–29.
74. Kappadath SC, Mikell J, Balagopal A, et al. Hepatocellular Carcinoma Tumor Dose Response After. Int J Radiat Oncol Biol Phys 2018;102(2):451–61.
75. Wei L, Cui C, Xu J, et al. Tumor response prediction in. EJNMMI Phys 2020; 7(1):74.
76. Luterstein E, Cao M, Lamb JM, et al. Clinical Outcomes Using Magnetic Resonance-Guided Stereotactic Body Radiation Therapy in Patients With Locally Advanced Cholangiocarcinoma. Adv Radiat Oncol 2020;5(2):189–95.
77. Boldrini L, Romano A, Mariani S, et al. MRI-guided stereotactic radiation therapy for hepatocellular carcinoma: a feasible and safe innovative treatment approach. J Cancer Res Clin Oncol 2021;147(7):2057–68.

A Review of Advances in Radiotherapy in the Setting of Esophageal Cancers

Joshua Cinicola, PharmD, RPh[a,1], Swati Mamidanna, MD[b,1],
Nikhil Yegya-Raman, MD[c], Kristen Spencer, DO, MPH[d],
Matthew P. Deek, MD[b], Salma K. Jabbour, MD, FASTRO[b,*]

KEYWORDS

- Esophageal cancer • Gastric cancer • Chemoradiotherapy • Targeted therapy
- Combination therapy • IMRT • PBT

KEY POINTS

- Treatment in the locally advanced setting includes multimodality approaches that include surgery, chemotherapy, radiotherapy, and targeted therapy.
- Advances in radiotherapy design through techniques have allowed for a reduction of clinical toxicities.
- Targeted therapies such as checkpoint inhibitors offer new options to improve treatment response.

INTRODUCTION

Esophageal cancer is the eighth most common cancer worldwide, accounting for approximately 20,640 cases in 2022 in the United States. Histologically, adenocarcinoma has seen a 2.5-fold increase in incidence and is observed predominantly among white men in the Western world.[1] Squamous cell carcinoma remains the prevalent histologic subtype among patients in underdeveloped countries. The aggressive nature of esophageal cancer associates with poor survival rates and is the sixth most common cause of cancer-related deaths. The prognosis relies heavily on factors such as the locoregional tumor extent, nodal involvement, and metastases to distant sites.

[a] Ernest Mario School of Pharmacy, Rutgers University, Piscataway, NJ, USA; [b] Department of Radiation Oncology, Rutgers Cancer Institute of New Jersey, Rutgers Robert Wood Johnson School of Medicine, Rutgers University, New Brunswick, NJ, USA; [c] Department of Radiation Oncology, University of Pennsylvania, Philadelphia, PA, USA; [d] New York Langone Perlmutter Cancer Center, New York, NY, USA
[1] Co-first authors.
* Corresponding author. Rutgers Cancer Institute of New Jersey, 195 Little Albany Street, New Brunswick, NJ 08903.
E-mail address: jabbousk@cinj.rutgers.edu

Surg Oncol Clin N Am 32 (2023) 433–459
https://doi.org/10.1016/j.soc.2023.03.004
1055-3207/23/© 2023 Elsevier Inc. All rights reserved.

surgonc.theclinics.com

Although the primary treatment paradigm often revolves around surgical resection, a multimodality approach with chemotherapy, radiation therapy (RT), and targeted therapies forms the standard of care. The aim of this review article is to examine data pertaining to the current management as well as advancements in radiotherapy and targeted therapies.

SURGICAL THERAPY

Early-stage esophageal cancers that have not invaded beyond the submucosa are amenable to endoscopic mucosal resection with curative intent. In other cases, esophagectomy can be considered via 2 main surgical approaches. Hulscher and colleagues compared randomized patients with adenocarcinoma to either transhiatal esophagectomy or transthoracic esophagectomy with extended en bloc lymphadenectomy.[2] The overall, disease-free survival (DFS) and quality-adjusted survival did not differ between the 2 surgical groups. Perioperative morbidity, but not in-hospital mortality, was higher with the transthoracic method. With improvements in surgical techniques, the 5-year survival has increased from ~4% in 1980 to ~25% in the 1990s, but surgery when considered as monotherapy continues to be insufficient to provide optimal outcomes.[3] Recurrence patterns were studied by Chen and colleagues and Nakagawa and colleagues and found that more than half of postesophagectomy patients progress to disease recurrence or metastases (commonly liver, bone, or lung) within 5 years, owing largely to the widespread and complicated lymphatic system, and the high incidence of skip metastasis.[4,5] These inadequate results of surgery alone prompted an increased interest in the addition of neoadjuvant systemic therapies and RT approaches (**Table 1**). The landmark CROSS trial provided a benchmark in comparing surgery alone with preoperative chemoradiotherapy (CRT) followed by surgery for patients with locally advanced disease. Neoadjuvant CRT improved overall survival (OS) over surgery alone (median OS 48.6 months vs 24 months, $P = .003$). Patients with squamous cell carcinoma can be considered for an observation approach should they achieve a complete response after neoadjuvant CRT; however, it is preferred for patients with esophageal adenocarcinoma to be operated after upfront chemoradiation. Newer approaches leverage recent advances in targeted therapies as an addition to traditional CRT approaches across multiple stages of treatment.

CHEMOTHERAPY/TARGETED THERAPY COMBINATIONS
Human Epidermal Growth Factor Receptor 2

One of the potential additions to combination radiotherapy treatment of patients with locally advanced esophagogastric cancers are agents targeted to human epidermal growth factor receptor 2 (HER2). HER2 is estimated to be amplified in 20% to 35% of gastroesophageal junction (GEJ) adenocarcinomas.[6–8] In addition, preclinical data have shown that trastuzumab sensitizes esophageal cancer cell lines to RT although the specific mechanism remains unclear.[7,9] Studies have attempted to combine HER2 therapy with RT with limited success. However, several combinations are still being explored.

The combination of trastuzumab with 5-fluorouracil (5-FU) and cisplatin chemotherapy improved OS in the ToGA trial for patients with metastatic disease and resulted in Food and Drug Administration (FDA) approval.[8] There was substantial interest in combining trastuzumab with radiotherapy following these positive results and existing preclinical data. In the RTOG 1010 phase III study (**Box 1**), investigators combined trastuzumab with the CROSS-like study regimen (paclitaxel, carboplatin, and

Table 1
Phase III trials in chemoradiotherapy for esophageal cancer

Title	Year	Trial	Patient Population	Study Arms	Median Follow-up	Results	PMID
Walsh et al[109] 1996	1990–1995	Phase III	102 patients with only esophageal adenocarcinoma AC n = 102	1. Surgery alone (n = 54) 2. Pre-op CRT to total of 40 Gy/15 fx with FU + cisplatin followed by surgery (n = 48)	10 mo	• Pre-op CRT improved 1-y OS (52% vs 32%) • Median OS was 16 mo in CRT group vs 11 mo in surgery alone	8672151
RTOG 85-01[110] 1999	1985–1990	Phase III	121 patients with locoregional thoracic esophageal cancers T1-3 N0-1 M0 SCC n = 107 AC n = 23	1. RT alone to 64 Gy/32fx (n = 62) 2. CRT to 50 Gy/25fx with FU + cisplatin (n = 59)	5 y	• Early termination due to clear benefit of CRT in improving OS • 5-y OS 26% in CRT arm vs 0% in RT alone (95% CI 15%–37%)	10235156
CALGB 9781[111] 2008	1997–2000	Phase III	56 patients with thoracic esophageal cancer to GEJ (<2 cm to cardia) Initially designed to randomize 500 patients but closed early due to poor accrual SCC n = 14 AC n = 42	1. Surgery alone (n = 26) 2. Preoperative CRT to total 50.4/28fx and cisplatin/5-FU followed by surgery (n = 30)	6 y	• pCR rate was 40% • Median OS better in trimodality group (4.5 y vs 1.8 y) • Five-year OS was 39% (95% CI, 21%–57%) vs 16% (95% CI, 5%–33%) for trimodality therapy vs surgery alone	18309943
RTOG 9405 (INT 0123) Kachnic et al[74] 2011	1995–1999	Phase III	218 patients with nonmetastatic esophageal cancer receiving concurrent cisplatin + FU SCC n = 185 AC n = 33	1. RT to total 50.4/28 fx 2. RT to total 64.8/36 fx	4 y	• 2-year OS was 31% in high-dose arm (64.8 Gy) vs 40% in the 50.4 Gy arm	21673875
Intergroup 0116 (INT-0116) Smalley et al[112] 2012	1991–1998	Phase III	559 patients with gastric (80%)/GEJ (20%) cancer s/p surgery with complete resection and at high risk for LRF (85% node positive)	1. Observation (n = 277) 2. Chemotherapy with 5-FU/leucovorin followed by CRT to total 45 Gy with 5-FU/leucovorin followed by 5-FU/leucovorin (n = 282)	10.3 y	• 3-y OS was improved in adjuvant CRT group (50% vs 42%) (95% CI, 1.10–1.60; P = .0046)	22585691

(continued on next page)

Table 1
(continued)

Title	Year	Trial	Patient Population	Study Arms	Median Follow-up	Results	PMID
POET[113] 2017	2009	Phase III	In 172 patients with locally advanced adenocarcinoma of lower esophageal cancer before surgical intervention AC n = 172	1. Induction CHT followed by surgery (n = 86) 2. Induction CHT with cisplatin/5-FU/leucovorin followed by CRT to total 30 Gy with cisplatin/etoposide followed by surgery (n = 86)	46 mo	• Closed early due to poor accrual • 5-y OS 40% in pre-op CRT arm vs 24% in pre-op chemo alone (95% CI 0.42–1.01, $P = .055$)	28628843
NEOCRTEC5010[114] 2018	2007–2014	Phase III	In 430 patients with potentially resectable thoracic esophageal SCC SCC n = 430	1. Surgery (n = 227) 2. Pre-op CRT to total 40 Gy/20fx with vinorelbine + cisplatin q3weekly (n = 224)	54 mo	• Compared with surgery alone, pre-op CRT had higher R0 resection rate (98% vs 91%) • Neoadjuvant therapy associated with better median OS 100 mo (95% CI, 74.6–125.6 mo) vs 67 mo (95% CI, 39.7–93.3 mo)	30089078
CROSS[115] 2021	2004–2008	Phase III	In 363 patients with resectable T1N1 and T2/3 N0/1 adeno (75%) or squamous (25%) of esophagus (75%) or GEJ (25%) SCC n = 84 AC n = 275	1. Surgery alone (n = 188) 2. Pre-op CRT to total 41.4 Gy/23 fx and weekly carboplatin/paclitaxel (n = 178)	147 mo in surviving patients	• Median OS was significantly higher in the CRT arm (49 vs 24 mo); (95% CI, 0.55–0.89) • 10-y OS 38% in CRT arm (95% CI, 31–45) vs 25% in surgery alone (95% CI, 19–32)	33891478

Abbreviations: AC, adenocarcinoma; CHT, chemotherapy; CRT, chemoradiotherapy; FU, fluorouracil; fx, fractions; GEJ, gastroesophageal junction; OS, overall survival; pCR, pathologic complete response; RT, radiation therapy; SCC, squamous cell carcinoma.

Box 1
Study spotlight: RTOG 1010[10]

- A phase III study enrolled 203 adults with locally advanced HER2-positive esophageal or gastroesophageal adenocarcinoma to receive weekly carboplatin, paclitaxel, and RT followed by surgery with (n = 98) or without trastuzumab (n = 96) with a primary endpoint of DFS.

- No significant difference in DFS or OS; grade 3 to 4 adverse events were comparable between groups; prespecified definition for excess cardiac adverse events were not met. Surgical outcomes also favored chemotherapy group.

- Thirty-nine percent of participants in the trastuzumab arm required chemotherapy dose reductions compared with 24% in the chemotherapy group. Regimens more like those used for systemic therapy studies may be more beneficial in future trimodality studies.

---

radiotherapy followed by esophagectomy) compared with the trimodality regimen alone.[10] A total of 194 participants received treatment on the study, and after a median follow-up of 2.8 years, the addition of trastuzumab to the CROSS-like regimen showed no significant increase in OS (hazard ratio [HR] 0.99, 95% confidence interval [CI] 0.71–1.39).[10] However, trastuzumab is still being explored in combination with other regimens in the perioperative and locally advanced space.[11–13] The phase II NEOHX study of a perioperative trastuzumab + XELOX regimen found promising improvements in DFS and OS.[11] XELOX has shown efficacy as a CRT regimen, so the addition of RT to the NEOHX regimen seems as a reasonable next step. The recent interim results of the ongoing KEYNOTE 811 study and completed AIO-INTEGA study suggest that combination of programmed death ligand 1 (PD-L1) and HER2 immunotherapy has signs of synergy in esophageal tumors (**Table 2**).[14,15] Both agents have been shown to enhance RT independently; therefore, the addition of radiotherapy to this immunotherapy combination may be reasonable in the future, as more data become available.

Another HER2-targeted therapy to be studied in combination with RT is the oral small molecule tyrosine kinase inhibitor lapatinib. Following negative results from the TRIO-013/LOGiC trial, where the addition of lapatinib to capecitabine and oxaliplatin did not improve OS, a phase II study examining lapatinib in combination with FOLFOX and 50.4 Gy of radiation was initiated, although it only enrolled 12 participants before termination due to a lack of accrual.[16,17] Of the 12 enrolled patients, 4 underwent surgery and 1 achieved pathologic complete response (pCR) with a reasonable toxicity profile.[17] Because of the low enrollment, no accurate comparison can be made, requiring additional studies to appreciate a role in therapy for lapatinib and RT. A phase II study of neoadjuvant lapatinib in head and neck squamous cell carcinomas (HNSCC) followed by surgery and risk-adapted adjuvant therapy was able to achieve a 36% pCR rate, suggesting further study in esophageal tumors may be warranted.[18]

Finally, following the DESTINY-Gastric01 study, trastuzumab deruxtecan (T-DXd), an antibody-drug conjugate (ADC), is an option to watch, as more data become available. The study showed promising results in participants with locally advanced or metastatic gastric or GEJ who had progressed on 2 prior therapies. In the study, 51% of patients achieved objective response, with 11 of 61 reaching a complete response compared with a 14% response rate in the investigators choice chemotherapy control ($P < .001$).[19] However, patients in the T-DXd arm experienced a higher rate of grade III and grade IV adverse events. Twelve participants experienced drug-related interstitial lung disease, with one instance leading to death. Preliminary data

Table 2
Relevant ongoing studies of diagnostic and treatment approaches in esophagogastric cancer

CT Identifier #	Study Name	Purpose	Modalities Studied	Primary Endpoint Completion Date	Design Characteristics	Primary Outcome	Expected Sample Size	Results?	PMID
NCT03615326	Pembrolizumab/Placebo Plus Trastuzumab Plus Chemotherapy in Human Epidermal Growth Factor Receptor 2 Positive (HER2+) Advanced Gastric or Gastroesophageal Junction (GEJ) Adenocarcinoma (MK-3475–811/KEYNOTE-811)[116]	Targeted combination	Pembrolizumab, trastuzumab, chemotherapy	15-Dec-23	2-arm active comparator trial of pembrolizumab as an add on to trastuzumab and chemotherapy in a first-line setting, enriched for HER2 overexpression	PFS, OS	732	Y	33167735
NCT03221426	Study of Pembrolizumab (MK-3475) Plus Chemotherapy vs Placebo Plus Chemotherapy in Participants with Gastric or Gastroesophageal Junction (GEJ) Adenocarcinoma (MK-3475–585/KEYNOTE-585)[116]	Perioperative combination therapy	Pembrolizumab, surgery, chemotherapy	28-Jun-24	4-arm active comparator trial of perioperative pembrolizumab in combination with chemotherapy	EFS, pCR, OS, Safety	1007	N	30777447
UMIN000034373	TENERGY: multicenter Phase II Study of Atezolizumab Monotherapy Following Definitive Chemoradiotherapy with 5-FU Plus Cisplatin in Patients with Unresectable Locally Advanced Esophageal Squamous Cell Carcinoma[116]	Definitive CRT combination	Atezolizumab, chemotherapy, RT	NA	Single-arm study to study atezolizumab following definitive CRT with cisplatin and 5-FU	cCR	50	N	32312286
NCT03474341	Preoperative Image-guided Identification of Response to Neoadjuvant Chemoradiotherapy in Esophageal Cancer[117]	Diagnostic	MRI, PET-CT, endoscopy, ctDNA	1-Sep-21	Single-arm study of patients receiving CROSS regimen CRT; the study explores the use of multimodal diagnostics to increase the ability to predict response	Histopathological response	200	N	30342494

NCT Number	Title	Category	Intervention	Date	Description	Primary Outcome	N	Y/N	ID
NCT03937362	Accuracy of Detecting Residual Disease After Neoadjuvant Chemoradiotherapy for Esophageal Squamous Cell Carcinoma[118]	Diagnostic	Endoscopy	8-Aug-22	Single-arm study to evaluate the ability of bite-on-bite biopsy, as well as PET-CT and EUS to predict clinical response	Clinical response accuracy	400	N	32143580
NCT03790553	A Phase III Study of Comparing 61.2 Gy Radiotherapy Dose vs 50.4 Gy Radiotherapy Dose for Locally Advanced Esophageal Carcinoma[119]	Diagnostic	PET-CT	15-Oct-23	2-arm study using 18F-FDG PET-CT response of tumor to guide titration of RT dose	OS in nonresponders, OS in ITT population	646	N	35906623
NCT03257163	A Phase II Study of Preoperative Pembrolizumab for Mismatch-Repair Deficient and Epstein-Barr Virus Positive Gastric Cancer Followed by Chemotherapy and Chemoradiation with Pembrolizumab	Preoperative treatment	Pembrolizumab, RT, capecitabine	31-Dec-22	Single-arm study, pembrolizumab with capecitabine, continued with radiation starting at course 4, biomarker enriched	RFS	40	N	NA
NCT04510285	A Single-Arm Pilot Study of Adjuvant Pembrolizumab Plus Trastuzumab in HER2+ Esophagogastric Tumors with Persistent Circulating Tumor DNA Following Curative Resection	Postoperative treatment	Pembrolizumab, trastuzumab	10-Aug-23	Single-arm pilot of trastuzumab pembrolizumab following curative resection. Enriched for HER2 overexpression, biomarker study	ctDNA clearance at 6 months	24	N	NA
NCT02730546	Phase 1b/2 Clinical Trial of Neoadjuvant Pembrolizumab Plus Concurrent Chemoradiotherapy with Weekly Carboplatin and Paclitaxel in Adult Patients With Resectable, Locally Advanced Adenocarcinoma of the Gastroesophageal Junction or Gastric Cardiac	Neoadjuvant combination therapy	Pembrolizumab, CRT, surgery	1-Jul-21	Single-arm study, pembrolizumab with CRT followed by surgery	pCR	31	Y	NA

(continued on next page)

Table 2
(continued)

CT Identifier #	Study Name	Purpose	Modalities Studied	Primary Endpoint Completion Date	Design Characteristics	Primary Outcome	Expected Sample Size	Results?	PMID
NCT03604991	Nivolumab and Ipilimumab in Treating Patients with Esophageal and Gastroesophageal Junction Adenocarcinoma Undergoing Surgery[35]	Perioperative combination therapy	Nivolumab, ipilimumab, carboplatin, paclitaxel, radiotherapy	31-Dec-2023	A multiarm, multistep study Step 1: nivolumab ± carboplatin, paclitaxel, and RT. Step 2: postoperative nivolumab ± ipilimumab	pCR, DFS	278	Y	NA
NCT03443856	Adjuvant Immunotherapy in Patients with Resected Gastric Cancer Following Preoperative Chemotherapy With High Risk for Recurrence (N+ and/or R1): an Open Label Randomized Controlled Phase-2-study	Postoperative treatment	Nivolumab, ipilimumab, chemotherapy, surgery	1-Sep-23	2-arm study of nivolumab and ipilimumab after resection vs perioperative SOC	DFS	197	N	NA
NCT03776487	Pilot Study of Dual Checkpoint Inhibition Followed by Immuno-Chemoradiation in Patients with Resectable Gastric Adenocarcinoma (Concept ID 2016-NIV-0551)	Perioperative combination therapy	Nivolumab, ipilimumab, chemotherapy, surgery	30-Jun-23	Single-arm pilot study, patients receive CRT or CRT and nivolumab/ipilimumab followed by resection and postoperative nivolumab	Safety	30	N	NA
NCT04014075	DS-8201a in HER2-positive Gastric Cancer That Cannot Be Surgically Removed or Has Spread (DESTINY-Gastric02)[20]	Targeted therapy	TDXd	9-Apr-2021	Single-arm phase II study of TDXd in patients with metastatic/unresectable gastric/GEJ cancer refractory to trastuzumab	ORR	79	Y	NA
NCT05034887	Phase 2 Study of Trastuzumab Deruxtecan (T-DXd) in the Neoadjuvant Treatment for Patients with HER2 Positive Gastric and Gastroesophageal Junction Adenocarcinoma	Neoadjuvant therapy	TDXd	31-Mar-24	Single-arm study of TDXd before surgery, enriched for HER2 overexpression	MPR	37	N	NA

NCT02205047	Integration of Trastuzumab, With or Without Pertuzumab, Into Perioperative Chemotherapy of HER-2 Positive Stomach Cancer	Perioperative combination therapy	Trastuzumab, pertuzumab, chemotherapy, surgery	31-Dec-22	3-arm study, trastuzumab/chemotherapy, trastuzumab/pertuzumab/chemotherapy, chemotherapy, enriched for HER2 overexpression	Near-pCR	171	N	NA
NCT05379972	Study of Induction SBRT and Olaparib Followed by Combination Pembrolizumab/Olaparib in Gastric and Gastroesophageal Junction (GEJ) Cancers	Targeted combination	SBRT, olaparib, pembrolizumab	1-Dec-25	2 arms—DNA repair deficient/proficient, both arms receive pembrolizumab, olaparib, and SBRT (25 Gy in 5 fractions daily for 5 days), participants can have metastatic disease and must have at least 1 line of prior treatment	ORR	26	N	NA
NCT04379596	A Phase 1b/2 Multicenter, Open-label, Dose-escalation and Dose-expansion Study to Evaluate the Safety, Tolerability, Pharmacokinetics, Immunogenicity, and Antitumor Activity of Trastuzumab Deruxtecan (T-DXd) Monotherapy and Combinations in Adult Participants with HER2 Overexpressing Gastric Cancer	Targeted combination	T-DXd, chemotherapy, pembrolizumab, durvalumab	29-Nov-24	Dose escalation and expansion study of TDXd in combination with chemotherapeutics and checkpoint inhibitors. Enriched for HER2 overexpression	ORR, safety	315	N	NA

from the follow-up study, DESTINY Gastric02 (see **Table 2**), which treated 79 patients with metastatic/unresectable gastric/GEJ tumors refractory to trastuzumab showed a decreased objective response rate (ORR) of 38%.[20] Safety data were consistent with previous studies and included 6 instances of interstitial lung disease, one of which was fatal.[20] Although the signs of efficacy are enticing, the toxicity profile could make it difficult to tolerate in combination with radiotherapy. There has been a study in breast cancer looking at trastuzumab emtansine (TDM-1), another HER-2 antibody drug conjugate, in combination with stereotactic radiation with a median of 25 Gy delivered in 3 to 5 fractions.[21] The study observed reasonable tolerability although concerns over increased risk of symptomatic radiation necrosis have been noted in the literature[21–23]; this is worth watching, as more safety data on T-DXd and other ADCs become available through ongoing clinical trials and organ-sparing radiotherapy techniques become better optimized.

Immune Checkpoints

Tumors expressing immune checkpoint ligands can downregulate immune responses in the tumor microenvironment, enabling further growth and proliferation. By blocking these receptor-ligand interactions, PD-(L)1 checkpoint inhibitors are able to induce durable response and improved outcomes, especially in patients with microsatellite instability and high PD-L1 expression.[24–26] In esophageal and gastric tumors, overexpression of these markers is correlated with a high mutational burden and poor prognosis.[27,28] Chemoradiation is associated with immunogenic changes including increase in interferon gamma signaling and CD28 stimulation. Increased neutrophil counts were detected in tumor tissue as well, suggesting a possible synergistic effect with radiation.[29,30]

Nivolumab has good efficacy data in esophageal and gastric cancers following the CheckMate 648 and ATTRACTION 3 study results, the latter of which recently published 3-year follow-up data.[24,31,32] These studies provided strong justification for exploration of nivolumab as an adjuvant to preoperative CRT. The CheckMate-577 study (**Box 2**), a phase III clinical trial, randomized 792 participants with esophageal or gastroesophageal tumor post-CRT with residual disease at time of resection in a 2:1 ratio to either nivolumab or placebo.[33] After a median follow-up 24.4 months, DFS was doubled to 22.4 months in the nivolumab arm compared with 11.0 months in the placebo arm with a 31% risk reduction in recurrence or death (HR 0.69; 96.4% CI, 0.56–0.86; $P < .001$).[33] Rates of serious adverse events and grade 3 to 4 adverse events were comparable between the placebo and the nivolumab groups. Events expected to be immune-related were primarily grades 1 and 2. Grade 3 and 4 immune-related adverse events occurred in 1% or less of the nivolumab group.[33]

Box 2
Study spotlight: CHECKMATE-577[33]

- A postoperative study of nivolumab in 792 participants with esophageal or GEJ tumors following CRT and an R0 resection with residual disease (non-pCR).

- The addition of nivolumab led to a 31% risk reduction of disease recurrence or death and improved outcomes in both histologies although those with squamous cell carcinoma showed improved DFS.

- Individuals with higher pathologic tumor status also seemed to benefit less from the addition of nivolumab, suggesting the success of CRT and surgery may be a driver of outcomes for this subgroup.

Additional evidence is available from the ROMONA trial, which examined nivolumab with and without ipilimumab in 22 and 44 participants, respectively.[34] The study enrolled adults aged 65 years and older with esophageal squamous cell carcinoma (ESCC) with disease refractory to first-line therapy, with 80% of the total study population having received prior CRT.[34] The participants who received immunotherapy had a median OS with 7.2 months, which was a significant improvement over a historical control treated with chemotherapy ($P = .0063$).[34] However, ipilimumab was associated with an increased risk of grade 3 to 5 adverse events including 4 instances of pneumonitis in the ipilimumab arm, one of which led to death.[34] This increase in toxicity is concerning and discourages the use of ipilimumab and nivolumab in conjunction with RT. Data from the AIO-INTEGA study suggest there may be a place in therapy for ipilimumab, but these data were not as impressive as the 70% 12-month survival rate seen in the trastuzumab plus nivolumab combination arm.[15] Based on this information, it seems reasonable to prioritize exploration of trastuzumab and nivolumab in combination with RT over ipilimumab. The addition of perioperative nivolumab and ipilimumab to a CROSS-like regimen in patients with localized esophageal/GEJ adenocarcinoma is being examined in the ongoing ECOG-ACRIN 2174 study.[35] Initial safety data did not indicate a marked increase in toxicity by adding nivolumab to an intensive neoadjuvant regimen, and the forthcoming efficacy data are highly anticipated (see **Table 2**).[35]

Pembrolizumab is approved in second-line metastatic ESCC and first-line locally advanced unresectable and metastatic GEJ adenocarcinoma based off KEYNOTE 180/181 and KEYNOTE 590, respectively.[25,36,37] Although it has not been studied much in a locally advanced population, it is worth noting that 10% of patients in KEYNOTE 590 had locally advanced disease.[37] Ongoing studies are examining pembrolizumab in combination with chemotherapy and trastuzumab (see **Table 2**).[14] These studies could be used to drive the exploration of novel RT combination options following the positive results of CheckMate-577. Other relevant checkpoint inhibitors include tislelizumab (PD-1 inhibitor), which received FDA approval in unresectable recurrent locally advanced or metastatic ESCC following previous systemic therapy following the results of the RATIONALE 302 study. In the study, 60% of the participants in both arms had progressed on CRT before treatment and had an acceptable safety profile that may support future combination exploration.[38]

Additional supportive data involve the PD-1 inhibitor camrelizumab in various combinations with volumetric arc intensity-modulated radiotherapy (IMRT) for locally advanced ESCC. Camrelizumab was studied by investigators as an addition to neoadjuvant CRT as well as a definitive regimen. The 2 studies enrolled 38 and 20 participants, respectively.[39,40] Participants received approximately 60 Gy (2.0 Gy/fx and 5fx/week).[39,40] In the neoadjuvant study, participants received carboplatin and paclitaxel. Both studies had encouraging results supporting further study.[39,40] In the neoadjuvant study, there were no serious treatment-related adverse events, and 94.7% of participants had an R0 resection, 39.5% had a pCR, and the 12-month survival rate was greater than 85%.[40] The definitive RT study had a 74% ORR and a 24-mo OS rate of 31.6%.[39] A phase 1b/2 study by Zhu and colleagues evaluated neoadjuvant pembrolizumab–containing chemoradiation (CROSS regimen) followed by surgical resection and adjuvant pembrolizumab, with a primary endpoint of tolerability and pCR. The primary endpoint of pCR was not significant at a rate of 22.6%. Patients with high combined positive score greater than or equal to 10 and baseline expression of PD-L1 had a significantly higher pCR rate than those with low expression (50.0% [4/8] vs 13.6% [3/22]; $P = .046$). Patients with high PD-L1 expression also experienced longer progression-free survival (PFS) and OS than propensity score–matched patients.[41]

These data as well as the design of studies, both past and pending, could be useful guides for further research. Finally, atezolizumab is being trialed in combination with definitive chemoradiation in the proof-of-concept TENERGY trial (see **Table 2**). Taken together with the data from the positive early phase camrelizumab studies, this treatment class continues to bring promise for patients with esophageal cancer.

Vascular Endothelial Growth Factor

Angiogenesis is a critical part of tumor growth. Triggered by hypoxia, vascular endothelial growth factor (VEGF) allows fresh nutrients and oxygen to reach the tumor, enables further development, and may potentiate metastasis. Because of this role, VEGF and its receptors have made an interesting target for potential anticancer therapy. Adjuvant VEGF targeting in the setting of CRT could potentially prevent the development of tumor vasculature and prevent prosurvival signaling mediated by VEGF interactions.[42]

The most well-studied VEGF/vascular endothelial growth factor receptors (VEGFR) agent in the setting of esophagogastric cancer is ramucirumab. The inhibitory VEGFR-2 monoclonal antibody has shown efficacy as second-line treatment in 2 phase III trials in advanced gastric and GEJ adenocarcinomas as both monotherapy and in combination with chemotherapy agents.[43–45] However, it has not improved OS as a first-line therapy, and data in combination with radiotherapy or in locally advanced disease in esophagogastric cancers are limited.[46] Most studies of VEGF inhibitors involve the use of bevacizumab in glioblastoma, rectal cancer, and colon cancer. A phase II study of bevacizumab and CRT was conducted in nasopharyngeal carcinoma and found a 90.9% 2-year OS and 83.7% 2-year locoregional progression-free interval and could provide additional justification for exploration.[47] Combinations of checkpoint inhibitors and VEGF therapy have been effective in other tumor types. A phase Ia/Ib study that treated 28 patients with refractory disease with durvalumab and ramucirumab provided intriguing results, although clinical data from bevacizumab studies combined with RT suggest toxicity may be a hurdle to combination with gastrointestinal side effects, thrombotic events, and pulmonary hemorrhage being major concerns.[48,49] However, the small study showed signals of activity, supporting the idea that further study may be worthwhile.

Epidermal Growth Factor Receptor

Similarly, EGFR also plays a role in angiogenesis, as well as cell survival and tumor progression. Preclinical research with the well-studied monoclonal antibody cetuximab suggested EGFR inhibition may have a radiosensitizing effect, and these data were confirmed by Bonner and colleagues where cetuximab and high-dose RT improved locoregional control in HNSCC[50–53]; this led to several studies looking to replicate these results in esophagogastric tumors but with limited success. Cetuximab has been studied in several phase III clinical studies, such as NRG Oncology RTOG 0436 for the management of nonoperable carcinoma of the esophagus in combination with definitive CRT, and in studies of preoperative CRT with no statistically significant improvement in OS.[54–56] Nimotuzumab and panitumumab, both EGFR-targeted monoclonal antibodies, have also been studied in combination with radiation modalities with no significant improvement over standard of care in large studies.[57,58] Small molecule EGFR inhibitors have also been studied in this population with similar results.[59] Recently, a Chinese study in adults 70 years and older with unresectable ESCC enrolled 127 participants who were treated with the oral EGFR tyrosine kinase inhibitor, icotinib, and RT versus RT alone. Icotinib improved response rates along with significant improvement in OS[60]; this is consistent with a few smaller studies in older adults given EGFR inhibitors and RT.[61–63] Perhaps there is a space in therapy for this combination in individuals who may not be able to tolerate intensive chemotherapy/ CRT regimens and have EGFR-positive disease. Further research is needed to confirm these results.

Poly (ADP-Ribose) Polymerase

Poly (ADP-ribose) polymerase (PARP) inhibitors are expected to be effective radiosen- sitizers because of their effect on DNA damage synergizing with RT. Olaparib garnered substantial interest in gastric and esophageal malignancies after its success targeting DNA base excision repair in other tumor types with defective homologous recombina- tion repair such as breast and ovarian cancer. Following a positive phase II study, a phase III superiority study of olaparib in combination with paclitaxel in gastric cancer was not able to show an OS benefit in the overall study population or the ataxia-telan- giectasia mutation (ATM)-negative population.[64] Interestingly, the phase II study was prospectively enriched for ATM-negative participants, whereas the phase III was not.[64,65] In addition, different ATM detection assays were used.[66,67] Combined, these factors may explain the negative results of the phase III trial.[68] Preclinical data sup- porting synergy between PARP-inhibitors and RT through the promotion of genomic instability and clinical data in other tumor types suggest this combination should not be abandoned quite yet.[69,70] In NSCLC, a phase I combination of olaparib, cisplatin, and high-dose RT observed a median OS of 28 months and 84% locoregional control rate, although severe pulmonary toxicity was observed.[71] A phase I study of RT, cetuximab, and olaparib in 16 heavy smokers with HNSCC also yielded signs of activ- ity with 72% 2-year survival rate.[72] Although small, these studies may suggest that further studies with PARP inhibitors in combination with RT and other modalities are worth exploring in esophagogastric tumors.

In summary, preclinical data have provided a basis for the study of several different targeted moieties in combination with RT and CRT across different phases of patient treatment. Although some of these efforts have not yielded a clear impact, evidence from landmark studies such as Checkmate-577 have shown that there is a clear path for further study in this space of PD-(L)1 checkpoint inhibitors. Preclinical evi- dence is needed to drive the study of emerging targets in esophagogastric cancer. Finally, well-designed clinical trials are needed to further study validated targets in combination with RT/CRT across the phases of patient treatment.

RADIATION THERAPY DOSE

Much debate has centered about the optimal RT dose for esophageal cancer. In the landmark CROSS study, patients received 4140 cGy with concurrent weekly carbo- platin and paclitaxel.[73] The radiation dose of 4140 cGy is a departure from earlier established doses of 5040 cGy in the definitive setting for a cohort of primarily squa- mous cell carcinoma histology.[74] Therefore, a dose range of 4140 to 5040 cGy has become acceptable in the setting of neoadjuvant therapy. The ARTDECO study also evaluated doses of RT for a variety of sublocations and included both adenocarci- nomas (39%) and squamous cell (61%) carcinomas of the esophagus. The standard dose (SD) of 50.4 Gy/1.8 Gy for 5.5 weeks to the tumor and regional lymph nodes was compared with a high-dose (HD) regimen up to a total dose of 61.6 Gy to the pri- mary tumor. The 3-year local PFS (LPFS) was 70% in the SD arm versus 73% in the HD arm (not significant). The LPFS for SCC and AC was 75% versus 79% and 61% versus 61% for SD and HD, respectively (not significant). The 3-year locoregional PFS was 52% and 59% for the SD and HD arms, respectively ($P = .08$). Limitations to this study include the very limited patients of cervical esophageal cancers, where the data are insufficient to interpret from this study, but nevertheless doses of 4140 to 5040 cGy remain standard at this time.[75] Higher RT doses have been studied in the setting of concurrent CRT; however, safety remains a barrier despite technological advances. Xu and colleagues randomized 319 patients in a 1:1 ratio to receive a conventional fractionated dose of 60 Gy or 50 Gy with concurrent chemotherapy.[76] They observed similar efficacy between the 2 study groups but with a statistically significant increase in grade 3+ pneumonitis in the 60 Gy group ($P = .03$).[76] Therefore, the role of RT dose escalation remains unclear and might need evaluation with novel techniques to minimize toxicities.

PERIOPERATIVE CHEMOTHERAPY VERSUS PREOPERATIVE CHEMORADIATION

Another controversial topic is the use of perioperative chemotherapy compared with chemoradiation for esophageal cancers. In the PreOperative therapy in Esophagogastric adenocarcinoma Trial (POET) study, 119 patients with locally advanced adenocarcinomas of the GEJ (Siewert types I–III) were randomized to chemotherapy using cisplatin, fluorouracil, and leucovorin (group A) or induction chemotherapy and CRT (group B) followed by surgery. Local PFS after tumor resection was significantly improved by CRT ($P = .01$) and 20 versus 12 patients were free of local tumor progression at 5 years ($P = .03$). Although the rate of postoperative inpatient mortality was higher with CRT (10.2% vs 3.8%, $P = .26$), more patients were alive at 3 and 5 years after CRT (46.7% and 39.5%) compared with chemotherapy (26.1% and 24.4%). Thus, OS showed a trend in favor of preoperative CRT (HR 0.65, 95% confidence interval [CI] 0.42 to 1.01, $P = .055$).

Another important study in this space is the Neo-AEGIS study presented in abstract form in 2023. This study randomized patients to perioperative FLOT (5-FU, leucovorin, oxaliplatin, docetaxel) chemotherapy compared with preoperative CROSS regimen therapy. Although this study suggested equivalence, there are significant issues when considering how best to counsel patients.[77] After the preoperative CROSS regimen, patients could receive nivolumab postoperatively as per the CheckMate-577 data, which doubles the DFS compared with observation. Therefore, preoperative chemoradiation followed by surgery and consolidative nivolumab may be superior to perioperative FLOT. Patients who received the perioperative chemotherapy alone had a higher chance to have an R1 resection implying positive margins/residual microscopic disease left after surgery. R1 resections predispose patients to higher rates of local and distant failures and are an indication for patients to need postoperative RT. The rates of downstaging are important and were improved with the CROSS regimen compared with perioperative chemotherapy. Studies such as the CALGB 80803 suggest that the patients who have better responses to chemoradiation can achieve improved outcomes, so maximizing the response rates from preoperative therapy is important for improving long-term outcomes for patients. Chemoradiation seems to have a better preoperative response rate compared with chemotherapy. Taken together, preoperative chemoradiation provides an important and effective method for downstaging that can allow for postoperative immunotherapy, downstaging, and decrease in local recurrences.

RADIATION TECHNIQUE AND TOXICITY CONSIDERATIONS

Given the efficacy of preoperative and definitive CRT for the treatment of stage II to III esophageal cancers, improving the toxicity profile of RT can improve tolerability and reduce long-term side effects. Because of the critical location of the esophagus adjacent to the lungs heart, and vertebra (ie, containing bone marrow), technological advancements in RT have aimed to achieve the highest probability of cure, while adopting a conscious approach to minimize toxicities. Before the availability of computed tomography (CT) scanning for treatment planning, 2-dimensional (2D) plans with simple treatment fields posed limitations, as the ability to minimize radiation doses to critical structures was more limited than modern approaches.[78] The advent of 3D conformal radiotherapy (3DCRT) in which several beams could be shaped around the target volume with subsequent dosimetric analysis with dose-volume histograms allowed more precise calculation of doses to nearby organs at risk (OARs). Data from multiple planning studies investigated improvements in dose conformality and better sparing of normal tissue using IMRT when compared with 3DCRT.[79–81] A further improvement is the use of proton beam therapy, which has the advantage of the characteristic proton beam therapy's (PBT) Bragg peak with a very narrow range of dose deposition prohibiting dose from spreading beyond the intended tumor target, proposing therapeutic advantages in sparing OARs.

In a single-institution analysis from MD Anderson evaluating definitive CRT using PBT versus IMRT, PBT had significantly better OS, PFS, distant metastasis–free survival, as well as marginally better locoregional failure-free survival. Analysis by clinical stage revealed considerably higher 5-year OS (34.6% vs 25.0%, $P = .038$) and PFS rates (33.5% vs 13.2%, $P = .005$) in the PBT group for patients with stage III disease but not with stage I/II disease.[82] Further work in the context of propensity matching between 3DCRT and IMRT in a cohort of patients with esophageal cancer treated with chemoradiation showed that 3DCRT patients had a higher risk of death and locoregional recurrence compared with IMRT, advancing the hypothesis that a high-toxicity profile could lead to worse survival outcomes, possibly related to cardiac and lung effects.[81,83]

Dosimetric analysis demonstrated that PBT resulted in significantly lowered whole heart doses and cardiac substructures including the coronary vessels compared with IMRT.[84] In a cohort of 355 patients with esophageal cancer, radiation dose to coronary substructures was associated with major coronary events and reduced OS.[85] Evaluation of 479 patients showed that grade 3 or higher (G3+) cardiac events occurred in 18% of patients at a median of 7 months, and preexisting cardiac disease and radiation modality (IMRT vs PBT) were significantly associated with G3+ cardiac events.[86] Furthermore, other studies suggest the importance of monitoring doses to the lungs. One study by Wang and colleagues evaluated postoperative complications after neoadjuvant chemoradiation and found that mean lung dose was an important factor in postoperative pulmonary complications.[87] In a study by Gibson and colleagues of the ECOG, E2205, that combined preoperative chemoradiation with cetuximab, of the 21 patients enrolled, there were significant pulmonary toxicities.[88] This experience speaks to the importance of careful field design. This work supported the concept that optimized radiation delivery by reducing doses to the lungs, coronary substructures, and heart results in reduced toxicities and improved survival rates.

Lin and colleagues conducted a phase IIB trial that randomized patients with locally advanced esophageal cancer to PBT or IMRT.[89] One innovative aspect of this trial was the endpoint of total toxicity burden (TTB), which was a composite of 11 distinct adverse events including common toxicities and postoperative complications up to 1 year following treatment. The posterior mean TTB was 2.3 times higher for IMRT (39.9) than PBT (17.4) with similar PFS. The mean postoperative complication score was 7.6 times higher for IMRT (19.1; 7.3–32.3) versus PBT (2.5; 0.3–5.2). The posterior probability that mean TTB was lower for PBT compared with IMRT was 0.9989, which

---

Box 3
Study spotlight: proton beam versus intensity-modulated radiotherapy trial using total toxicity burden endpoint[89]

- A phase II trial enrolled patients with stage II to III squamous cell carcinoma/adenoid cystic carcinoma and esophageal cancer and eligible to receive concurrent CRT with radiation delivered using either PBT (passive scatter) or IMRT (static or VMAT) with PFS and TTB as the coprimary endpoints.

- TTB is the calculated cumulative severity of 11 distinct adverse effects and postoperative complications that patients experience after CRT with or without surgery on completing of CRT.

- The mean TTB was 2.3 times higher for IMRT (39.9; 95% density interval 26.2–54.9), compared with PBT (17.4; 95% density interval 7.3–32.3), with the PBT arm experiencing fewer cardiopulmonary toxicities and POCs. No differences noted in the PFS and quality of life between IMRT and PBT.

- First randomized trial to elucidate the benefits of PBT in the treatment of esophageal cancer.

---

exceeded the trial's stopping boundary at the 67% interim analysis; however, there were no differences in PFS or OS at 3 years (**Box 3**).[89]

Because of the sensitivity of circulating lymphocytes to radiation exposure, evaluation of a cohort of patients with esophageal cancer treated with neoadjuvant IMRT versus PBT showed a doubling in the of grade 4 lymphopenia with IMRT (40.4%) compared with PBT (17.6%).[90] Increasing radiation dose to the thoracic vertebra, which encompasses approximately 20% of bone marrow, can increase the risk of lymphopenia, as shown by Deek and colleagues.[91] Adjusting for chemotherapy-induced effects, Lee and colleagues aimed to study the possible dose constraints that may be associated with hematologic toxicity (HT) owing to radiation of esophageal cancers using IMRT plans.[92] It was determined that the mean vertebral dose, mean rib dose (V5-V20), V20, and V30 of the thoracic vertebra were associated with an increased risk of leukopenia, and with every 2 Gy increase in mean vertebral dose, there was an associated 22% increase in the risk of developing leukopenia, grade 3 and higher. A study by Warren and colleagues selected a cohort of 21 patients who received treatment with 3D conformal plans for midesophageal cancer and were also analyzed using volumetric modulated arc therapy (VMAT) and proton therapy plans using the dose–volume parameters used in predicting HT in thoracic malignancies.[93–95] There was a significantly higher mean dose to the thoracic vertebra in 3D plans when compared with the VMAT and proton techniques; however, there was greatest potential to spare the mean bone dose and the low-dose region (V10) with the use of PBT, especially in the setting of larger treatment fields (planning target volume). Therefore, proton therapy plays an influential role in potentially decreasing the hematological toxicity associated with incidental bone marrow irradiation.

These studies demonstrate that proton therapy can have a dosimetric benefit in reducing the risk of HT. When further comparing IMRT, passive-scattering proton therapy (PSPT), and intensity-modulated proton therapy (IMPT), a study by Ebrahimi and colleagues used prediction models for lymphocyte depletion based on radiation doses and found that the average mean body doses were 14.44, 7.37, and 6.12 Gy for IMRT, PSPT, and IMPT treatments, respectively, suggesting that IMPT provides an additional advantage over PSPT.[96] However, IMPT is more sensitive to motion and setup uncertainties, and efforts must be made to limit these variations to achieve a highly reproducible treatment. There have also been studies in which severe lymphopenia has been shown to be associated with a poorer prognosis in patients with esophageal cancer.[97] When treating with combined CRT, there may be an element of contribution to HT from chemotherapy; therefore, any possible reduction in bone marrow toxicity owing to radiation could help tolerance of chemotherapy.

ASSESSING TREATMENT RESPONSE

An approach that has been seeing increased interest in recent years is the use of various imaging techniques to augment ongoing CRT regimens. Approaches such as PET with fludeoxyglucose F18 [(18)F-FDG PET]/CT scans and diffusion-weighted MRI have allowed clinicians to measure the metabolic activity of a tumor and use it to assess response. Efforts to use FDG-PET scans to select induction chemotherapy is not an entirely new concept, with the MUNICON I and MUNICON II studies being notable and influential examples of the exploration of image-guided algorithms.[98,99] Retrospectively developed algorithms and small prospective studies have suggested that PET-guided decision-making could affect patient outcomes by identifying patients who may benefit most for esophagectomy, predicting pCR, detecting interval metastasis, and guiding radiotherapy dose escalation.[100–102] However, the results of the CALBG 80803 (**Box 4**) are particularly noteworthy. CALGB 80803 used a 35% decrease in standardized uptake value to identify responders and nonresponders to induction chemotherapy before chemoradiation in 225 participants. Responders remained on the initial regimens, whereas nonresponders were switched to the other regimen. Responders had median 48.8-month OS and nonresponders a 27.4-month median OS, which was found not to be statistically significant.[103] Nonresponders also achieved pCR rate of 20% when crossing from carboplatin/paclitaxel to FOLFOX and 18% when changing from FOLFOX to carboplatin/paclitaxel, a substantial improvement over the expected 5% pCR typically seen from nonresponders.[103]

In the setting of assessing response after chemoradiation, recent models in development have incorporated diffusion-weighted MRI in the FDG-PET approach and achieved algorithms with better specificity and sensitivity to predict pCR than either imaging approach alone.[104,105] Combining diagnostic tools to improve prediction power seems to be gaining traction. The preSANO study used a multidiagnostic model to guide decision-making during and after CRT using a combination of endoscopy, biopsy (bite on bite and traditional), fine-needle aspiration, PET scan, and ultrasound.[106] The primary endpoint was the correlation between the clinical evaluations and the final pathologic evaluation following resection. The final analysis found that fine-needle aspiration and bite-on-bite biopsy had best predictive values and could be used to predict residual disease and stratify patients for surgery with a role for

---

Box 4
Study spotlight: CALGB 80803[103]

- A study examining the use of PET scans to guide chemotherapy selection during CRT induction before surgery. The primary endpoint was pCR rate following surgery.

- The pCR rate was observed to be improved over the expected rate of 5% for the nonresponders (18% for FOLFOX nonresponders and 20% for carboplatin nonresponders).

- Although FOLFOX responders had a higher pCR rate of 40.3%, there was no observed statistical difference in median OS between the pooled responders and nonresponders.

- Predictive biomarkers can have a significant impact on a patient's likelihood of achieving pCR and associated improved outcomes.

PET scans to detect new interval metastasis.[106] Several clinical trials have been designed seeking to replicate the results of the preSANO and the CALGB 80803 study, with some even including newer biomarkers such as circulating tumor DNA (ctDNA) (see **Table 2**).

The utility of ctDNA could be to monitor long-term outcomes after definitive therapy to evaluate for recurrences in advance of imaging findings. One example of the use of ctDNA in esophageal cancer by Azad and colleagues studied deep sequencing (CAncer Personalized Profiling by deep Sequencing [CAPP-Seq]) analyses of plasma cell–free DNA collected from 45 patients before and after chemoradiation, as well as DNA from leukocytes and fixed esophageal tumor biopsy samples collected during esophagogastroduodenoscopy. Detection of ctDNA after chemoradiation was associated with tumor progression (HR 18.7; $P < .0001$), formation of distant metastases (HR 32.1; $P < .0001$), and shorter disease-specific survival times (HR 23.1; $P < .0001$). Detection of ctDNA after CRT preceded radiographic evidence of tumor progression by an average of 2.8 months. Among patients who received CRT without surgery, combined ctDNA and metabolic imaging analysis was superior to cDNA and metabolic imaging alone and predicted progression in 100% of patients with tumor progression.[107]

The use of biomarkers may inform another method to select individualized patient management paradigms. To risk stratify patients, Sihag and colleagues evaluated the TP53 pathway in 238 patients with esophageal adenocarcinoma of the lower esophagus or GEJ who were treated with neoadjuvant multimodal therapy with curative intent. MDM2 amplification was independently associated with poor response to neoadjuvant therapy ($P = .032$), when accounting for significant clinicopathologic variables. Moreover, TP53 pathway alterations, grouped according to inferred severity of TP53 dysfunction, were significantly associated with response to neoadjuvant therapy ($P = .004$). Using MDM2 amplification and TP53 status to gauge therapies going forward may improve outcomes in patients with esophageal adenocarcinoma.[108] The data from these studies could provide clinicians with new ways to maximize benefit while reducing treatment burden for patients.

SUMMARY

The understanding of the molecular subtypes of esophageal cancers has provided a strong basis for the development of the next generation of potential targets. In addition, combinations of targeted pharmacotherapy to RT and CRT represents an opportunity for improved outcomes in the treatment of esophagogastric tumors. Preclinical evidence of mechanistic synergy has been observed between RT and many types of targeted therapy. In several instances, these data have translated into positive results in clinical studies. Although more studies are required to determine how targeted systemic therapy can potentiate RT therapy, recent data from studies with checkpoint inhibitors forecast a substantial potential for clinical benefit. Technological advances have also paved the way for an increase in local tumor control by allowing higher dose to be delivered with the aid of modern techniques. Ultimately, the complexity lies in striking a balance between the toxicity profile and curative intent. The careful dosimetry consideration of the lung, cardiac, and bone marrow structures when comparing various external beam radiation plans provides patients with a considerable degree of protection from avoidable toxicities while maintaining the equilibrium between efficacy and safety. Together, these advances offer clinicians a wider variety of options when treating patients, with new imaging, and biopsy-guided response assessment could allow for a more patient-specific approach to treatment planning and optimization of initial treatment efforts. Early detection, formulation of multimodality treatment design, and close surveillance with attention to treatment response may lead to a shift in the paradigm of esophageal cancer management.

DISCLOSURES

J.Cinicola reports employment as a contractor for Merck, Sharp & Dohme (MSD). S. Jabbour reports grant funding from Merck & Co, Inc., Beigene; Consultant for Merck & Co, Inc, Novocure, Radialogica, IMX Medical; Adjudication Committee: Syntactx; DSMB: Advarra. This study was supported by NIH P30CA072720.

REFERENCES

1. Zhang Y. Epidemiology of esophageal cancer. World J Gastroenterol 2013; 19(34):5598–606.
2. Hulscher JB, van Sandick JW, de Boer AG, et al. Extended transthoracic resection compared with limited transhiatal resection for adenocarcinoma of the esophagus. N Engl J Med 2002;347(21):1662–9.
3. Herskovic A, Russell W, Liptay M, et al. Esophageal carcinoma advances in treatment results for locally advanced disease: review. Ann Oncol 2012;23(5): 1095–103.
4. Nakagawa S, Kanda T, Kosugi S, et al. Recurrence pattern of squamous cell carcinoma of the thoracic esophagus after extended radical esophagectomy with three-field lymphadenectomy. J Am Coll Surg 2004;198(2):205–11.
5. Chen G, Wang Z, Liu XY, et al. Recurrence pattern of squamous cell carcinoma in the middle thoracic esophagus after modified Ivor-Lewis esophagectomy. World J Surg 2007;31(5):1107–14.
6. Network CGAR, University AWGA, Agency BC, et al. Integrated genomic characterization of oesophageal carcinoma. Nature 2017;541(7636):169–75.
7. Sato S, Kajiyama Y, Sugano M, et al. Monoclonal antibody to HER-2/neu receptor enhances radiosensitivity of esophageal cancer cell lines expressing HER-2/ neu oncoprotein. Int J Radiat Oncol Biol Phys 2005;61(1):203–11.
8. Bang YJ, Van Cutsem E, Feyereislova A, et al. Trastuzumab in combination with chemotherapy versus chemotherapy alone for treatment of HER2-positive advanced gastric or gastro-oesophageal junction cancer (ToGA): a phase 3, open-label, randomised controlled trial. Lancet 2010;376(9742):687–97.
9. Jabbour SK, Williams TM, Sayan M, et al. Potential Molecular Targets in the Setting of Chemoradiation for Esophageal Malignancies. J Natl Cancer Inst 2021;113(6):665–79.
10. Safran HP, Winter K, Ilson DH, et al. Trastuzumab with trimodality treatment for oesophageal adenocarcinoma with HER2 overexpression (NRG Oncology/ RTOG 1010): a multicentre, randomised, phase 3 trial. Lancet Oncol 2022; 23(2):259–69.
11. Rivera F, Izquierdo-Manuel M, García-Alfonso P, et al. Perioperative trastuzumab, capecitabine and oxaliplatin in patients with HER2-positive resectable gastric or gastro-oesophageal junction adenocarcinoma: NEOHX phase II trial. Eur J Cancer 2021;145:158–67.
12. Rivera F, Romero C, Jimenez-Fonseca P, et al. Phase II study to evaluate the efficacy of Trastuzumab in combination with Capecitabine and Oxaliplatin in first-line treatment of HER2-positive advanced gastric cancer: HERXO trial. Cancer Chemother Pharmacol 2019;83(6):1175–81.
13. Hofheinz RD, Hegewisch-Becker S, Kunzmann V, et al. Trastuzumab in combination with 5-fluorouracil, leucovorin, oxaliplatin and docetaxel as perioperative

treatment for patients with human epidermal growth factor receptor 2-positive locally advanced esophagogastric adenocarcinoma: A phase II trial of the Arbeitsgemeinschaft Internistische Onkologie Gastric Cancer Study Group. Int J Cancer 2021;149(6):1322–31.

14. Janjigian YY, Maron SB, Chatila WK, et al. First-line pembrolizumab and trastuzumab in HER2-positive oesophageal, gastric, or gastro-oesophageal junction cancer: an open-label, single-arm, phase 2 trial. Lancet Oncol 2020;21(6): 821–31.

15. Tintelnot J, Goekkurt E, Binder M, et al. Ipilimumab or FOLFOX with Nivolumab and Trastuzumab in previously untreated HER2-positive locally advanced or metastatic EsophagoGastric Adenocarcinoma - the randomized phase 2 IN-TEGA trial (AIO STO 0217). BMC Cancer 2020;20(1):503.

16. Hecht JR, Bang YJ, Qin SK, et al. Lapatinib in Combination With Capecitabine Plus Oxaliplatin in Human Epidermal Growth Factor Receptor 2-Positive Advanced or Metastatic Gastric, Esophageal, or Gastroesophageal Adenocarcinoma: TRIO-013/LOGiC–A Randomized Phase III Trial. J Clin Oncol 2016; 34(5):443–51.

17. Shepard G, Arrowsmith ER, Murphy P, et al. A Phase II Study with Lead-In Safety Cohort of 5-Fluorouracil, Oxaliplatin, and Lapatinib in Combination with Radiation Therapy as Neoadjuvant Treatment for Patients with Localized HER2-Positive Esophagogastric Adenocarcinomas. Oncol 2017;22(10):1152-e98.

18. Weiss JM, Grilley-Olson JE, Deal AM, et al. Phase 2 trial of neoadjuvant chemotherapy and transoral endoscopic surgery with risk-adapted adjuvant therapy for squamous cell carcinoma of the head and neck. Cancer 2018;124(14): 2986–92.

19. Shitara K, Bang YJ, Iwasa S, et al. Trastuzumab Deruxtecan in Previously Treated HER2-Positive Gastric Cancer. N Engl J Med 2020;382(25):2419–30.

20. Van Cutsem E, Di Bartolomeo M, Smyth E, et al. LBA55 - Primary analysis of a phase II single-arm trial of trastuzumab deruxtecan (T-DXd) in western patients (Pts) with HER2-positive (HER2+) unresectable or metastatic gastric or gastro-esophageal junction (GEJ) cancer who progressed on or after a trastuzumab-containing regimen. Ann Oncol 2021;32(suppl_5):S1283–346.

21. Mills MN, Walker C, Thawani C, et al. Trastuzumab Emtansine (T-DM1) and stereotactic radiation in the management of HER2+ breast cancer brain metastases. BMC Cancer 2021;21(1):223.

22. Stumpf PK, Cittelly DM, Robin TP, et al. Combination of Trastuzumab Emtansine and Stereotactic Radiosurgery Results in High Rates of Clinically Significant Radionecrosis and Dysregulation of Aquaporin-4. Clin Cancer Res 2019;25(13): 3946–53.

23. Id Said B, Chen H, Jerzak KJ, et al. Trastuzumab emtansine increases the risk of stereotactic radiosurgery-induced radionecrosis in HER2 + breast cancer. J Neurooncol. Aug 2022;159(1):177–83.

24. Kato K, Cho BC, Takahashi M, et al. Nivolumab versus chemotherapy in patients with advanced oesophageal squamous cell carcinoma refractory or intolerant to previous chemotherapy (ATTRACTION-3): a multicentre, randomised, open-label, phase 3 trial. Lancet Oncol. Nov 2019;20(11):1506–17.

25. Kojima T, Shah MA, Muro K, et al. Randomized Phase III KEYNOTE-181 Study of Pembrolizumab Versus Chemotherapy in Advanced Esophageal Cancer. J Clin Oncol 2020;38(35):4138–48.

26. Marabelle A, Le DT, Ascierto PA, et al. Efficacy of Pembrolizumab in Patients With Noncolorectal High Microsatellite Instability/Mismatch Repair-Deficient

Cancer: Results From the Phase II KEYNOTE-158 Study. J Clin Oncol 2020; 38(1):1–10.

27. Loos M, Langer R, Schuster T, et al. Clinical significance of the costimulatory molecule B7-H1 in Barrett carcinoma. Ann Thorac Surg 2011;91(4):1025–31.

28. Secrier M, Li X, de Silva N, et al. Mutational signatures in esophageal adenocarcinoma define etiologically distinct subgroups with therapeutic relevance. Nat Genet 2016;48(10):1131–41.

29. Nomi T, Sho M, Akahori T, et al. Clinical significance and therapeutic potential of the programmed death-1 ligand/programmed death-1 pathway in human pancreatic cancer. Clin Cancer Res 2007;13(7):2151–7.

30. Park S, Joung JG, Min YW, et al. Paired whole exome and transcriptome analyses for the Immunogenomic changes during concurrent chemoradiotherapy in esophageal squamous cell carcinoma. J Immunother Cancer 2019;7(1):128.

31. Janjigian YY, Shitara K, Moehler M, et al. First-line nivolumab plus chemotherapy versus chemotherapy alone for advanced gastric, gastro-oesophageal junction, and oesophageal adenocarcinoma (CheckMate 649): a randomised, open-label, phase 3 trial. Lancet 2021;398(10294):27–40.

32. Okada M, Kato K, Cho BC, et al. Three-Year Follow-Up and Response-Survival Relationship of Nivolumab in Previously Treated Patients with Advanced Esophageal Squamous Cell Carcinoma (ATTRACTION-3). Clin Cancer Res 2022; 28(15):3277–86.

33. Kelly RJ, Ajani JA, Kuzdzal J, et al. Adjuvant Nivolumab in Resected Esophageal or Gastroesophageal Junction Cancer. N Engl J Med 2021;384(13): 1191–203.

34. Ebert MP, Meindl-Beinker NM, Gutting T, et al. Second-line therapy with nivolumab plus ipilimumab for older patients with oesophageal squamous cell cancer (RAMONA): a multicentre, open-label phase 2 trial. Lancet Healthy Longev 2022;3(6):e417–27.

35. Eads JR, Weitz M, Catalano PJ, et al. A phase II/III study of perioperative nivolumab and ipilimumab in patients (pts) with locoregional esophageal (E) and gastroesophageal junction (GEJ) adenocarcinoma: Results of a safety run-in—A trial of the ECOG-ACRIN Cancer Research Group (EA2174). J Clin Oncol 2021;39(15_suppl):4064.

36. Shah MA, Kojima T, Hochhauser D, et al. Efficacy and Safety of Pembrolizumab for Heavily Pretreated Patients With Advanced, Metastatic Adenocarcinoma or Squamous Cell Carcinoma of the Esophagus: The Phase 2 KEYNOTE-180 Study. JAMA Oncol 2019;5(4):546–50.

37. Sun JM, Shen L, Shah MA, et al. Pembrolizumab plus chemotherapy versus chemotherapy alone for first-line treatment of advanced oesophageal cancer (KEYNOTE-590): a randomised, placebo-controlled, phase 3 study. Lancet 2021;398(10302):759–71.

38. Shen L, Kato K, Kim SB, et al. Tislelizumab Versus Chemotherapy as Second-Line Treatment for Advanced or Metastatic Esophageal Squamous Cell Carcinoma (RATIONALE-302): A Randomized Phase III Study. J Clin Oncol 2022; 40(26):3065–76.

39. Zhang W, Yan C, Gao X, et al. Safety and Feasibility of Radiotherapy Plus Camrelizumab for Locally Advanced Esophageal Squamous Cell Carcinoma. Oncologist 2021;26(7):e1110–24.

40. Chen F, Qiu L, Mu Y, et al. Neoadjuvant chemoradiotherapy with camrelizumab in patients with locally advanced esophageal squamous cell carcinoma. Front Surg 2022;9:893372.

41. Zhu M, Chen C, Foster NR, et al. Pembrolizumab in Combination with Neoadjuvant Chemoradiotherapy for Patients with Resectable Adenocarcinoma of the Gastroesophageal Junction. Clin Cancer Res 2022;28(14):3021–31.
42. El Kaffas A, Tran W, Czarnota GJ. Vascular strategies for enhancing tumour response to radiation therapy. Technol Cancer Res Treat 2012;11(5):421–32.
43. Wilke H, Muro K, Van Cutsem E, et al. Ramucirumab plus paclitaxel versus placebo plus paclitaxel in patients with previously treated advanced gastric or gastro-oesophageal junction adenocarcinoma (RAINBOW): a double-blind, randomised phase 3 trial. Lancet Oncol 2014;15(11):1224–35.
44. Fuchs CS, Tomasek J, Yong CJ, et al. Ramucirumab monotherapy for previously treated advanced gastric or gastro-oesophageal junction adenocarcinoma (REGARD): an international, randomised, multicentre, placebo-controlled, phase 3 trial. Lancet 4 2014;383(9911):31–9.
45. Klempner SJ, Maron SB, Chase L, et al. Initial Report of Second-Line FOLFIRI in Combination with Ramucirumab in Advanced Gastroesophageal Adenocarcinomas: A Multi-Institutional Retrospective Analysis. Oncologist 2019;24(4):475–82.
46. Fuchs CS, Shitara K, Di Bartolomeo M, et al. Ramucirumab with cisplatin and fluoropyrimidine as first-line therapy in patients with metastatic gastric or junctional adenocarcinoma (RAINFALL): a double-blind, randomised, placebo-controlled, phase 3 trial. Lancet Oncol 2019;20(3):420–35.
47. Lee NY, Zhang Q, Pfister DG, et al. Addition of bevacizumab to standard chemoradiation for locoregionally advanced nasopharyngeal carcinoma (RTOG 0615): a phase 2 multi-institutional trial. Lancet Oncol 2012;13(2):172–80.
48. Bang YJ, Golan T, Dahan L, et al. Ramucirumab and durvalumab for previously treated, advanced non-small-cell lung cancer, gastric/gastro-oesophageal junction adenocarcinoma, or hepatocellular carcinoma: An open-label, phase Ia/b study (JVDJ). Eur J Cancer 2020;137:272–84.
49. Ahn PH, Machtay M, Anne PR, et al. Phase I Trial Using Induction Ciplatin, Docetaxel, 5-FU and Erlotinib Followed by Cisplatin, Bevacizumab and Erlotinib With Concurrent Radiotherapy for Advanced Head and Neck Cancer. Am J Clin Oncol 2018;41(5):441–6.
50. Kim K, Wu HG, Jeon SR. Epidermal growth factor-induced cell death and radiosensitization in epidermal growth factor receptor-overexpressing cancer cell lines. Anticancer Res 2015;35(1):245–53.
51. Nijkamp MM, Span PN, Bussink J, et al. Interaction of EGFR with the tumour microenvironment: implications for radiation treatment. Radiother Oncol 2013;108(1):17–23.
52. Milas L, Fan Z, Andratschke NH, et al. Epidermal growth factor receptor and tumor response to radiation: in vivo preclinical studies. Int J Radiat Oncol Biol Phys 2004;58(3):966–71.
53. Bonner JA, Harari PM, Giralt J, et al. Radiotherapy plus cetuximab for squamous-cell carcinoma of the head and neck. N Engl J Med 2006;354(6):567–78.
54. Suntharalingam M, Winter K, Ilson D, et al. Effect of the Addition of Cetuximab to Paclitaxel, Cisplatin, and Radiation Therapy for Patients With Esophageal Cancer: The NRG Oncology RTOG 0436 Phase 3 Randomized Clinical Trial. JAMA Oncol 2017;3(11):1520–8.
55. Crosby T, Hurt CN, Falk S, et al. Chemoradiotherapy with or without cetuximab in patients with oesophageal cancer (SCOPE1): a multicentre, phase 2/3 randomised trial. Lancet Oncol 2013;14(7):627–37.

56. Ruhstaller T, Thuss-Patience P, Hayoz S, et al. Neoadjuvant chemotherapy followed by chemoradiation and surgery with and without cetuximab in patients with resectable esophageal cancer: a randomized, open-label, phase III trial (SAKK 75/08). Ann Oncol 2018;29(6):1386–93.

57. de Castro Junior G, Segalla JG, de Azevedo SJ, et al. A randomised phase II study of chemoradiotherapy with or without nimotuzumab in locally advanced oesophageal cancer: NICE trial. Eur J Cancer 2018;88:21–30.

58. Lockhart AC, Reed CE, Decker PA, et al. Phase II study of neoadjuvant therapy with docetaxel, cisplatin, panitumumab, and radiation therapy followed by surgery in patients with locally advanced adenocarcinoma of the distal esophagus (ACOSOG Z4051). Ann Oncol 2014;25(5):1039–44.

59. Wu SX, Wang LH, Luo HL, et al. Randomised phase III trial of concurrent chemoradiotherapy with extended nodal irradiation and erlotinib in patients with inoperable oesophageal squamous cell cancer. Eur J Cancer 2018;93:99–107.

60. Luo H, Jiang W, Ma L, et al. Icotinib With Concurrent Radiotherapy vs Radiotherapy Alone in Older Adults With Unresectable Esophageal Squamous Cell Carcinoma: A Phase II Randomized Clinical Trial. JAMA Netw Open 2020;3(10):e2019440.

61. Iyer R, Chhatrala R, Shefter T, et al. Erlotinib and radiation therapy for elderly patients with esophageal cancer - clinical and correlative results from a prospective multicenter phase 2 trial. Oncology 2013;85(1):53–8.

62. Li G, Hu W, Wang J, et al. Phase II study of concurrent chemoradiation in combination with erlotinib for locally advanced esophageal carcinoma. Int J Radiat Oncol Biol Phys 2010;78(5):1407–12.

63. Yang X, Zhai Y, Bi N, et al. Radiotherapy combined with nimotuzumab for elderly esophageal cancer patients: A phase II clinical trial. Chin J Cancer Res 2021;33(1):53–60.

64. Bang YJ, Xu RH, Chin K, et al. Olaparib in combination with paclitaxel in patients with advanced gastric cancer who have progressed following first-line therapy (GOLD): a double-blind, randomised, placebo-controlled, phase 3 trial. Lancet Oncol 2017;18(12):1637–51.

65. Bang YJ, Im SA, Lee KW, et al. Randomized, Double-Blind Phase II Trial With Prospective Classification by ATM Protein Level to Evaluate the Efficacy and Tolerability of Olaparib Plus Paclitaxel in Patients With Recurrent or Metastatic Gastric Cancer. J Clin Oncol 2015;33(33):3858–65.

66. Kim HS, Kim MA, Hodgson D, et al. Concordance of ATM (ataxia telangiectasia mutated) immunohistochemistry between biopsy or metastatic tumor samples and primary tumors in gastric cancer patients. Pathobiology 2013;80(3):127–37.

67. Miller RM, Nworu C, McKee L, et al. Development of an Immunohistochemical Assay to Detect the Ataxia-Telangiectasia Mutated (ATM) Protein in Gastric Carcinoma. Appl Immunohistochem Mol Morphol 2020;28(4):303–10.

68. Smyth E. Missing a GOLDen opportunity in gastric cancer. Lancet Oncol 2017;18(12):1561–3.

69. Noël G, Godon C, Fernet M, et al. Radiosensitization by the poly(ADP-ribose) polymerase inhibitor 4-amino-1,8-naphthalimide is specific of the S phase of the cell cycle and involves arrest of DNA synthesis. Mol Cancer Ther 2006;5(3):564–74.

70. Guillot C, Favaudon V, Herceg Z, et al. PARP inhibition and the radiosensitizing effects of the PARP inhibitor ABT-888 in in vitro hepatocellular carcinoma models. BMC Cancer 2014;14:603.

71. de Haan R, van den Heuvel MM, van Diessen J, et al. Phase I and Pharmacologic Study of Olaparib in Combination with High-dose Radiotherapy with and without Concurrent Cisplatin for Non-Small Cell Lung Cancer. Clin Cancer Res 2021;27(5):1256–66.

72. Karam SD, Reddy K, Blatchford PJ, et al. Final Report of a Phase I Trial of Olaparib with Cetuximab and Radiation for Heavy Smoker Patients with Locally Advanced Head and Neck Cancer. Clin Cancer Res 2018;24(20):4949–59.

73. van Hagen P, Hulshof MC, van Lanschot JJ, et al. Preoperative chemoradiotherapy for esophageal or junctional cancer. N Engl J Med 2012;366(22):2074–84.

74. Kachnic LA, Winter K, Wasserman T, et al. Longitudinal Quality-of-Life Analysis of RTOG 94-05 (Int 0123):A Phase III Trial of Definitive Chemoradiotherapy for Esophageal Cancer. Gastrointest Cancer Res 2011;4(2):45–52.

75. Hulshof M, Geijsen ED, Rozema T, et al. Randomized Study on Dose Escalation in Definitive Chemoradiation for Patients With Locally Advanced Esophageal Cancer (ARTDECO Study). J Clin Oncol 2021;39(25):2816–24.

76. Xu Y, Dong B, Zhu W, et al. A Phase III Multicenter Randomized Clinical Trial of 60 Gy versus 50 Gy Radiation Dose in Concurrent Chemoradiotherapy for Inoperable Esophageal Squamous Cell Carcinoma. Clin Cancer Res 2022;28(9):1792–9.

77. Reynolds JV, Preston SR, O'Neill B, et al. Neo-AEGIS (Neoadjuvant trial in Adenocarcinoma of the Esophagus and Esophago-Gastric Junction International Study): Preliminary results of phase III RCT of CROSS versus perioperative chemotherapy (Modified MAGIC or FLOT protocol). (NCT01726452). J Clin Oncol 2021;39(15_suppl):4004.

78. Bucci MK, Bevan A, Roach M 3rd. Advances in radiation therapy: conventional to 3D, to IMRT, to 4D, and beyond. CA Cancer J Clin. Mar-Apr 2005;55(2):117–34.

79. Fenkell L, Kaminsky I, Breen S, et al. Dosimetric comparison of IMRT vs. 3D conformal radiotherapy in the treatment of cancer of the cervical esophagus. Radiother Oncol 2008;89(3):287–91.

80. Xi M, Lin SH. Recent advances in intensity modulated radiotherapy and proton therapy for esophageal cancer. Expert Rev Anticancer Ther. Jul 2017;17(7):635–46.

81. Lin SH, Wang L, Myles B, et al. Propensity score-based comparison of long-term outcomes with 3-dimensional conformal radiotherapy vs intensity-modulated radiotherapy for esophageal cancer. Int J Radiat Oncol Biol Phys 2012;84(5):1078–85.

82. Xi M, Xu C, Liao Z, et al. Comparative Outcomes After Definitive Chemoradiotherapy Using Proton Beam Therapy Versus Intensity Modulated Radiation Therapy for Esophageal Cancer: A Retrospective, Single-Institutional Analysis. Int J Radiat Oncol Biol Phys 2017;99(3):667–76.

83. Boyce-Fappiano D, Nguyen QN, Chapman BV, et al. Single Institution Experience of Proton and Photon-based Postoperative Radiation Therapy for Non-small-cell Lung Cancer. Clin Lung Cancer 2021;22(5):e745–55.

84. Shiraishi Y, Xu C, Yang J, et al. Dosimetric comparison to the heart and cardiac substructure in a large cohort of esophageal cancer patients treated with proton beam therapy or Intensity-modulated radiation therapy. Radiother Oncol 2017;125(1):48–54.

85. Wang X, Palaskas NL, Hobbs BP, et al. The Impact of Radiation Dose to Heart Substructures on Major Coronary Events and Patient Survival after

Chemoradiation Therapy for Esophageal Cancer. Cancers (Basel) 2022;14(5). https://doi.org/10.3390/cancers14051304.

86. Wang X, Palaskas NL, Yusuf SW, et al. Incidence and Onset of Severe Cardiac Events After Radiotherapy for Esophageal Cancer. J Thorac Oncol 2020;15(10): 1682–90.

87. Wang J, Wei C, Tucker SL, et al. Predictors of postoperative complications after trimodality therapy for esophageal cancer. Int J Radiat Oncol Biol Phys 2013; 86(5):885–91.

88. Gibson MK, Catalano P, Kleinberg LR, et al. Phase II Study of Preoperative Chemoradiotherapy with Oxaliplatin, Infusional 5-Fluorouracil, and Cetuximab Followed by Postoperative Docetaxel and Cetuximab in Patients with Adenocarcinoma of the Esophagus: A Trial of the ECOG-ACRIN Cancer Research Group (E2205). Oncologist 2020;25(1):e53–9.

89. Lin SH, Hobbs BP, Verma V, et al. Randomized Phase IIB Trial of Proton Beam Therapy Versus Intensity-Modulated Radiation Therapy for Locally Advanced Esophageal Cancer. J Clin Oncol 2020;38(14):1569–79.

90. Shiraishi Y, Fang P, Xu C, et al. Severe lymphopenia during neoadjuvant chemoradiation for esophageal cancer: A propensity matched analysis of the relative risk of proton versus photon-based radiation therapy. Radiother Oncol 2018; 128(1):154–60.

91. Deek MP, Benenati B, Kim S, et al. Thoracic Vertebral Body Irradiation Contributes to Acute Hematologic Toxicity During Chemoradiation Therapy for Non-Small Cell Lung Cancer. Int J Radiat Oncol Biol Phys 2016;94(1):147–54.

92. Lee J, Lin JB, Sun FJ, et al. Dosimetric predictors of acute haematological toxicity in oesophageal cancer patients treated with neoadjuvant chemoradiotherapy. Br J Radiol 2016;89(1066):20160350.

93. Warren S, Hurt CN, Crosby T, et al. Potential of Proton Therapy to Reduce Acute Hematologic Toxicity in Concurrent Chemoradiation Therapy for Esophageal Cancer. Int J Radiat Oncol Biol Phys 2017;99(3):729–37.

94. Zhang Y, Jabbour SK, Zhang A, et al. Proton beam therapy can achieve lower vertebral bone marrow dose than photon beam therapy during chemoradiation therapy of esophageal cancer. Med Dosim. Autumn 2021;46(3):229–35.

95. Fang P, Shiraishi Y, Verma V, et al. Lymphocyte-Sparing Effect of Proton Therapy in Patients with Esophageal Cancer Treated with Definitive Chemoradiation. Int J Part Ther. Winter 2018;4(3):23–32.

96. Ebrahimi S, Lim G, Liu A, et al. Radiation-Induced Lymphopenia Risks of Photon Versus Proton Therapy for Esophageal Cancer Patients. Int J Part Ther. Fall 2021;8(2):17–27.

97. Davuluri R, Jiang W, Fang P, et al. Lymphocyte Nadir and Esophageal Cancer Survival Outcomes After Chemoradiation Therapy. Int J Radiat Oncol Biol Phys 2017;99(1):128–35.

98. Lordick F, Ott K, Krause BJ, et al. PET to assess early metabolic response and to guide treatment of adenocarcinoma of the oesophagogastric junction: the MUNICON phase II trial. Lancet Oncol 2007;8(9):797–805.

99. zum Büschenfelde CM, Herrmann K, Schuster T, et al. 18)F-FDG PET-guided salvage neoadjuvant radiochemotherapy of adenocarcinoma of the esophagogastric junction: the MUNICON II trial. J Nucl Med 2011;52(8):1189–96.

100. Xi M, Liao Z, Hofstetter WL, et al. F-FDG PET Response After Induction Chemotherapy Can Predict Who Will Benefit from Subsequent Esophagectomy After Chemoradiotherapy for Esophageal Adenocarcinoma. J Nucl Med 2017; 58(11):1756–63, 18.

101. Pöttgen C, Gkika E, Stahl M, et al. Dose-escalated radiotherapy with PET/CT based treatment planning in combination with induction and concurrent chemotherapy in locally advanced (uT3/T4) squamous cell cancer of the esophagus: mature results of a phase I/II trial. Radiat Oncol 2021;16(1):59.

102. Goense L, Ruurda JP, Carter BW, et al. Prediction and diagnosis of interval metastasis after neoadjuvant chemoradiotherapy for oesophageal cancer using (18)F-FDG PET/CT. Eur J Nucl Med Mol Imaging 2018;45(10):1742–51.

103. Goodman KA, Ou FS, Hall NC, et al. Randomized Phase II Study of PET Response-Adapted Combined Modality Therapy for Esophageal Cancer: Mature Results of the CALGB 80803 (Alliance) Trial. J Clin Oncol 2021;39(25): 2803–15.

104. Xu X, Sun ZY, Wu HW, et al. Diffusion-weighted MRI and (18)F-FDG PET/CT in assessing the response to neoadjuvant chemoradiotherapy in locally advanced esophageal squamous cell carcinoma. Radiat Oncol 2021;16(1):132.

105. Borggreve AS, Goense L, van Rossum PSN, et al. Preoperative Prediction of Pathologic Response to Neoadjuvant Chemoradiotherapy in Patients With Esophageal Cancer Using (18)F-FDG PET/CT and DW-MRI: A Prospective Multicenter Study. Int J Radiat Oncol Biol Phys 2020;106(5):998–1009.

106. Noordman BJ, Spaander MCW, Valkema R, et al. Detection of residual disease after neoadjuvant chemoradiotherapy for oesophageal cancer (preSANO): a prospective multicentre, diagnostic cohort study. Lancet Oncol 2018;19(7): 965–74.

107. Azad TD, Chaudhuri AA, Fang P, et al. Circulating Tumor DNA Analysis for Detection of Minimal Residual Disease After Chemoradiotherapy for Localized Esophageal Cancer. Gastroenterology 2020;158(3):494–505.e6.

108. Sihag S, Nussenzweig SC, Walch HS, et al. The Role of the TP53 Pathway in Predicting Response to Neoadjuvant Therapy in Esophageal Adenocarcinoma. Clin Cancer Res 2022;28(12):2669–78.

109. Walsh TN, Noonan N, Hollywood D, et al. A comparison of multimodal therapy and surgery for esophageal adenocarcinoma. N Engl J Med 1996;335(7):462–7.

110. Cooper JS, Guo MD, Herskovic A, et al. Chemoradiotherapy of locally advanced esophageal cancer: long-term follow-up of a prospective randomized trial (RTOG 85-01). Radiation Therapy Oncology Group. JAMA 1999;281(17): 1623–7.

111. Tepper J, Krasna MJ, Niedzwiecki D, et al. Phase III trial of trimodality therapy with cisplatin, fluorouracil, radiotherapy, and surgery compared with surgery alone for esophageal cancer: CALGB 9781. J Clin Oncol 2008;26(7):1086–92.

112. Smalley SR, Benedetti JK, Haller DG, et al. Updated analysis of SWOG-directed intergroup study 0116: a phase III trial of adjuvant radiochemotherapy versus observation after curative gastric cancer resection. J Clin Oncol 2012;30(19): 2327–33.

113. Stahl M, Walz MK, Riera-Knorrenschild J, et al. Preoperative chemotherapy versus chemoradiotherapy in locally advanced adenocarcinomas of the oesophagogastric junction (POET): Long-term results of a controlled randomised trial. Eur J Cancer 2017;81:183–90.

114. Yang H, Liu H, Chen Y, et al. Neoadjuvant Chemoradiotherapy Followed by Surgery Versus Surgery Alone for Locally Advanced Squamous Cell Carcinoma of the Esophagus (NEOCRTEC5010): A Phase III Multicenter, Randomized, Open-Label Clinical Trial. J Clin Oncol 2018;36(27):2796–803.

115. Eyck BM, van Lanschot JJB, Hulshof M, et al. Ten-Year Outcome of Neoadjuvant Chemoradiotherapy Plus Surgery for Esophageal Cancer: The Randomized Controlled CROSS Trial. J Clin Oncol 2021;39(18):1995–2004.
116. Chung HC, Bang YJ, C SF, et al. First-line pembrolizumab/placebo plus trastuzumab and chemotherapy in HER2-positive advanced gastric cancer: KEYNOTE-811. Future Oncol 2021;17(5):491–501.
117. Borggreve AS, Mook S, Verheij M, et al. Preoperative image-guided identification of response to neoadjuvant chemoradiotherapy in esophageal cancer (PRIDE): a multicenter observational study. BMC Cancer 2018;18(1):1006.
118. Zhang X, Eyck BM, Yang Y, et al. Accuracy of detecting residual disease after neoadjuvant chemoradiotherapy for esophageal squamous cell carcinoma (preSINO trial): a prospective multicenter diagnostic cohort study. BMC Cancer 2020;20(1):194.
119. Zhu H, Liu Q, Xu H, et al. Dose escalation based on (18)F-FDG PET/CT response in definitive chemoradiotherapy of locally advanced esophageal squamous cell carcinoma: a phase III, open-label, randomized, controlled trial (ESO-Shanghai 12). Radiat Oncol 2022;17(1):134.

Advances in Radiotherapy for Rectal Cancer

Timothy Lin, MD, MBA[a], Amol Narang, MD[a],*

KEYWORDS

- Rectal adenocarcinoma • Short-course radiotherapy • Total neoadjuvant therapy
- Watch-and-wait • Nonoperative management

KEY POINTS

- Total neoadjuvant therapy (TNT) has emerged as the preferred standard of care for patients with locally advanced rectal cancer due to improvements in pathologic complete response and distant failure compared with standard of care involving chemoradiotherapy and adjuvant chemotherapy.
- Acceptable TNT regimens include short-course radiotherapy followed by full-dose chemotherapy or chemoradiotherapy with induction versus consolidation chemotherapy; notably, consolidation chemotherapy has been associated with improved pathologic complete response in the surgical setting and total mesorectal excision-free survival in the nonoperative setting compared with induction chemotherapy.
- Nonoperative management may be considered in patients with near complete or clinical complete response to neoadjuvant therapy, although randomized data comparing outcomes between nonoperative and operative management are lacking.

INTRODUCTION

Colorectal cancer is the third most commonly occurring cancer worldwide and the second-leading cause of cancer death.[1] Historically, the definitive management of rectal adenocarcinoma has involved total mesorectal excision (TME), following studies by Heald and colleagues[2] in the 1980s reporting excellent locoregional control with this surgical technique. Around the same time, trials began to demonstrate the benefit of the addition of chemoradiotherapy to surgery, first in the postoperative setting,[3,4] with later trials demonstrating the superior efficacy of preoperative chemoradiotherapy.[5,6] More recently, the standard of care management of locally advanced rectal adenocarcinoma has shifted again, with the emergence of total neoadjuvant therapy (TNT) consisting of either neoadjuvant short-course radiotherapy (SCRT) with full-dose chemotherapy before surgery, or long-course chemoradiotherapy (LCCRT) with either induction or consolidative chemotherapy before surgery.[7] The optimal TNT regimen remains an area of continued investigation, with the sequencing of

[a] Department of Radiation Oncology & Molecular Radiation Sciences, Johns Hopkins University School of Medicine, 401 N Broadway, Baltimore, MD 21287, USA
* Corresponding author.
E-mail address: anarang2@jhmi.edu

Surg Oncol Clin N Am 32 (2023) 461–473
https://doi.org/10.1016/j.soc.2023.02.003
surgonc.theclinics.com

chemotherapy as induction or consolidation in the setting of LCCRT as well as the comparative efficacy of SCRT and LCCRT. Finally, owing to the morbidity associated with TME, the feasibility of nonoperative management (NOM) in patients with (near) clinical complete response to neoadjuvant therapy also continues to be explored as an avenue to preserve quality of life.

HISTORICAL CONTEXT

The benefit of the addition of chemoradiation to surgery was demonstrated in the GITSG 7175 trial, which showed that the addition of postoperative chemoradiotherapy reduced local recurrence rates and improved overall survival (OS).[8] However, TME was not standard. The subsequent trials of radiation therapy in the setting of TME demonstrated a local recurrence benefit but no difference in OS. For instance, the Dutch TME trial showed that the addition of preoperative SCRT (**Fig. 1**) delivered in 25 Gy in 5 fractions before TME resulted in a reduction in 10-year local recurrence from 11% to 5% (*P* < .0001) but no difference in disease-free or OS.[9] Despite excellent local control rates, distant failure occurred in a significant proportion of patients in both cohorts (25% vs 28%, *P* = .21). Subsequent chemoradiotherapy trials including the German Rectal Study demonstrated that despite excellent local control, distant failure continued to occur in close to one-third of all patients.[6] A meta-analysis of trials failed to demonstrate an added benefit to the addition of adjuvant chemotherapy to preoperative (chemo)radiotherapy and surgery in terms of distant recurrence, or OS, potentially in part due to challenges with compliance to chemotherapy as a result of treatment-related adverse effects.[10]

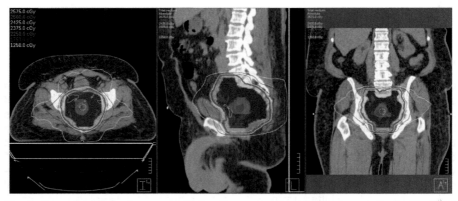

Fig. 1. Example of a short-course radiation therapy treatment plan for a patient with cT3N2 high rectal adenocarcinoma. Axial, sagittal, and coronal sections from the planning computed tomography scan used for radiotherapy treatment planning. Patient received neoadjuvant chemotherapy followed by short-course radiation therapy (25 Gy in 5 fractions) and surgical resection. Radiation therapy was delivered using intensity modulated radiation therapy. Gross tumor volume (*shaded red*) representing the grossly involved rectal primary (grossly involved nodes not shown); clinical target volume (*shaded royal blue*) encompassing gross tumor volume and nodal regions at risk of subclinical disease; planning target volume (*shaded turquoise*) consisting of the clinical target volume with a 7 mm uniform margin to account for positional set-up uncertainty. Isodose lines in centiGray (cGy) representing the distribution of the cumulative radiation dose, with the prescription dose of 2500 cGy (ie, 25 Gy, *thick red line*) ideally encompassing at least 95% of the planning target volume (shaded turquoise). The *yellow line* represents the 50% isodose line (ie, 1250 cGy) as indicated in the legend in the top left hand corner of each image, and is there only for reference.

In response, TNT, the sequencing of all radiotherapy and chemotherapy before potential TME, began to emerge as a potential therapeutic option. The potential benefits of TNT include increased chemotherapy compliance compared with adjuvant chemotherapy,[11] improvements in pathologic complete response (pCR) rates, which has been associated with improved outcomes,[12] as well as early treatment of micrometastatic disease, reducing the probability of subsequent distant failure.

TOTAL NEOADJUVANT THERAPY COMPARED WITH NEOADJUVANT CHEMORADIOTHERAPY WITH ADJUVANT CHEMOTHERAPY

Randomized trials directly comparing TNT to preoperative and postoperative chemotherapy regimens demonstrated improved rates of completion of chemotherapy with neoadjuvant as compared with adjuvant chemotherapy.[13] The GCR-3 trial was a phase 2 study of patients with T3–T4 or node-positive rectal cancer randomized to treatment with induction chemotherapy followed by chemoradiotherapy and TME versus chemoradiotherapy followed by TME and adjuvant chemotherapy. Induction and adjuvant chemotherapy consisted of four cycles of capecitabine and oxaliplatin (CAPOX). Radiation therapy was delivered to a dose of 50.4 Gy in 28 fractions with concurrent chemotherapy. There was no statistically significant difference in 5-year local recurrence (2% vs 5%), distant failure (64% vs 62%), or OS (78% vs 75%) between the two arms. However, patients who received induction chemotherapy had significantly improved adherence to chemotherapy (94% vs 57%, $P < .0001$). In addition, the rates of grade 3 to 4 toxicity were significantly lower for the induction chemotherapy arm compared with the adjuvant chemotherapy arm (19% vs 54%, $P = .0004$).[13]

More recently, the RAPIDO trial[14] compared SCRT (25 Gy in 5 fractions) followed by six cycles of CAPOX or nine cycles of 5-fluorouracil, leucovorin, and oxaliplatin (FOLFOX4) to standard of care chemoradiotherapy to 50 to 50.4 Gy in 25 to 28 fractions with concurrent capecitabine in addition to eight cycles of adjuvant CAPOX or 12 cycles of adjuvant FOLFOX. Patients were eligible if they had one of the following "high risk" factors: cT4a–b disease, extramural vascular invasion, cN2 disease, involved mesorectal fascia, or enlarged lateral lymph nodes. The TNT arm demonstrated an improvement in the primary endpoint of 3-year disease-related treatment failure (23.7% vs 30.4%, hazard ratio [HR] 0.75, 95% CI 0.60–0.95, $P = .019$). Similar rates of serious adverse events occurred in the TNT (38%) and the standard of care (34%) arms. Based on superior treatment outcomes in the TNT arm, the authors concluded that TNT should be considered the new standard of care in patients with high-risk locally advanced rectal adenocarcinoma. Additional phase 3 trials include Polish II,[15] STELLAR,[16] and PRODIGE-23[17] trials (**Table 1**) which similarly showed improvements in treatment-related outcomes with intensification of neoadjuvant therapy compared with standard of care chemoradiotherapy, though notably in the latter two trials, adjuvant chemotherapy was also administered in the "TNT" arm. Also of note in the PRODIGE-23 trial, which tested the addition of neoadjuvant modified leucovorin, fluorouracil, irinotecan, and oxaliplatin (mFOLFIRINOX) to chemoradiotherapy (50 Gy in 25 fractions with concurrent capecitabine) followed by TME and adjuvant chemotherapy, there was a 28% pCR rate and 83% distant metastasis-free survival rate in the experimental arm, similar to the 28% pCR rate and 20% distant failure rate (ie, 80% freedom from distant metastases rate) of the TNT arm of the RAPIDO trial. Although a direct comparison of separate studies is limited by differences in patient population, the numerical similarity of these results raises important questions regarding the optimal TNT regimen, particularly as it pertains to the sequencing of

Table 1
Phase 3 trials comparing total neoadjuvant therapy to standard of care chemoradiotherapy

Study	STELLAR[16]		Polish II[15,41]		RAPIDO[14]		PRODIGE-23[17]	
Year	2022		2016		2021		2021	
Inclusion criteria	Distal/middle 1/3 cT3–4 or N+		Fixed cT3; cT4		>1 high-risk feature: cT4a–b, EMVI, cN2, tumor/node <1 mm from MRF, enlarged lateral LNs		cT3–4	
PEP	DFS		R0 resection		3-y Disease-related treatment failure		3-y DFS	
Treatment	*TNT:* SCRT (25 Gy/5 fx) → CAPOX x4c	*SOC:* LCRT 50 Gy/25 fx with capecitabine	*TNT:* SCRT (25 Gy/5 fx) →FOLFOX4 X3c	*SOC:* LCRT (50.4 Gy/28 fx) with concurrent FOLFOX x2c (Week 1 and week 5); weekly oxaliplatin (optional)	*TNT:* SCRT (25Gy/5 fx) → CAPOX x6c or FOLFOX x9c	*SOC:* LCCRT (50–50.4 Gy/ 25–28 fx) with capecitabine→TME -> adjuvant CAPOX x8c or FOLFOX4 x12c (per hospital policy)	*TNT:* FOLFIRINOX (2, 4, or 6c) →LCCRT	*SOC:* LCCRT
N	302	297	261	254	462	450	231	230
TME timing	6–8 wk after NAT	6–8 wk after NAT	12 wk after RT start/6 wk after NAT	12 wk after RT start/6 wk after NAT	2–4 wk after ChT completion	6–10 wk after RT completion	6–8 wk after NAT	6–8 wk after NAT
Adjuvant ChT	CAPOX x2c	CAPOX x6c	None	None	None	adjuvant CAPOX x8c or FOLFOX4 x12c (per hospital policy)	Capecitabine or mFOLFOX6	Capecitabine or mFOLFOX6
PEP result	3-y DFS 64.5% vs 62.3%, $P < .001$ for non-inferiority		R0 resection 77% vs 71% ($P = .007$) favoring TNT		3-y disease-related treatment failure 23.7% vs 30.4% ($P = .019$) favoring TNT		3-y DFS 76% vs 69% ($P = .034$) favoring TNT	

pCR	21.8%[a,b]	12.3%[b]	16%	12%	28%[a]	14%	28%[a]	12%
3-y DFS	64.50%	62.30%	53%	52%	NR	NR	76%[a]	69%
3-y OS	86.5%[a]	75.10%	73%[a]	65%	89.10%	88.80%	91%	88%
3-y DF	HR 0.88 (95% CI .63–1.24)[c]		30%	27%	20%[a]	26.80%	DMFS: 79%	DMFS: 77%
3-y LRR	HR 0.80 (95% CI .45–1.44)[c]		22%	21%	8.30%	6.00%	NR	NR

Abbreviations: CAPOX, capecitabine/oxaliplatin; cCR, clinical complete response; ChT, chemotherapy; cT, clinical tumor stage; DF, distant failure; DFS, disease-free survival; DMFS, distant metastases-free survival; EMVI, extramural vascular invasion; FOLFIRINOX, leucovorin/fluorouracil/irinotecan /oxaliplatin; FOLFOX, fluorouracil, leucovorin, and oxaliplatin; fx, fraction; HR, hazard ratio; LCCRT, long-course chemoradiotherapy; LN, lymph node; LRR, locoregional recurrence; MRF, mesorectal fascia; N+, node-positive; NR, not reported; OS, overall survival; pCR, pathologic complete response; PEP, primary endpoint; SCRT, short-course radiotherapy; SOC, standard of care; TME, total mesorectal excision; TNT, total neoadjuvant therapy.

[a] Statistically significant.
[b] Represents combined pathologic and clinical complete response per article reporting.
[c] 3-year rates not available.

chemotherapy as well as the choice of SCRT versus LCCRT. An additional question that remains unanswered is the value of TNT in patients with clinical stage (c) T3N0 disease, as these patients were eligible for inclusion in both studies, but few were enrolled, making it difficult to draw conclusions about this low-risk population.

TOTAL NEOADJUVANT THERAPY: OPTIMAL SEQUENCING OF CHEMOTHERAPY

The optimal sequencing of chemotherapy in the context of TNT remains debated, based on multiple randomized control trials that have investigated this question.

The CAO/ARO/AIO-12 study[18,19] was a phase 2 trial of 311 patients with rectal adenocarcinoma randomized to chemoradiotherapy to 50.4 Gy in 28 fractions delivered with induction versus consolidation chemotherapy consisting of six doses of FOLFOX, followed by TME. Eligible patients included those with cT3 disease less than 6 cm from the anal verge, greater than cT3b disease, or node-positive disease. TME was to take place on day 123 following initiation of TNT for all patients regardless of tumor response to TNT. The primary endpoint was pathologic complete response as compared with a historical control, using a pick-the-winner design with an expected 15% rate of pCR with standard chemoradiotherapy. Pathologic complete response was observed in 27/156 (17%; 95% CI 12–24%; $P = .210$) patients in the induction arm compared with 38/150 patients (25%, 95% CI 18–32%; $P < .001$) in the consolidation arm; thus only the consolidation arm showed a significantly improved rate of pCR compared with the expected rates with standard chemoradiotherapy.[18] In long-term follow-up, there were no significant differences between the induction and consolidation arms in terms of 3-year disease-free survival (DFS; 73% vs 73% HR 0.95, 95% CI 0.63–1.45; $P = .82$), 3-year cumulative incidence of locoregional recurrence (6% vs 5%; $P = .67$) and 3-year distant failure (18% vs 16%; $P = .52$). There were no differences between the induction and consolidation arms with respect to chronic grade 3 to 4 toxicity (11.8% vs 9.9%), global health status, and quality of life score at 1 year after randomization, or stool incontinence as measured by the Wexner questionnaire.[19]

Perhaps the most direct comparison of induction and consolidation chemotherapy was performed in the OPRA trial,[20] a randomized phase 2 study of patients with stage II/III rectal adenocarcinoma who received concurrent chemoradiotherapy with either induction or consolidation chemotherapy, followed by either TME or watch-and-wait surveillance. The primary outcome was DFS, with comparison of each arm to a historical control, with a secondary outcome of TME-free survival. Radiotherapy was delivered to 45 Gy in 25 fractions to the pelvic nodes with a boost to gross primary and nodal disease to a total of 50–56 Gy. Concurrent chemotherapy consisted of capecitabine or continuous infusion fluorouracil. Induction or consolidation chemotherapy consisted of eight cycles of FOLFOX or five cycles of CAPOX per medical oncologist preference. Tumor restaging occurred within 4 to 12 weeks of completion of TNT and consisted of digital rectal examination, endoscopic examination, MRI, and CT of the chest, abdomen, and pelvis; those with an incomplete clinical response underwent TME, whereas those with at least a near complete response were offered watch-and-wait. Ultimately, 105/146 (71%) and 120/158 (76%) of patients in the induction and consolidation arms were offered watch-and-wait. There was no difference in 3-year DFS between the induction (76%; 95% CI 69–84) and consolidation (76%; 95% CI 69–83) arms and the historical 3-year DFS rate of 75%. However, TME-free survival was improved for patients who received consolidation (3-year rate of 53%, 95% CI 45–62) versus induction (3-year rate of 41%, 95% CI 33–50; log-rank $P = .016$).

The reasons for the observed improvement in TME-free survival in the consolidation arm are not immediately clear. Of note, the rates of clinical complete response (cCR) and near cCR were similar between the two arms, suggesting that any benefit in terms of TME-free survival is not related to differences in the proportion of patients undergoing NOM. In addition, the suggestion of benefit to consolidation generally aligns with the observation from CAO/ARO/AIO-12 of a higher pCR rate with consolidation chemotherapy as compared with induction. Given these findings, for patients in whom a watch-and-wait approach is being considered, selecting a consolidation chemotherapy regimen may be preferred over induction chemotherapy.

TOTAL NEOADJUVANT THERAPY: SHORT-COURSE RADIOTHERAPY VERSUS LONG-COURSE CHEMORADIOTHERAPY?

Another question surrounding TNT is the choice between SCRT versus LCCRT. This remains an area lacking in randomized data. No published randomized trials have directly compared SCRT and LCCRT both delivered in the context of TNT. The existing data to support TNT delivered with SCRT come from comparisons to LCCRT with adjuvant chemotherapy showing similar outcomes between the two regimens,[14–16] though there may be a cost-effectiveness justification for SCRT.[21] The STELLAR trial[16] was a phase 3 trial of non-inferiority comparing SCRT (25 Gy in 5 fractions) followed by two cycles of CAPOX versus LCCRT (50 Gy in 25 fractions) with capecitabine. Both groups received adjuvant CAPOX, with two cycles in the SCRT group and six cycles in the concurrent chemoradiotherapy group. SCRT was non-inferior to LCCRT in terms of 3-year DFS (64.5% vs 62.3%, HR 0.883, $P < .001$ for non-inferiority). In addition, 3-year OS was 86.5% vs 75.1% ($P = .033$) favoring SCRT. Acute grade 3 to 5 toxicity was higher for SCRT (26.5%) compared with LCCRT (12.6%; $P < .001$). The Polish II study compared SCRT (25 Gy in 5 fractions) followed by FOLFOX4 to chemoradiotherapy to 50.4 Gy/28 fx with concurrent FOLFOX2 (weekly oxaliplatin made optional with protocol amendment) followed by TME. There were no differences in 3-year DFS (53% vs 52%, not statistically significant) but 3-year OS was higher in the SCRT arm (73% vs 65%, $P = .046$). Preoperative acute toxicity was lower for SCRT than LCCRT ($P = .006$). The Polish II study[15] is perhaps a more apt comparison of SCRT and LCCRT in the context of TNT given that all chemotherapy was delivered in the preoperative setting. Its results suggest that TNT delivered with SCRT may have similar DFS (53% vs 52%, $P = .85$) and potentially improved OS (77% vs 71%, $P = .07$) at 3 years, compared with LCCRT with adjuvant chemotherapy, in addition to decreased acute preoperative toxicities ($P = .006$), making it a reasonable alternative treatment option. More recently, the PRODIGE 42-GERICO 12 NACRE study,[22] compared LCCRT (50 Gy in 25 fractions with capecitabine) and delayed surgery to SCRT (25 Gy in 5 fractions) with delayed surgery in elderly patients (age *75 years or older*) diagnosed with cT3–4 rectal adenocarcinoma or cT2 disease of the low rectum. The preliminary results suggest that the R0 resection rate for SCRT is non-inferior to that of LCCRT and that SCRT may provide an OS in this patient population compared with LCCRT (log-rank $P = .04$), though the final results from a published article remain pending.

Studies to date have not directly addressed the comparative efficacy of TNT delivered with SCRT versus with LCCRT and either induction or consolidative chemotherapy. Fortunately, the ACO/ARO/AIO-18 trial[23] is designed to answer this question. In that trial, patients will be randomized to receive SCRT (25 Gy in 5 fractions) followed by nine cycles of mFOLFOX6 or six cycles of CAPOX versus concurrent chemoradiotherapy to 45 Gy in 25 fractions to the whole pelvis followed by a 9 Gy boost to the gross tumor, followed by consolidation chemotherapy with six cycles of mFOLFOX6 or four cycles of CAPOX. Patients achieving a clinical complete response (cCR) will be eligible for watch-and-wait, whereas all others will proceed to TME. In the absence of clear randomized evidence to guide this choice and given the advantages of SCRT with respect to cost and patient convenience as compared with LCCRT, the burden of proof would seem to fall more heavily on demonstrating the superiority of LCCRT over SCRT rather than the converse.

TOTAL NEOADJUVANT THERAPY: DOES TIMING OF SURGERY AFTER RADIOTHERAPY INFLUENCE OUTCOMES?

The majority of phase 3 trials comparing TNT to standard of care chemoradiotherapy specified TME to take place 6 to 8 weeks after the completion of neoadjuvant therapy (see **Table 1**). However, given that pathologic complete response to neoadjuvant therapy in rectal cancer has been associated with improved treatment outcomes,[24,25] as well as the continued study of organ preservation, factors that may influence pathologic or clinical response to therapy are of great interest. Multiple trials have investigated the influence of timing of surgery following neoadjuvant therapy in rectal adenocarcinoma but have yielded mixed results. The Stockholm III study[26] compared patients treated with SCRT in 25 Gy/5 followed by immediate (ie, within 1 week) versus delayed (ie, within 4–8 weeks) surgery, with a third arm of long-course radiotherapy (50 Gy/25 fx) also with delayed (ie, within 4–8 weeks) surgery. Pathologic complete response rates were significantly improved in the SCRT with delayed surgery compared with SCRT with immediate surgery or long-course radiotherapy (10.4% vs 2.2% vs 0.3%, $P < .0001$). Further subgroup analyses suggest that patients with pCR in this study had improved OS and time to recurrence compared with those without pCR.[27] However, local recurrence rates were similar across the three arms, whereas postoperative complications were lower for SCRT with delayed surgery compared with SCRT with immediate surgery (41% vs 53%, $P = .001$).[26] In contrast, GRECCAR-6[28] compared chemoradiotherapy followed by surgery at 7 versus 11 weeks and found that delayed surgery did not result in improved pathologic complete response rates or overall and DFS, but was associated with worse surgical complication rates. Patients in GRECCAR-6, however, received chemotherapy only concurrent with radiotherapy. A separate randomized-controlled trial[29] of locally advanced rectal adenocarcinoma patients demonstrated increased pCR (18.6% vs 10%, $P = .027$) and disease regression ($P = .004$) in patients who underwent TME 8 or more weeks after chemoradiotherapy compared with those who underwent TME within 8 weeks. The results of the latter two trials discussed are more concordant with the TIMING trial,[30] which was a phase 2 study comparing chemoradiotherapy to 50.4 Gy with concurrent 5-FU followed by mFOLFOX given in 2, 4, or 6 cycles followed 4 weeks later by TME, which showed an increasing rate of pathologic complete response with more cycles of mFOLFOX ($P = .0036$), with no differences in the surgical technical difficulty or complication rates, despite increasing pelvic fibrosis as measured by the surgeon performing resection. Overall, these data suggest that increasing the intensity of neoadjuvant chemotherapy and/or the duration from radiotherapy to surgery may affect response rates.

NONOPERATIVE MANAGEMENT OF RECTAL CANCER

Given the excellent local recurrence rates with preoperative radiation and chemotherapy followed by TME and the significant morbidity associated with surgical resection, including decreased quality of life and the potential need for permanent colostomy, NOM of rectal adenocarcinoma has been increasingly investigated. NOM has been associated with a reduction in low anterior resection syndrome symptoms as well as improvement in defecation, sexual, and urinary tract function.[31] NOM is currently included in the National Comprehensive Cancer Network guidelines for consideration at experienced multidisciplinary centers as an alternative to surgery in the management of locally advanced rectal adenocarcinoma patients with complete clinical response to neoadjuvant therapy on digital rectal examination, rectal MRI, and endoscopic evaluation.[7] Although randomized data directly comparing operative and NOM are currently lacking,[23,32,33] a number of retrospective[31,34–36] and prospective[20,37,38] studies have suggested that NOM may be offered to rectal adenocarcinoma patients with cCR or near cCR after neoadjuvant therapy as a means to preserve quality of life without an adverse impact on survival outcomes. For instance in the OPRA trial, as previously discussed, patients with at least near cCR were offered watch-and-wait surveillance, resulting in nearly three-quarters of patients being offered watch-and-wait surveillance after TNT, with superior TME-free survival in the consolidation chemotherapy cohort.[20]

Other landmark studies exploring NOM include the International Watch and Wait Database (IWWD),[31] which was a multicenter registry of patients with rectal cancer who opted for NOM following neoadjuvant therapy. Patients with a cCR were analyzed, with 2-year cumulative incidence of local recurrence of 25.2% (95% CI 22.2–28.5%). Distant failure occurred in 71/880 (8%) of patients overall, and in 38/213 (18%) and 33/634 (5%) of patients with and without local regrowth, respectively. Five-year OS and DFS were 85% (95% CI 80.9–87.7%) and 94% (91–96%), respectively.[31] Using conditional survival analysis modeling, the authors estimated that patients who maintained a cCR at 1, 3, and 5 years posttreatment would have an expected 2-year local-regrowth free interval of 88.1% (95% CI 85.8–90.9%), 97.3% (95.2–98.6%), and 98.6% (97.6–100.0%), respectively.[39] Taken together, these findings suggest that patients maintaining a clinical complete response may be able to reduce the frequency of surveillance after 3 years of follow-up.

A question still remains whether NOM may compromise distant metastatic failure rates by missing a window for surgical control of the primary tumor, given the higher rate of distant metastases observed in the IWWD study in those with local regrowth compared with those without. This finding mirrors a similar trend from another large retrospective study from Memorial Sloan Kettering Cancer Center, in which patients with locally advanced rectal adenocarcinoma who underwent NOM with and without subsequent local regrowth had a 5-year distant metastasis rate of 36% versus 1%.[36] However, the IWWD study's investigators suggest that the similar rates of OS and distant metastasis among patients with local regrowth in the IWWD study and those without pathologic complete response in a pooled analysis of patients treated with preoperative chemoradiotherapy followed by TME[12] suggest that inherent tumor biology and not the presence or absence of upfront TME may be more predictive of subsequent distant failure.

SURVEILLANCE STRATEGIES FOR WATCH-AND-WAIT

A variety of surveillance strategies have been used in the NOM of patients with rectal cancer after neoadjuvant therapy, though all consist of rectal MRI, endoscopic surveillance, and digital rectal examination at a frequency that typically decreases after 2 years of surveillance.[20,31] Similarly, definitions of clinical complete response and near clinical complete response have varied across studies. Given this heterogeneity, expert international consensus guidelines on watch-and-wait surveillance were recently produced that include recommendations for response assessment time points, definitions of clinical response by mode of assessment, and definitions of treatment endpoints.[40]

SUMMARY

For patients with locally advanced rectal adenocarcinoma, the preferred standard of care management involves TNT followed by TME. Questions remain regarding the optimal TNT regimen as it relates to chemotherapy sequencing and radiotherapy regimen as well as the use of NOM. The available evidence suggests concurrent chemoradiotherapy followed by consolidative chemotherapy may produce superior outcomes in terms of TME-free survival compared with an induction chemotherapy approach, though the reasons for such a difference are not well understood. SCRT followed by full-dose chemotherapy and TME is an acceptable TNT option alongside LCCRT that has been prospectively studied. A randomized trial comparing TNT using short-course versus long-course radiotherapy is ongoing, though in the interim SCRT may be preferable when feasible given considerations of cost-effectiveness and patient convenience. Finally, NOM of patients who receive neoadjuvant therapy and achieve a (near) clinical complete response continues to be studied, suggesting that a clinically significant proportion of patients may be able to delay or avoid altogether surgical resection. Nonetheless, judgment should be exercised given observed higher rates of distant failure in those with local regrowth and given that no randomized comparison to operative management has been performed. Efforts to standardize watch-and-wait surveillance strategies continue, though generally consist of a combination of digital rectal examination and endoscopy every 3 to 4 months, and rectal MRI every 6 months at minimum for the first 2 years.

DISCLOSURES

The authors report no commercial or financial conflicts of interest.

CLINICS CARE POINTS

- The standard of care management of locally advanced rectal cancer is total neoadjuvant therapy followed by total mesorectal excision (TME).
- Radiotherapy for total neoadjuvant therapy may be delivered as short-course radiation therapy to a total dose of 25 Gy in 5 fractions, or long-course chemoradiotherapy to a total dose of 50 Gy in 25 fractions.
- Long-course chemoradiotherapy may be delivered either with induction or consolidation chemotherapy. Consolidation chemotherapy may be preferred if non-operative management is being considered due to higher rates of TME-free survival following treatment.
- Non-operative management may be considered in carefully selected patients with near complete or clinical complete response to total neoadjuvant therapy.

REFERENCES

1. Bray F, Ferlay J, Soerjomataram I, et al. Global cancer statistics 2018: GLOBOCAN estimates of incidence and mortality worldwide for 36 cancers in 185 countries. CA Cancer J Clin 2018;68(6):394–424.

2. Heald RJ, Ryall RDH. Recurrence and survival after total mesorectal excision for rectal cancer. Lancet 1986;1(8496):1479–82.

3. Prolongation of the disease-free interval in surgically treated rectal carcinoma. N Engl J Med 1985;312(23):1465–72.

4. Krook JE, Moertel CG, Gunderson LL, et al. Effective surgical adjuvant therapy for high-risk rectal carcinoma. N Engl J Med 1991;324(11):709–15.

5. Roh MS, Colangelo LH, O'Connell MJ, et al. Preoperative multimodality therapy improves disease-free survival in patients with carcinoma of the rectum: NSABP R-03. J Clin Oncol 2009;27(31):5124–30.

6. Sauer R, Becker H, Hohenberger W, et al. Preoperative versus postoperative chemoradiotherapy for rectal cancer. N Engl J Med 2004;351(17):1731–40.

7. NCCN Clinical Practice Guidelines in Oncology (NCCN Guidelines) for Rectal, In: Cancer, 1, All rights reserved.

8. Thomas PRM, Lindblad AS. Adjuvant postoperative radiotherapy and chemotherapy in rectal carcinoma: a review of the Gastrointestinal Tumor Study Group experience. Radiother Oncol 1988;13(4):245–52.

9. van Gijn W, Marijnen CAM, Nagtegaal ID, et al. Preoperative radiotherapy combined with total mesorectal excision for resectable rectal cancer: 12-year follow-up of the multicentre, randomised controlled TME trial. Lancet Oncol 2011;12(6):575–82.

10. Breugom AJ, Swets M, Bosset JF, et al. Adjuvant chemotherapy after preoperative (chemo)radiotherapy and surgery for patients with rectal cancer: a systematic review and meta-analysis of individual patient data. Lancet Oncol 2015; 16(2):200–7.

11. van der Valk MJM, Marijnen CAM, van Etten B, et al. Compliance and tolerability of short-course radiotherapy followed by preoperative chemotherapy and surgery for high-risk rectal cancer - results of the international randomized RAPIDO-trial. Radiother Oncol 2020;147:75–83.

12. Maas M, Nelemans PJ, Valentini V, et al. Long-term outcome in patients with a pathological complete response after chemoradiation for rectal cancer: a pooled analysis of individual patient data. Lancet Oncol 2010;11(9):835–44.

13. Fernández-Martos C, Garcia-Albeniz X, Pericay C, et al. Chemoradiation, surgery and adjuvant chemotherapy versus induction chemotherapy followed by chemoradiation and surgery: long-term results of the Spanish GCR-3 phase II randomized trial. Ann Oncol 2015;26(8):1722–8.

14. Bahadoer RR, Dijkstra EA, van Etten B, et al. Short-course radiotherapy followed by chemotherapy before total mesorectal excision (TME) versus preoperative chemoradiotherapy, TME, and optional adjuvant chemotherapy in locally advanced rectal cancer (RAPIDO): a randomised, open-label, phase 3 trial. Lancet Oncol 2021;22(1):29–42.

15. Bujko K, Wyrwicz L, Rutkowski A, et al. Long-course oxaliplatin-based preoperative chemoradiation versus 5 × 5 Gy and consolidation chemotherapy for cT4 or fixed cT3 rectal cancer: results of a randomized phase III study. Ann Oncol 2016; 27(5):834–42.

16. Jin J, Tang Y, Hu C, et al. Multicenter, Randomized, Phase III Trial of Short-Term Radiotherapy Plus Chemotherapy Versus Long-Term Chemoradiotherapy in Locally Advanced Rectal Cancer (STELLAR). J Clin Oncol 2022;40(15):1681–92.

17. Conroy T, Bosset JF, Etienne PL, et al. Neoadjuvant chemotherapy with FOLFIRINOX and preoperative chemoradiotherapy for patients with locally advanced rectal cancer (UNICANCER-PRODIGE 23): a multicentre, randomised, open-label, phase 3 trial. Lancet Oncol 2021;22(5):702–15.

18. Fokas E, Allgäuer M, Polat B, et al. Randomized phase II trial of chemoradiotherapy plus induction or consolidation chemotherapy as total neoadjuvant therapy for locally advanced rectal cancer: CAO/ArO/AIO-12. J Clin Oncol 2019;37(34): 3212–22.

19. Fokas E, Schlenska-Lange A, Polat B, et al. Chemoradiotherapy Plus Induction or Consolidation Chemotherapy as Total Neoadjuvant Therapy for Patients With Locally Advanced Rectal Cancer: Long-term Results of the CAO/ARO/AIO-12 Randomized Clinical Trial. JAMA Oncol 2022;8(1). https://doi.org/10.1001/JAMAONCOL.2021.5445.

20. Garcia-Aguilar J, Patil S, Gollub MJ, et al. Organ preservation in patients with rectal adenocarcinoma treated with total neoadjuvant therapy. J Clin Oncol 2022;18. https://doi.org/10.1200/JCO.22.00032.

21. Raldow AC, Chen AB, Russell M, et al. Cost-effectiveness of short-course radiation therapy vs long-course chemoradiation for locally advanced rectal cancer. JAMA Netw Open 2019;2(4):e192249.

22. FRANCOIS E, Pernot M, Ronchin P, et al. NACRE: A randomized study comparing short course radiotherapy with radiochemotherapy for locally advanced rectal cancers in the elderly—Preliminary results. J Clin Oncol 2021; 39(3_suppl):4.

23. Short-course radiotherapy versus chemoradiotherapy, followed by consolidation chemotherapy, and selective organ preservation for MRI-defined Intermediate and high-risk rectal cancer patients - full text view - ClinicalTrials.gov. Available at: https://clinicaltrials.gov/ct2/show/NCT04246684. Accessed September 19, 2022.

24. Zorcolo L, Rosman AS, Restivo A, et al. Complete pathologic response after combined modality treatment for rectal cancer and long-term survival: a meta-analysis. Ann Surg Oncol 2012;19(9):2822–32.

25. Yeo SG, Kim DY, Kim TH, et al. Pathologic complete response of primary tumor following preoperative chemoradiotherapy for locally advanced rectal cancer: Long-term outcomes and prognostic significance of pathologic nodal status (KROG 09-01). Ann Surg 2010;252(6):998–1004.

26. Erlandsson J, Holm T, Pettersson D, et al. Optimal fractionation of preoperative radiotherapy and timing to surgery for rectal cancer (Stockholm III): a multicentre, randomised, non-blinded, phase 3, non-inferiority trial. Lancet Oncol 2017;18(3): 336–46.

27. Erlandsson J, Lörinc E, Ahlberg M, et al. Tumour regression after radiotherapy for rectal cancer – Results from the randomised Stockholm III trial. Radiother Oncol 2019;135:178–86.

28. Lefevre JH, Mineur L, Cachanado M, et al. Does a longer waiting period after neoadjuvant radio-chemotherapy improve the oncological prognosis of rectal cancer?: three years' follow-up results of the greccar-6 randomized multicenter trial. Ann Surg 2019;270(5). https://doi.org/10.1097/SLA.0000000000003530.

29. Akgun E, Caliskan C, Bozbiyik O, et al. Randomized clinical trial of short or long interval between neoadjuvant chemoradiotherapy and surgery for rectal cancer. Br J Surg 2018;105(11):1417–25.

30. Garcia-Aguilar J, Chow OS, Smith DD, et al. Effect of adding mFOLFOX6 after neoadjuvant chemoradiation in locally advanced rectal cancer: a multicentre, phase 2 trial. Lancet Oncol 2015;16(8):957–66.

31. van der Valk MJM, Hilling DE, Bastiaannet E, et al. Long-term outcomes of clinical complete responders after neoadjuvant treatment for rectal cancer in the

International Watch & Wait Database (IWWD): an international multicentre registry study. Lancet 2018;391(10139):2537–45.

32. Curative Chemoradiation of Low Rectal Cancer - Full Text View - ClinicalTrials.gov. Available at: https://clinicaltrials.gov/ct2/show/NCT02438839. Accessed September 19, 2022.

33. Bach SP, Wilt JHW de, Peters F, et al. STAR-TREC phase II: can we save the rectum by watchful waiting or transanal surgery following (chemo)radiotherapy versus total mesorectal excision for early rectal cancer? J Clin Oncol 2022; 40(16_suppl):3502.

34. Habr-Gama A, Perez RO, Nadalin W, et al. Operative versus nonoperative treatment for stage 0 distal rectal cancer following chemoradiation therapy: long-term results. Ann Surg 2004;240(4):711–8.

35. Chin RI, Roy A, Pedersen KS, et al. Clinical complete response in patients with rectal adenocarcinoma treated with short-course radiation therapy and nonoperative management. Int J Radiat Oncol Biol Phys 2022;112(3):715–25.

36. Smith JJ, Strombom P, Chow OS, et al. Assessment of a watch-and-wait strategy for rectal cancer in patients with a complete response after neoadjuvant therapy. JAMA Oncol 2019;5(4):e185896.

37. Appelt AL, Pløen J, Harling H, et al. High-dose chemoradiotherapy and watchful waiting for distal rectal cancer: a prospective observational study. Lancet Oncol 2015;16(8):919–27.

38. Maas M, Beets-Tan RGH, Lambregts DMJ, et al. Wait-and-see policy for clinical complete responders after chemoradiation for rectal cancer. J Clin Oncol 2011; 29(35):4633–40.

39. Fernandez LM, São Julião GP, Figueiredo NL, et al. Conditional recurrence-free survival of clinical complete responders managed by watch and wait after neoadjuvant chemoradiotherapy for rectal cancer in the International Watch & Wait Database: a retrospective, international, multicentre registry study. Lancet Oncol 2021;22(1):43–50.

40. Fokas E, Appelt A, Glynne-Jones R, et al. International consensus recommendations on key outcome measures for organ preservation after (chemo)radiotherapy in patients with rectal cancer. Nat Rev Clin Oncol 2021;18(12):805–16.

41. Ciseł B, Pietrzak L, Michalski W, et al. Long-course preoperative chemoradiation versus 5 × 5 Gy and consolidation chemotherapy for clinical T4 and fixed clinical T3 rectal cancer: long-term results of the randomized Polish II study. Ann Oncol 2019;30(8):1298–303.

Modern Radiation for Hematologic Stem Cell Transplantation
Total Marrow and Lymphoid Irradiation or Intensity-Modulated Radiation Therapy Total Body Irradiation

Claire Hao, BS, Colton Ladbury, MD, Jeffrey Wong, MD, Savita Dandapani, MD, PhD*

KEYWORDS

- IMRT TBI • VMAT • Helical TomoTherapy • TMI • TMLI • SIB • Boost
- Acute leukemia

KEY POINTS

- Total marrow irradiation and total marrow and lymphoid irradiation allow safe dose escalation to 20 Gy while sparing organs at risk to acceptable levels.
- Numerous feasibility and retrospective studies have demonstrated that both helical TomoTherapy-based and volumetric-modulated arc therapy-based intensity-modulated radiation therapy (IMRT) total body irradiation (TBI) are feasible and can reduce the dose to organs at risk; however, prospective studies are limited.
- Boosting active bone marrow and extramedullary disease sites in IMRT TBI may help augment disease control.

INTRODUCTION

Historically, radiation therapy (RT) has played an important role in hematologic malignancies including leukemia. Total body irradiation (TBI) has been used since the 1970s for patients with acute myeloid leukemia (AML) or acute lymphoblastic leukemia (ALL) as a myeloablative element of the conditioning regimen for allogeneic hematopoietic stem cell transplant (allo-HSCT).[1] TBI helps facilitate HSCT through the cytotoxic elimination of leukemic cells from blood, bone marrow, and lymph nodes and through immunosuppressive effects to prevent rejection of donor cells.[2] The multi-institutional

Department of Radiation Oncology, City of Hope, 1500 East Duarte Road, Duarte, CA 91010, USA
* Corresponding author.
E-mail address: sdandapani@coh.org

Surg Oncol Clin N Am 32 (2023) 475–495
https://doi.org/10.1016/j.soc.2023.03.001
1055-3207/23/© 2023 Elsevier Inc. All rights reserved.

surgonc.theclinics.com

Phase III FORUM trial demonstrated TBI-based conditioning regimens to be significantly superior in survival, relapse rates, and treatment-related mortality (TRM) compared with chemotherapy-only conditioning regimens,[3] supporting findings from earlier studies.[4–6] One advantage to RT is that RT is not affected by blood supply, drug absorption, metabolism, biodistribution, and clearance kinetics. Additionally, RT can treat sanctuary sites not reached by chemotherapy.[2]

However, conventional TBI (cTBI) is associated with significant long-term toxicities, which is of primary concern considering the prevalence of this disease in children and relatively favorable cure rates for patients in first remission receiving HSCT. Long-term toxicities seen after cTBI-based conditioning regimens correlate with increased radiation dose and include interstitial pneumonitis, mucositis, nephropathy, chronic kidney disease, veno-occlusive disease of the liver, thyroid disease, gonadal dysfunction, cognitive deficiencies, cataract formation, and secondary malignant neoplasia.[7–9] These toxicities influence quality of life and contribute to TRM. Prospective studies have reported that while higher radiation doses greater than 13.2 Gy reduce relapse rates, they also increase TRM, negating any benefit.[10] TBI needs further optimization to lower the risk of relapse while mitigating toxicities.

The development of image-guided intensity-modulated radiation therapy (IMRT) dramatically improved control over RT dose delivery by permitting the delivery of highly conformal dose distributions to large complex target shapes while minimizing doses to organs at risk (OARs). This enabled the development of more targeted forms of TBI: total marrow irradiation (TMI), total marrow and lymphoid irradiation (TMLI), and IMRT TBI. This review will explore the safety and efficacy of these targeted methods and discuss the clinical potential of a hybrid approach of TMLI and TBI.

Total Body Irradiation-Induced Toxicities

Treatment-related toxicities significantly contribute to morbidity after allo-HSCT. Lung toxicities are a major cause of TRM and occur in up to 60% of patients.[11] A study by the Children's Oncology Group (COG) found that a mean lung dose of 8 Gy or greater is significantly associated with inferior overall survival (OS) on multivariable analysis (hazard ratio 1.85, $P = .04$).[12] Furthermore, ocular toxicities and severe mucositis were significantly increased ($P = .013$ and $P < .001$, respectively) in 322 patients who received TBI when 12 Gy total dose was used instead of 8 Gy.[13] Renal toxicities are also observed.[14] The risk of secondary malignancies, particularly hematologic or skin cancers, is again of significant concern, with a recent long-term analysis of 285 patients reporting that the cumulative incidence of secondary malignancies was 12.3% after a median follow-up of 8.5 years (range 3.0–20.9 years).[15]

As cTBI uses radiation beams of uniform intensity, large-dose heterogeneity occurs throughout the target volume due to variations in body thickness, contouring, and tissue densities.[16,17] Tissue compensators may be used but are imprecise. The lungs may receive more radiation because of their reduced tissue density, requiring the use of 2D lung blocks for shielding. Dose heterogeneity contributes to morbidity associated with TBI at doses greater than 13.2 Gy, which inhibits dose escalation. Large-field IMRT permits highly conformal radiation doses while sparing OARs, which is beneficial for radiation-based conditioning regimens for HSCT.

DISCUSSION
Total Marrow Irradiation and Total Marrow and Lymphoid Irradiation

TMI and TMLI have been used since 2004 to achieve full coverage of malignant sites while sparing healthy tissues and OARs and improving dose homogeneity

(Table 1).[18–21,22–24] In TMI, RT targets the skeletal bone, and in TMLI, the lymph nodes, spleen, liver, and sanctuary sites (ie, brain and testes) are additional targets **(Fig. 1)**. TMI and TMLI are indicated for relapsed or refractory (R/R) patients and elderly patients who have poor responses to cTBI, have increased toxicities on dose escalation of cTBI needed to reduce risk of relapse, or are unable to tolerate cTBI. Wong and colleagues (2020) conducted an excellent review of the development of TMI/TMLI and findings from clinical trials on the safety, feasibility, and efficacy of TMI/TMLI.[2] The first feasibility studies and treatment planning methods for TMI/TMLI were reported by our group at City of Hope (COH) in 2004.[22,23] Following this, the first clinical experience using TMI/TMLI was reported by our group in 2006.[24,25] Clinical trials utilizing TMI/TMLI for acute leukemia have focused on dose escalation to improve disease control while limiting toxicities or using it as an alternative to TBI. Long-term toxicities up to 8 years after TMI/TMLI have been found to be less than historical reports for cTBI, and investigators have demonstrated that the higher dose rate used by TMI/TMLI is not associated with organ dysfunction or nonengraftment.[26,27] Moreover, organ sparing has not been shown to affect relapse rates and sites of relapse were demonstrated to be dose independent.[28]

In the last 2 years since the review by Wong and colleagues (2020) was published, some important advancements have been made in TMI/TMLI **(Table 1)**. Stein and colleagues (2022) at COH recently reported the results of their pilot study using a chemotherapy-free allo-HSCT conditioning regimen of 20 Gy TMLI and posttransplantation prophylactic cyclophosphamide (PTCy) treatment of 18 patients with AML in first remission with negative minimum residual disease.[29] The study intended to reduce the rate of graft-versus-host disease (GVHD) using PTCy while preventing increased relapses using TMLI dose escalation. Stein and colleagues (2022) reported mean RT to nontarget organs was significantly lower compared with cTBI, including doses of 7 to 8 Gy to lungs, kidneys, heart, and thyroid, and ~4 Gy to eyes; GI tract and oral cavity were also spared. No patients experienced toxicities greater than Grade 2. OS at 2 years was 86.7% and relapse-free survival (RFS) was 83.3%. A 2-year nonrelapse mortality (NRM) was 0%, substantially improved from the 1-year NRM rate of 10% reported in historical TBI patients.[30] The decrease in NRM may be attributed to sparing of the GI tract and oral cavity from radiation, which may have reduced incidence of infections. Furthermore, they also observed a 2-year GVHD-free/relapse-free survival (GRFS) of 59.3%, increased compared with the 1-year GRFS rate of 45% in the historical TBI patients. Despite the small sample size, this study provides encouraging results for the use of TMLI to offset the increased risk of relapse associated with PTCy-based GVHD prophylaxis, ultimately limiting GVHD and NRM while maintaining efficacy of leukemia transplants.[29]

Our group at COH has also conducted a dose-escalation phase I trial using 12 to 20-Gy TMLI, cyclophosphamide, and etoposide as a conditioning regimen for R/R patients with acute leukemia. A 20-Gy TMLI (the maximum tolerated dose) was safe and effective with similar rates of GVHD and extramedullary relapse compared with published data[28] and low rates of NRM (8.1% at 1 year).[31] Preliminary results from the ongoing phase II trial using the same conditioning regimen and patient population but with 20-Gy TMLI for all patients have so far demonstrated similarly low NRM (6% at 1 year) and potentially improved OS compared with the phase I trial (1-year OS 67% vs 55.5%, respectively).[32] A recent review of all TMLI treatment plans at COH found that even at 20 Gy, the dose to OARs was kept at cTBI doses with no change in safety or efficacy.[19]

Another point of consideration is whether TMLI could reduce risk of secondary malignancies. Ladbury and colleagues' analysis of early follow-up data from COH has

Table 1
Summary of studies exploring total marrow irradiation or total marrow and lymphoid irradiation

Author	Objective	N	Median Age (Range)	Disease Status	Dose	Result	Notes
Schultheiss et al,[22,23] 2004	Pre-clinical feasibility of HT for TMI/TMLI	1	NR	NR	12 Gy in 6 fx	For all OARs, ~50% of organ volume receives <50% of target dose. Lungs D_{median} = 6.3–6.7 Kidneys D_{median} = 5.4–6.0 Thyroid D_{median} = 4.2–6.4	TMI target: bones TMLI: bones, spleen, LNs Treatment time ~20 mins for 25mm slice thickness and pitch 0.5
Hui et al,[18] 2005	Preclinical feasibility of HT for TBI and TMI	1	NR	NR	13.2 Gy in 8 fx	Mean dose to lungs, kidneys, heart, eyes reduced by 40%–60% compared with prescribed dose	Target: bones BOT 31 min
Han et al,[19] 2022	Report tx planning experience of 12 Gy and 20 Gy TMLI	108 (12 Gy cohort) 120 (20 Gy cohort)	12 Gy: 54 (10–71) 20 Gy: 40 (17–64)	NR	12 Gy in 8 fx or 20 Gy in 10 fx	Average mean dose for normal organs = 18.3%–78.3% and 13.0%–76.0% for 12 Gy and 20 Gy cohorts, respectively	Target: bones, LNs, spleen, spinal canal (brain and liver included and treated to 12 Gy for 20 Gy cohort) Dosimetric data provided to aid clinical implementation at other institutions
Aydogan et al,[20] 2006	Preclinical feasibility of linac-based TMI	1	NR	NR	12 Gy in 6 fx	1.3–4.5-fold reduction in median dose to OARs compared with cTBI	Target: bones BOT 14.5 min

Study	Purpose	N	Median age (range)	Disease status	Dose	Outcomes	Target/BOT
Aydogan et al,[21] 2011	Preclinical feasibility of VMAT-TMI	6	NR	NR	12 Gy in 6 fx	Average median doses to OARs were mostly <50% except in brain and lungs. Lungs D_{median} = 7.2, Kidneys D_{median} = 5.4, Lenses D_{median} = 4.1	Target: bones BOT 18 min
Wong et al,[25] 2006	Feasibility of HT TMI/TMLI	3 (1 pt w/ MM treated)	20 (5–53)	NR	12 Gy in 10 fx Treated pt: 10 Gy in 5 fx	1.7-7.5-fold reduction in median dose to OARs compared with cTBI. Dose escalation to 20 Gy possible while maintaining OAR doses lower than cTBI. Treated pt engrafted. AEs: G2 nausea, G1 emesis	TMI target: bones TMLI target: bones, LNs, liver, spleen, brain BOT 50 min
Schultheiss et al,[24] 2007	Report results of 6 pts treated with HT TMI on a clinical trial	6 (MM)	53 (42-65)	NR	10-14 Gy in 5-7 fx	Median doses to OARs reduced by average 65-70%. Lungs D_{median} = 6.4, Kidneys D_{median} = 6.9-7.4, Lenses D_{median} = 2.3	BOT 50.5 min Total in-room time 1.5-2 h
Shinde et al,[26] 2019	Report pulmonary, renal, thyroid, and cataract toxicities	142 (36 MM, 106 AML/ALL)	52 (9-70)	NR; ALL and AML pts were R/R w/or w/o	10-19 Gy in 8-10 fx	Lung D_{mean} = 7.0, Kidneys D_{mean} = 7.1, Thyroid D_{mean} = 6.7, Lens D_{mean} = 2.8	TMI target: bones TMLI target: bones, LNs, and spleen.

(continued on next page)

Table 1
(continued)

Author	Objective	N	Median Age (Range)	Disease Status	Dose	Result	Notes
	from 3 prospective trials of TMI			active disease, and ineligible for standard HSCT		Median f/u 2 y (0–8) Radiation pneumonitis (RP) 0.7% Infection/RP (I/RP) 22.7% at 2-y Mean lung dose ≤8 Gy predicted for less I/RP (P = .012) Hypothyroidism 6.0% Cataracts 7.0% No renal toxicities	Liver and brain in some pts
Kim et al,[28] 2014	Retrospective evaluation of EM relapse in TMLI pts	101	47 (10–70)	16 CR1 6 CR2 2 PR 77 RL, IF, or other	12–15 Gy in 8–10 fx	Median f/u 12.8 mo EM relapse 12.9% Bone marrow relapse 25.7% EM relapse was similar in regions treated ≥10 Gy and <10 Gy Pretransplant EM disease was the only predictor of EM relapse	Target: bones, LNs, liver, spleen, testes, brain
Stein et al,[29] 2022	Pilot study of safety/ feasibility of novel conditioning regimen using posttransplant cyclophosphamide GVHD prophylaxis	18	40 (19–56)	18 CR1	20 Gy in 10 fx	Median f/u 24.5 mo No > G2 Bearman toxicities G2-4 aGVHD 11.1% Moderate-to-severe cGVHD 11.9% 2-y OS 86.7% 2-y RFS 83.3%	Target: bones, LNs, spleen, testes, liver, brain

Study	Description	N	Median age (range)	Disease status	Dose	Outcomes	Target/Comments
	and 20 Gy TMLI in CR1 or CR2 pts					2-y NRM 0% 2-y GRFS 59.3%	
Stein et al,[31] 2017	Phase I dose escalation trial of TMLI conditioning with cyclophosphamide and etoposide	51	34 (16–57)	14 RL1 3 RL2 34 IF All w/active disease	12–20 Gy in 8–10 fx	Median f/u 24.6 mo Max tolerated dose 20 Gy 1-y NRM 8.1% G2-4 aGVHD 43.1% 1-y OS 55.5% 2-y OS 41.5% Relapse in 64.7%	Target: 20 Gy to bones, LNs, spleen, testes, 12 Gy to brain, liver
Wong et al,[32] 2020	Phase II study of 20 Gy TMLI with cyclophosphamide and etoposide	57	40 (16–59)	18 RL1 4 RL2 35 IF 52 Active disease	20 Gy in 10 fx	Median f/u 12.5 mo 1-y NRM 6% 1-y PFS 48% 1-y OS 67% Relapse in 60%	Target: 20 Gy to bone, LNs, spleen and 12 Gy to brain, liver
Ladbury et al,[33] 2022	Retrospective matched-pair analysis comparing rate of subsequent malignant neoplasms (SMNs) in TBI vs TMI pts	171 TMI 171 TBI	NR	139 CR1 43 CR2 8 CR3+ 129 IF/RL 23 Other	TMI 12–20 Gy TBI 12–13.2 Gy	Median f/u 2.0 y No significant difference in rate of SMNs (P = .81) SMNs after TBI 5.3% SMNs after TMI 5.8%	Patients in the TMI cohort did receive a significantly higher radiation dose (median, 16.0 Gy vs 13.2 Gy; P < .001)
Han et al,[34] 2020	Predict and compare secondary-solid tumor occurrence risks between cTBI and TMI	20	48 (21–69)	NR	TMI 12 or 20 Gy in 8–10 fx TBI 12 Gy	Secondary-solid tumor risk per 10,000 people per year 12 Gy TMI: 159.3 (men) and 221.5 (women) = 38.8% and 32.9% reduction from cTBI 20 Gy TMI: 220.3 (men) and 298.5 (women) = 14.6% and 9.2% reduction from cTBI	Target: 12 or 20 Gy to bone, LNs, spleen. 20 Gy pts also received 12 Gy to brain, liver

(continued on next page)

Table 1
(continued)

Author	Objective	N	Median Age (Range)	Disease Status	Dose	Result	Notes
Kong et al,[35] 2022	Safety/efficacy of TMLI	17	17 (8–35)	16 CR 1 NotR	10–12 Gy in 5–6 fx	Median f/u 9 mo No > G2 toxicities 1-y OS 69.8% 1-y cumulative recurrence 19.5% 1-y DFS 54.2%	Average treatment time 29.9 min
Haraldsson et al,[36] 2021	Prospective observational study comparing toxicities and engraftment of TMI pts to TBI pts	37 TMI 33 TBI	TMI 29 (5–57) TBI 28 (10–53)	TMI vs TBI: 16 vs 20 CR1 21 vs 13 ≥CR2 (or MDS)	8–12 Gy in 4–6 fx	TMI vs TBI: Median f/u 13 mo and 72 mo 1-y GRFS 67.5% vs 39.4% (P = .027) Engraftment was significantly faster for TMI group	No significant difference in OS, TRM, or relapse
Zhao et al,[37] 2020	Retrospective comparison of high-risk ALL pts receiving TMLI or non-TMLI conditioning regimens	29 TMLI 41 Non-TMLI	TMLI 26 (15–46) Non-TMLI 28 (14–54)	TMI vs non-TMLI: 21 vs 37 CR1 4 vs 2 ≥CR2 4 vs 2 NotR	8 Gy in 2 fx	TMLI vs non-TMLI Median f/u 13.3 vs 10.3 mo 1-y cumulative incidence of relapse 25% vs 46.5% (P = .018) 1-y OS 73.1% vs 52.6% (P = .033) 1-y DFS 65.2% vs 48.2% (P = .026)	No significant difference in TRM

Abbreviations: BOT, beam-on time; CR, complete remission; DFS, disease-free survival; D_{mean}, mean dose; EM, extramedullary; Fx, fraction; GRFS, GVHD-free relapse-free survival; IF, induction failure; Mo, months; NotR, not in remission; NR, not reported; NRM, nonrelapse mortality; OS, overall survival; PFS, progression-free survival; PR, partial remission; Pts, patients; RFS, relapse-free survival; RL, relapsed; R/R, released or refractory; TRM, treatment-related mortality.

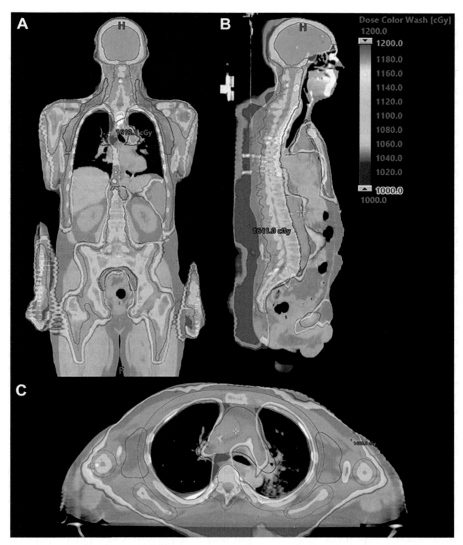

Fig. 1. Isodose distribution for one 12-Gy TMLI plan in a coronal view (*A*), sagittal view (*B*), and axial view (*C*).

shown that while TMI patients receive a significantly higher RT dose (median 16.0 Gy) compared with TBI patients (13.2 Gy), they have similar risks of developing secondary malignancies (~5%) in the short term.[33] Han and colleagues' modeling study predicted that using a 12-Gy TMI instead of TBI plan reduced the total risk of RT-induced secondary solid tumors for major organs by 38.8% in men and 32.9% in women. When 20-Gy TMI plans were compared with 12-Gy cTBI plans, the decrease in risk was 14.6% in men and 9.2% in women, demonstrating that even at escalated dose levels, TMI could be associated with reduced secondary solid-tumor risks compared with cTBI.[34] Through numerous clinical trials, our COH group has demonstrated that TMLI dose escalation to 20 Gy is safe with favorable normal organ sparing, low NRM, and potential improvement in survival outcomes. Our dosimetric report provides useful reference data for the clinical implementation of TMI/TMLI at other institutions.[19]

The work of other RT groups has also provided valuable insight into the use of TMI/TMLI for pretransplant conditioning. Kong and colleagues (2022) recently reported a 1-year OS and disease-free survival (DFS) of 69.8% and 54.2%, respectively, in a retrospective review of 17 patients conditioned with 12-Gy TMLI,[35] which are comparable results to Stein and colleagues' phase II study using 20-Gy TMLI. Haraldsson and colleagues (2021) sought to compare outcomes of patients who received 12-Gy TMI versus TBI conditioning before HSCT.[36] Thrity-seven TMI patients were prospectively observed and compared with a historical TBI cohort. About 43.2% of TMI patients and 60.6% of TBI patients were in first complete remission. One-year GRFS was significantly improved for TMI patients compared with TBI patients (67.5% vs 39.4%, respectively, $P = .027$). The benefit of TMI over TBI was significant with the matched unrelated donor subgroup (80.5% vs 42.3%, respectively, $P = .003$). Engraftment times were similar but notably platelet recovery to less than 20 K/μL and greater than 50 K/μL was significantly faster in the TMI cohort ($P = .01$ and $P = .03$, respectively). Although there were no significant differences in acute GVHD between patients who received TMI compared with TBI (10.8% vs 18.2%, respectively, $P = .35$), there was a trend toward a reduction in incidences of moderate-to-severe chronic GVHD (8.3% vs 25.0%, respectively, $P = .11$) with TMI.[36] Zhao and colleagues (2020) also examined outcomes of adult high-risk patients with ALL who received either TMLI or non-TMLI conditioning before allo-HSCT.[37] Clinicians used a novel hypofractionated TMLI regimen consisting of 8 to 10 Gy in 2 fractions, which provides an approximately equal biologically effective dose as a typical 12 Gy in 6 fractions regimen. The TMLI cohort demonstrated significant improvement in the 1-year cumulative incidence of relapse ($P = .018$), 1-year OS ($P = .033$), and DFS ($P = .026$), with no difference in TRM ($P = .619$).[37] These promising results reinforce findings from Stein and colleagues that a potential benefit may be gained with TMI/TMLI.

Helical TomoTherapy or Volumetric-Modulated Arc Therapy-Based Total Body Irradiation

Although the goal of IMRT TMLI is to dose escalate over cTBI in patients with advanced leukemia, large-field IMRT has also led to advancements in modernizing TBI. In cTBI,[38] cerrobend lung blocks have long been used to reduce the mean lung dose (MLD). However, pulmonary toxicities are seen in as many as 71% of patients and idiopathic pneumonia syndrome in up to 60%.[11] MLDs still reach unacceptable levels greater than 8 Gy, which as noted above, is predictive of inferior survival.[12] IMRT TBI presents the opportunity to use highly conformal radiation techniques to limit the dose to the lungs and is a focus of a current clinical trial (NCT04281199).

IMRT TBI feasibility was evaluated by Hui and colleagues (2005) who simultaneously assessed both IMRT TBI and TMI in a preclinical simulation study (**Table 2**). RT was simulated with HT and methods to reduce dose to the lung, eyes, heart, kidney, and liver (range 34%–70%) were reported.[18] In 2008, Zhuang and colleagues' dosimetric study noted that the average dose received by 90% of the target volume was 12.3 Gy with TomoTherapy, and 10.3 Gy when the conventional method was used ($P < .001$). TomoTherapy also decreased lung doses to ~5 to 6 Gy compared with ~8 to 9 Gy with cTBI.[39]

The first analysis of IMRT TBI in patients was reported in 2011.[17] Peñagarícano and colleagues explored the clinical feasibility of TBI with HT in 4 patients with AML receiving allo-HSCT. Lung RT ranged from 6.5 to 7.4 Gy, and kidney RT ranged

Table 2
Summary of studies exploring the feasibility, safety, and efficacy of IMRT TBI using VMAT or helical TomoTherapy

Author	Objective	N	Median Age (Range)	Disease Status	Prescribed Dose and Dose Constraints	Result	Notes
Hui et al,[18] 2005	Preclinical feasibility of HT for TBI and TMI	1	NR	NR	13.2 Gy in 8 fx	Total body D_{mean} = 14.34–14.78 Gy OAR dose reduced to 35%–70% Lungs D_{mean} = 7.84–8.72 Gy Kidneys D_{mean} = 6.33–7.15 Gy Eyes D_{mean} = 3.19–3.88 Gy	HI = 0.93 Methods to reduce dose to OARs (lungs, eyes, heart, liver, kidneys) reported. BOT = 31 min
Zhuang et al,[39] 2010	Preclinical Feasibility of HT-TBI vs conventional extended source-to-surface distance (X-SSD) TBI	4	NR	NR	12 Gy in 10 fx	HT vs X-SSD: D90% = 12.3 vs 10.3 Gy, $P < .001$ Lt lung D_{mean} = 5.44 vs 8.34 Gy Rt lung D_{mean} = 5.40 vs 8.95 Gy	Tx planning time similar. BOT longer for HT
Peñagarícano et al,[17] 2011	Feasibility of HT-TBI	4	44 (31–51)	2 CR 1 NotR 1 Refractory	12 Gy in 6 fx	CTV dose = 11.9–12.3 Gy Lungs = 6.5–7.4 Gy Lt kidney = 7.2–8.6 Gy Rt kidney = 7.3–8.5 Gy Median f/u 7 mo 2 pts alive disease-free, 2 died from GVHD but disease-free	HI = 0.90–0.95 Difference between planned and delivered dose = 2.7% BOT = 19–23 min AEs: grade 1 dermatitis and grade 1 headache

(continued on next page)

Table 2
(continued)

Author	Objective	N	Median Age (Range)	Disease Status	Prescribed Dose and Dose Constraints	Result	Notes

Corvò et al,[51] 2011	Retrospective of pts treated with conventional TBI + TMI	15	35 (18–55)	8 RL
				6 CR2
				1 CR3
					12 Gy in 6 fx conventional TBI + subsequent boost of 2 Gy in 1 fx TMI	PTV D95% = 93.3%
						Lungs
						  D_{median} = 11.02 Gy
						Kidneys
						  D_{median} = 12.74 Gy
						Median f/u 10.2 mo. All pts reached CR, 2 relapsed, 2 died from GVHD, 1 died from infection
							Median OAR dose reduction with TMI ranged from 30% to 65%

Gruen et al,[40] 2013	Feasibility of HT-TBI	10	12.5 (4–22)	4 CR1 5 CR2 1 CR3	12 Gy in 6 fx D95% = 95% Lung D_{mean} = 8–10 Gy	PTV D95% = 11.7 Gy Lungs D_{mean} = 9.14 Gy F/u range 1–15 mo, 8 pts alive in remission. 1 died from infection, 1 died from GVHD.	BOT = 13.6–20.6 min No $\geq$ G3 AEs
Springer et al,[41] 2016	Feasibility of VMAT-TBI	7	30.6 (20–52)	3 CR1 2 CR2 1 PR 1 RL	13.2 Gy in 8 fx for 4 pts 9.9 Gy for 1 pt 8 Gy for 2 pts Lungs D_{mean} <10 Gy	D95% = 8.3–13.1 Gy Rt lung D_{mean} = 6.8–10.7 Gy Lt lung D_{mean} = 6.9–10.7 Gy Median f/u = 8 mo 5 pts alive disease-free, 1 pt died of refractory disease and 1 from relapse	Difference between planned and delivered dose 3.6%–4.3% AEs: fatigue, G3 mucositis, bladder inflammation

Study	Purpose	No.	Median age (range)	Status	Dose/Constraints	Dosimetry/Outcomes	AEs/Results
Tas et al,[42] 2018	Feasibility of VMAT-TBI	30	18.5 (6–63)	NR	12 Gy in 6 fx, D90% = 100%, Lungs and kidneys D_{mean} <10 Gy, Lens D_{max} <6 Gy	PTV D_{mean} = 12.7 Gy, Lungs D_{mean} = 9.7 Gy, Kidneys D_{mean} = 9.6 Gy, Lens D_{max} = 4.5 Gy	HI = 1.16, Difference between planned and delivered dose = 3.3%, 1.1%, 0.9% for kidneys, lungs and PTV, No ≥ G3 AEs
Jiang et al,[52] 2018	Feasibility of HT-TBI with SIB to BM, CNS leukemia, and EM disease	14	22.5 (12–50)	8 CR1, 1 CR2, 1 PR, 4 Refractory	10 Gy + SIB 2 Gy to bone marrow and extramedullary disease, D80% = 100%, Lung D_{mean} = 6–8 Gy	PTV D80% = 12.01 Gy, Skeletal bone D_{median} = 12.7 Gy, Lungs D_{mean} = ~7.4 Gy, Kidneys D_{mean} = ~11.1 Gy, Median f/u 14.6 mo, OS and RFS = 71.4%, NRM = 28.6%	Median HI = 0.475, Pts alive still are in complete remission, including remission of extramedullary leukemic
Konishi et al,[46] 2020	Single-center pilot study to evaluate safety of IMRT TBI	10	45.5 (20–53)	7 CR1, 1 CR2, 2 CP2	12 Gy in 6 fx	PTV D80% = 12.01 Gy, Lungs D80% = 7.50 Gy, Kidneys D80% = 9.03 Gy, Lens D80% = ~4.0–4.4 Gy, Median f/u = 18.8 mo 9 pts alive disease-free	AEs: 8 pts oral mucositis and GI toxicities. 1 pt had G3 kidney/liver toxicities. No G3-4 acute GVHD or late AEs
Guo et al,[43] 2021	Feasibility of automatic scripts for VMAT-TBI	25	NR (9–59)	NR	12–13.2 Gy in 8 fx, V95% = 95%, Lung D_{mean} ≤10 Gy (adults) or 8 Gy (peds), Kidney D_{mean} ≤6 Gy	VMAT vs conventional TBI: PTV V95% = 94.8% vs 87.7% (P < .001), Lung D_{mean} = 9.4 Gy vs 10.8 Gy (P < .001), Kidney D_{mean} = 6.1 Gy vs 5.8 Gy (P = .09)	VMAT planning time 8–12 h

(continued on next page)

Table 2
(continued)

Author	Objective	N	Median Age (Range)	Disease Status	Prescribed Dose and Dose Constraints	Result	Notes
Simiele et al,[45] 2021	Feasibility of automizing treatment planning VMAT TBI and comparing manual vs autoplans	10	NR	NR	2 Gy in 1 fx or 12 Gy in 6 fx D100% = 90%	Manual vs autoplan: Global D_{max} ($P < .893$) PTV V110% ($P < .734$) Kidneys D_{mean} ($P < .351$) Bowel D_{max} ($P < .473$) Lungs D_{mean} ($P < .024$)	Planning time for manual plans 2–3 d vs 3–5 h for autoplans. Autoplans selected as equivalent or superior to manual 77% of the time by blinded physicians
Kobyzeva et al,[47] 2021	Retrospective review of pediatric pts who received VMAT or HT-TBI	HT-TBI = 151 VMAT-TBI = 40 IMRT-TBI + SIB to BM = 29	10.2 (3–21)	53 CR1 128 CR2/3 39 Active diseases	12 Gy in 4-6 fx For SIB group, boost to BM up to 15 Gy	Median f/u 2.8 y, OS = 63%, EFS = 58%, TRM = 10.7%	Lungs, kidneys, lenses spared
Kovalchuk et al,[44] 2022	To describe their institutional VMAT TBI technique using autoplans	35 pts	10 (1–56)	NR	2–13.2 Gy D100% = 90%	Lungs spared to 57.6% of prescription Kidneys spared to 70.0% of prescription	Treatment time (patient set-up + BOT) = 47.5 min Myeloablative regimens spared lungs, kidneys, lenses Nonmyeloablative regimens spared lungs, kidneys, lenses, gonads, brain, thyroid

| Zhang-Velten et al,[48] 2022 | Retrospective review of pts who received VMAT-TBI | Myeloablative = 32 Nonmyeloablative = 12 | 21 (3–68) | NR | Myeloablative = 12–13.2 Gy in 6–8 fx Nonmyeloablative = 2–4 Gy in 1 fx PTV coverage >90% | PTV coverage = 93.9% Lung D$_{mean}$ = 69.8% (~8.3 Gy myeloablative, ~1.5 Gy nonmyeloablative) Median f/u = 2.17 y, 1-y OS = 90%, RFS = 88%, 2-y OS = 79%, RFS = 71% | ≥G3 Aes: mucositis (71%), nephrotoxicity (13%), RT-induced pneumonitis (2%) |
| Marquez et al,[49] 2022 | Retrospective review of pediatric and AYA pts who received VMAT-TBI | Myeloablative = 16 Nonmyeloablative = 22 | 7.2 (NR) | NR | 2–13.2 Gy in 1–8 fx PTV coverage >90% | Lungs D$_{mean}$ = 58.5% Kidneys D$_{mean}$ = 71.4% Median f/u = 8.7 mo. For all pts, OS = 89.5%, RFS = 94.7%. For myeloablative pts OS = 100%, RFS = 100% | VMAT planned using automated planning scripts G1-2 AEs: nausea (68.4%), fatigue (55.3%); G3-4 AEs: mucositis (39.5%); G3 GVHD = 1 (2.6%) |

Abbreviations: BOT, beam-on time; CP, chronic phase; CR, complete remission; CTV, clinical target volume; D90% = 100%, dose received by 90% of the target volume is 100% of prescription dose; D$_{mean}$, mean dose; EFS, event-free survival; EM, extramedullary; F/u, follow-up; Fx, fraction; HI, homogeneity index; Mo, months; NotR, not in remission; NR, not reported; NRM, nonrelapse mortality; OAR, organs at risk; OS, overall survival; PR, partial remission; Pts, patients; PTV, planning target volume; RFS, relapse-free survival; RL, relapsed; TRM, treatment-related mortality; V8<40%, volume of each lung receiving 8 Gy is not to exceed 40% of whole lung volume.

from 7.2 to 8.6 Gy. Other than grade 1 dermatitis and grade 1 headache, no other toxicities were reported; however, 2 patients died of GVHD within 6 months of transplantation.[17] Similar results were reported in a 2013 study of 10 high-risk AML or ALL pediatric and young-adult patients (see **Table 2**).[40]

In addition to TomoTherapy, VMAT can be implemented for IMRT TBI (**Fig. 2**). Springer and colleagues (2016) reported the first clinical experience using VMAT for myeloablative TBI in 7 patients receiving allo-HSCT. They aimed to optimize dose homogeneity of the PTV while reducing MLD. Although treatment planning times were very high (greater than 36 hours), investigators achieved adequate dose coverage and were able to decrease the MLD to 50% to 80% of the prescribed dose (6.7–10.7 Gy).[41] No pulmonary toxicities were reported but all patients experienced fatigue and grade 3 mucositis. Tas and colleagues (2018) reported on VMAT-TBI in 30 AML and ALL patients; mean lung dose was 9.7 Gy, mean kidney dose was 9.6 Gy and maximum lens dose was 4.5 Gy. The mean PTV dose was 12.7 Gy.[42] These studies indicate that favorable dose distribution is achievable using VMAT but the time-intensive treatment planning process limits its clinical implementation. Studies are underway to automate this process and dramatically reduce VMAT-TBI and TMLI treatment planning times (see **Table 2**).[43–45]

Following a report by COG, which demonstrated that MLD greater than 8 Gy was significantly predictive of inferior survival,[12] a pilot IMRT TBI trial was conducted in 2020.[46] Mean doses to the lungs and kidneys were 7.50 Gy and 9.03 Gy, respectively, and the mean minimum dose received by 80% of the left and right lenses were 4.03 and 4.41 Gy, respectively. Patients displayed an acceptable toxicity profile. After a median 18-month follow-up, 9 out of 10 patients were alive and disease-free, with 1 patient passing from sinusoidal obstruction syndrome before achieving platelet recovery. Four patients experienced grade I and II acute GVHD, and 1 patient developed mild chronic GVHD. This first pilot study provides insights for developing future clinical trials with IMRT TBI.

Kobyzeva and colleagues (2021) published a large retrospective analysis of 220 patients who received either VMAT-TBI or HT-TBI for allo-HSCT conditioning.[47] A total of

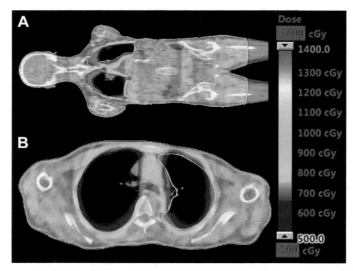

Fig. 2. Isodose distribution for one 13.2-Gy VMAT TBI plan in a coronal view (A) and axial view (B).

151 patients received HT, 40 patients received VMAT, and 29 patients received either VMAT-TBI or HT-TBI with a simultaneous integrated boost (SIB) up to 15 Gy to the bone marrow. After a median follow-up of 2.8 years (range 0.3–6.4 years), OS was 63%, event-free survival was 58%, and TRM was 10.7% for all patients. Acute toxicities included nausea and vomiting, the frequency of which correlated with the amount of a single radiation dose, headache, parotitis, and enteritis. One patient experienced interstitial pneumonia and died from respiratory failure, and no patients experienced radiation-induced kidney toxicity.

Zhang-Velten and colleagues (2022) reported their 6-year clinical experience using myeloablative and nonmyeloablative VMAT-TBI in a retrospective analysis of 44 patients. One-year and 2-year OS was 90% and 79%, and RFS was 88% and 71%, respectively. Grade 3+ mucositis was observed in 71% of patients, and grade 3+ nephrotoxicity was seen in 13% of patients. One patient (2%) developed grade 3+ pneumonitis probably attributed to TBI.[48] Marquez and colleagues (2022) conducted a similar study on the early outcomes of 38 VMAT-TBI patients.[49] MLD was 7.3 Gy and no pneumonitis or nephrotoxicity attributable to TBI was reported. After a short median follow-up of 8.7 months, OS and RFS were both 100% for patients who received myeloablative conditioning but 81.8% and 90.9% for patients who received nonmyeloablative conditioning, respectively. Grade I GVHD was observed in 10 patients (26.3%) and Grade III GVHD was observed in one (2.6%) patient. These favorable results demonstrate the ability of VMAT-TBI to effectively spare OARs, with acceptable toxicity profiles.

Although data suggest that using TMI or TMLI for radiation conditioning in place of cTBI is not associated with an increased risk of extramedullary recurrence, the evidence is relatively sparse and some clinicians are still hesitant to implement these organ-sparing strategies for fear of increasing relapse rates. In this scenario, IMRT TBI or a hybrid IMRT TBI/TMLI approach may be a more favorable option. This was first proposed in 2006 by Aydogan and colleagues, who suggested that IMRT-facilitated dose escalation to the whole skeletal system or only to hematopoietically active bone marrow (ABM) sites may augment the efficiency of TBI without increasing organ damage.[20] Jaccard and colleagues have reported on the feasibility of adding a SIB of 4 Gy to ABM during 12 Gy TMI for 5 patients.[50] Corvò and colleagues retrospectively reported on their clinical experience treating patients with acute leukemia with TMI after cTBI for allo-HSCT conditioning. Their method involves treating patients with conventional 12 Gy TBI using a linear accelerator, and then boosting patients with 2 Gy TMI in a single fraction using helical TomoTherapy the following day, with subsequent cyclophosphamide 60 mg/kg for 2 days.[51] Ten AML and 5 patients with ALL either in relapse or in second or third complete remission were treated, and a median 30% to 65% dose reduction to OARs was achieved using TMI. The boost treatment was well tolerated (see **Table 2**). Jiang and colleagues developed a novel myeloablative regimen consisting of using HT to simultaneously deliver 10-Gy TBI and a targeted dose boost to 12 Gy to the bone marrow, central nervous system leukemia and extramedullary disease sites, for 14 high-risk or relapsed/refractory patients with ALL receiving haploidentical allo-HSCT with favorable outcomes (see **Table 2**)[52] suggesting a pathway for a novel TBI/TMI hybrid approach to HSCT.

SUMMARY

Technological progress in radiation oncology, in particular the development of large-field IMRT, has enabled the implementation of TMI, TMLI, and IMRT TBI. Although still sparingly used, these techniques have demonstrated promise in reducing the adverse effects of TBI while maintaining and potentially improving survival outcomes. Unlike cTBI, IMRT allows for dose escalation to malignant sites while still sparing OARs to acceptable levels and thus preventing an increase in toxicities and organ damage. Multiple clinical trials have already demonstrated that dose escalation of TMI and TMLI to 20 Gy is safe, feasible, and effective, and several studies have shown that IMRT TBI is able to spare organ doses to favorable levels, particularly in the lungs, kidneys, and lenses, which are vulnerable to toxicities. Future studies comparing the outcomes of using dose-escalated TMLI is needed to understand the potential benefit for high-risk patients with leukemia, and research in IMRT TBI should explore the addition of a simultaneous boost to malignant sites.

CLINICS CARE POINTS

- TMI/TMLI for patients with acute leukemia receiving allo-HSCT can be safely dose escalated to 20 Gy and has been associated with promising NRM, decreased GVHD, and improved RFS.
- IMRT TBI is a safe and feasible treatment to reduce dose to OARs compared with cTBI.
- Both HT and VMAT can be used for TMI, TMLI, and IMRT TBI treatment plans.
- A hybrid approach, where TMI/TMLI dose escalation of ABM and extramedullary disease sites is combined with IMRT TBI, could be beneficial for high-risk patients with leukemia, and can be facilitated by using a SIB.

DISCLOSURE

Dr S. Dandapani has research funding from Bayer. Dr J. Wong has research funding from Varian. Dr C. Ladbury has research funding from Reflexion.

REFERENCES

1. Wong JYC, Filippi AR, Dabaja BS, et al. Total Body Irradiation: Guidelines from the International Lymphoma Radiation Oncology Group (ILROG). Int J Radiat Oncol Biol Phys 2018;101(3):521–9.
2. Wong J.Y.C., Filippi A.R., Scorsetti M., et al., Total marrow and total lymphoid irradiation in bone marrow transplantation for acute leukaemia, Lancet Oncol, 21 (10), 2020, e477–e487.
3. Peters C Dalle JH, Locatelli F,, et al. Total Body Irradiation or Chemotherapy Conditioning in Childhood ALL: A Multinational, Randomized, Noninferiority Phase III Study. J Clin Oncol 2021;39(4):295–307.
4. Davies SM, Ramsay NK, Klein JP, et al. Comparison of preparative regimens in transplants for children with acute lymphoblastic leukemia. J Clin Oncol 2000; 18(2):340–7.
5. Bunin N, Aplenc R, Kamani N, et al. Randomized trial of busulfan vs total body irradiation containing conditioning regimens for children with acute lymphoblastic leukemia: a Pediatric Blood and Marrow Transplant Consortium study. Bone Marrow Transplant 2003;32(6):543–8.
6. Gupta T, Kannan S, Dantkale V, t, et al. Cyclophosphamide plus total body irradiation compared with busulfan plus cyclophosphamide as a conditioning regimen prior to hematopoietic stem cell transplantation in patients with leukemia: a systematic review and meta-analysis, Hematology/Oncology and Stem Cell. Therapy 2011;4(1):17–29.

7. Saglio F., Zecca M., Pagliara D.,et al., Occurrence of long-term effects after hematopoietic stem cell transplantation in children affected by acute leukemia receiving either busulfan or total body irradiation: results of an AIEOP (Associazione Italiana Ematologia Oncologia Pediatrica) retrospective study, *Bone Marrow Transplant*, 55 (10), 2020, 1918–1927.

8. Lawitschka A, Peters C. Long-term Effects of Myeloablative Allogeneic Hematopoietic Stem Cell Transplantation in Pediatric Patients with Acute Lymphoblastic Leukemia. Curr Oncol Rep 2018;20(9):74.

9. Baker K.S., Leisenring W.M., Goodman P.J., et al., Total body irradiation dose and risk of subsequent neoplasms following allogeneic hematopoietic cell transplantation, *Blood*, 133 (26), 2019, 2790–2799.

10. Clift RA, Buckner CD, Appelbaum FR, et al. Allogeneic Marrow Transplantation in Patients With Acute Myeloid Leukemia in First Remission: A Randomized Trial of Two Irradiation Regimens. Blood 1990;76(9):1867–71.

11. Vogel J, Hui S, Hua CH, et al. Pulmonary Toxicity After Total Body Irradiation - Critical Review of the Literature and Recommendations for Toxicity Reporting. *Front Oncol* 2021;11:708906.

12. Esiashvili N, Lu X, Ulin K, et al. Higher Reported Lung Dose Received During Total Body Irradiation for Allogeneic Hematopoietic Stem Cell Transplantation in Children With Acute Lymphoblastic Leukemia Is Associated With Inferior Survival: A Report from the Children's Oncology Group. Int J Radiat Oncol Biol Phys 2019; 104(3):513–21.

13. Oertel M., Martel J., Mikesch J.H., et al., The Burden of Survivorship on Hematological Patients-Long-Term Analysis of Toxicities after Total Body Irradiation and Allogeneic Stem Cell Transplantation, *Cancers*, 13 (22), 2021, 5640.

14. Esiashvili N, et al. Renal toxicity in children undergoing total body irradiation for bone marrow transplant. Radiother Oncol 2009;90(2):242–6.

15. Sieker K., Fleischmann M., Trommel M., et al., Twenty years of experience of a tertiary cancer center in total body irradiation with focus on oncological outcome and secondary malignancies, *Strahlenther Onkol*, 198 (6), 2022, 547–557.

16. Salhotra A, Stein AS. Role of Radiation Based Conditioning Regimens in Patients With High-Risk AML Undergoing Allogenic Transplantation in Remission or Active Disease and Mechanisms of Post-Transplant Relapse. Front Oncol 2022;12: 802648.

17. Peñagarícano JA, Chao M, Van Rhee F, et al. Clinical feasibility of TBI with helical tomotherapy. *Bone Marrow Transplant* 2011;46(7):929–35.

18. Hui SK, Kapatoes J, Fowler J, et al. Feasibility study of helical tomotherapy for total body or total marrow irradiation. *Med Phys* 2005;32(10):3214–24.

19. Han C, Liu A, Wong JYC. Target Coverage and Normal Organ Sparing in Dose-Escalated Total Marrow and Lymphatic Irradiation: A Single-Institution Experience. Front Oncol 2022;12:946725.

20. Aydogan B, Mundt AJ, Roeske JC. Linac-based intensity modulated total marrow irradiation (IM-TMI). Technol Cancer Res Treat 2006;5(5):513–9.

21. Aydogan B, et al. Total marrow irradiation with RapidArc volumetric arc therapy. Int J Radiat Oncol Biol Phys 2011;81(2):592–9.

22. Schultheiss TE, Liu A, Wong J,, et al. Total marrow and total lymphatic irradiation with helical tomotherapy. Med Phys 2004;31(6):1845–1845.

23. Schultheiss T.E., Wong J., Liu A., et al., *Normal tissue sparing in total marrow and total lymphatic irradiation with helical tomotherapy*, Int J Radiat Oncol Biol Phys, 60 (1), 2004, S544–S545.

24. Schultheiss TE, et al. *Image-guided total marrow and total lymphatic irradiation using helical tomotherapy.* Int J Radiat Oncol Biol Phys 2007;67(4):1259–67.
25. Wong JYC, et al. Targeted Total Marrow Irradiation Using Three-Dimensional Image-Guided Tomographic Intensity-Modulated Radiation Therapy: An Alternative to Standard Total Body Irradiation. Biol Blood Marrow Transplant 2006;12(3): 306–15.
26. Shinde A, et al. Radiation-Related Toxicities Using Organ Sparing Total Marrow Irradiation Transplant Conditioning Regimens. Int J Radiat Oncol Biol Phys 2019;105(5):1025–33.
27. Shinde A, Wong JYC. Acute and Late Toxicities with Total Marrow Irradiation. In: Wong JYC, Hui SK, editors. Total marrow irradiation: a comprehensive review. Cham: Springer International Publishing; 2020. p. 187–96.
28. Kim J.H., Stein A., Tsai N., et al., Extramedullary relapse following total marrow and lymphoid irradiation in patients undergoing allogeneic hematopoietic cell transplantation, *Int J Radiat Oncol Biol Phys*, 89 (1), 2014, 75–81.
29. Stein AS, et al. Total Marrow and Lymphoid Irradiation with Post-Transplantation Cyclophosphamide for Patients with AML in Remission. Transplant Cell Ther 2022;28(7):368.e1–7.
30. Salhotra A, et al. Long-Term Outcomes of Patients with Acute Myelogenous Leukemia Treated with Myeloablative Fractionated Total Body Irradiation TBI-Based Conditioning with a Tacrolimus- and Sirolimus-Based Graft-versus-Host Disease Prophylaxis Regimen: 6-Year Follow-Up from a Single Center. Biol Blood Marrow Transplant 2020;26(2):292–9.
31. Stein A, et al. Phase I Trial of Total Marrow and Lymphoid Irradiation Transplantation Conditioning in Patients with Relapsed/Refractory Acute Leukemia. Biol Blood Marrow Transplant 2017;23(4):618–24.
32. Wong JYC, et al. Phase II Study of Dose Escalated Total Marrow and Lymphoid Irradiation (TMLI) in Combination with Cyclophosphamide and Etoposide in Patients with Poor-Risk Acute Leukemia. Int J Radiat Oncol Biol Phys 2020;108(3): S155.
33. Ladbury C., Armenian S., Bosworth A., et al., Risk of subsequent malignant neoplasms following hematopoietic stem cell transplantation with total body irradiation or total marrow irradiation: insights from early follow-up, *Transplant Cell Ther*, 28 (12), 2022, 860.e1-860.e6.
34. Han C, Liu A, Wong JYC. Estimation of radiation-induced, organ-specific, secondary solid-tumor occurrence rates with total body irradiation and total marrow irradiation treatments. Pract Radiat Oncol 2020;10(5):e406–14.
35. Kong F, Liu S, Liu L, et al. Clinical study of total bone marrow combined with total lymphatic irradiation pretreatment based on tomotherapy in hematopoietic stem cell transplantation of acute leukemia. *Front Oncol* 2022;12:936985.
36. Haraldsson A., Wichert S., Engström P.E., et al., Organ sparing total marrow irradiation compared to total body irradiation prior to allogeneic stem cell transplantation, *Eur J Haematol*, 107 (4), 2021, 393–407.
37. Zhao X, et al. Comparing the outcomes between TMLI and non-TMLI conditioning regimens for adult high-risk acute lymphoblastic leukemia patients undergoing allogeneic hematopoietic stem cell transplantation: a single-center experience. Leuk Lymphoma 2020;61(12):2859–67.
38. Bailey DW, et al. TBI lung dose comparisons using bilateral and anteroposterior delivery techniques and tissue density corrections. J Appl Clin Med Phys 2015; 16(2):5293.

39. Zhuang AH, et al. Dosimetric study and verification of total body irradiation using helical tomotherapy and its comparison to extended SSD technique. Med Dosim 2010;35(4):243–9.

40. Gruen A, et al. Total Body Irradiation (TBI) using Helical Tomotherapy in children and young adults undergoing stem cell transplantation. Radiat Oncol 2013;8:92.

41. Springer A., Hammer J., Winkler E., et al., Total body irradiation with volumetric modulated arc therapy: Dosimetric data and first clinical experience, *Radiat Oncol*, 11 (1), 2016, 46.

42. Tas B, et al. Total-body irradiation using linac-based volumetric modulated arc therapy: Its clinical accuracy, feasibility and reliability. Radiother Oncol 2018; 129(3):527–33.

43. Guo B, et al. Image-guided volumetric-modulated arc therapy of total body irradiation: An efficient workflow from simulation to delivery. J Appl Clin Med Phys 2021;22(10):169–77.

44. Kovalchuk N., Simiele E., Skinner L., et al., The Stanford Volumetric Modulated Arc Therapy Total Body Irradiation Technique, *Pract Radiat Oncol*, 12 (3), 2022, 245–258.

45. Simiele E, et al. A Step Toward Making VMAT TBI More Prevalent: Automating the Treatment Planning Process. Pract Radiat Oncol 2021;11(5):415–23.

46. Konishi T., Ogawa H., Najima Y., et al., Safety of total body irradiation using intensity-modulated radiation therapy by helical tomotherapy in allogeneic hematopoietic stem cell transplantation: a prospective pilot study, *J Radiat Res*, 61 (6), 2020, 969–976.

47. Kobyzeva D, et al. Optimized Conformal Total Body Irradiation Among Recipients of TCRαβ/CD19-Depleted Grafts in Pediatric Patients With Hematologic Malignancies: Single-Center Experience. Front Oncol 2021;11:785916.

48. Zhang-Velten ER, et al. Volumetric Modulated Arc Therapy Enabled Total Body Irradiation (VMAT-TBI): Six-year Clinical Experience and Treatment Outcomes. Transplant Cell Ther 2022;28(2):113.e1–8.

49. Marquez C., Hui C., Simiele E., et al., Volumetric modulated arc therapy total body irradiation in pediatric and adolescent/young adult patients undergoing stem cell transplantation: Early outcomes and toxicities, *Pediatr Blood Cancer*, 69 (6), 2022, e29689.

50. Jaccard M, et al. Dose-escalated volumetric modulated arc therapy for total marrow irradiation: A feasibility dosimetric study with 4DCT planning and simultaneous integrated boost. Phys Med 2020;78:123–8.

51. Corvò R, et al. Helical tomotherapy targeting total bone marrow after total body irradiation for patients with relapsed acute leukemia undergoing an allogeneic stem cell transplant. Radiother Oncol 2011;98(3):382–6.

52. Jiang Z, et al. Haploidentical hematopoietic SCT using helical tomotherapy for total-body irradiation and targeted dose boost in patients with high-risk/refractory acute lymphoblastic leukemia. Bone Marrow Transplant 2018;53(4):438–48.

The Emerging Role of Radiotherapy in Oligoprogressive Non-Small Cell Lung Cancer

Andrew Tam, MD[a], Nicholas Eustace, MD, PhD[a],
Ari Kassardjian, MD[a], Howard West, MD[b],
Terence M. Williams, MD, PhD[a], Arya Amini, MD[a],*

KEYWORDS

- Non-small cell lung cancer • Oligoprogressive disease • Local ablative treatment
- Stereotactic body radiation treatment • Stereotactic ablative radiotherapy

KEY POINTS

- Oligoprogressive disease is a new clinical entity classification that describes metastatic disease with limited sites of progression.
- Early data suggest that the local ablation of oligoprogressive sites improves progression-free survival and overall survival.
- High-quality data from randomized controlled trials are needed before the adoption of radiotherapy, or other local ablative therapies, as the standard of care.

INTRODUCTION

Recent advances in targeted therapies have made significant progress in improving survival outcomes in patients with many types of cancer. In non-small cell lung cancer (NSCLC) specifically, patients with epidermal growth factor receptor (EGFR) mutations or anaplastic lymphoma kinase (ALK) gene rearrangements have shown to have great responses and prolonged survival when treated with EGFR-tyrosine kinase inhibitors (TKIs) or ALK inhibitors, respectively.[1–4] **Fig. 1** provides a summary of gene mutations detectable in lung adenocarcinoma. However, most of these patients acquire resistance to these agents over time and often first develop progression in a few metastatic sites. For example, the most commonly acquired resistance to EGFR-TKIs is the secondary mutation in codon 790 with the substitution of threonine to methionine (T790 M).[5] This base pair change introduces a bulkier amino acid side chain to the

[a] Department of Radiation Oncology, City of Hope National Medical Center, 1500 East Duarte Road, Duarte, CA, USA; [b] Department of Medical Oncology, City of Hope National Medical Center, 1500 East Duarte Road, Duarte, CA, USA
* Corresponding author.
E-mail address: aamini@coh.org

Surg Oncol Clin N Am 32 (2023) 497–514
https://doi.org/10.1016/j.soc.2023.02.004
surgonc.theclinics.com

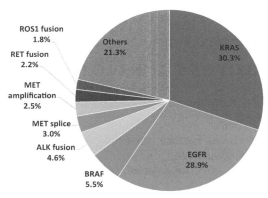

Fig. 1. Oncogenic divers in advanced or metastatic lung adenocarcinoma ($n = 5262$). A pie chart summarizes the gene alterations in advanced or metastatic lung adenocarcinoma. Data are based on next-generation sequencing results collected from MSK-IMPACT ($n = 860$), FoundationOne ($n = 4402$), and Dall'Olio and colleagues ($n = 537$).[46–48]

TKI-binding region, resulting in resistance to erlotinib.[6] The subset of patients who progress typically in three or fewer sites of disease with otherwise controlled widespread metastatic disease is now commonly referred to as having "oligoprogressive disease" (OPD).

In recent years, there is a growing recognition that metastatic NSCLC exists on a spectrum. New disease paradigms have emerged, including the concepts of oligometastatic disease (OMD) and OPD. OMD was first coined by Hellman and Weichselbaum in 1995 to describe a disease state detected "early in the chain of progression."[7] The European Society of Radiotherapy and Oncology and American Society for Radiation Oncology consensus recommended the definition of OMD to be the presence of one to five metastatic lesions, where all metastatic sites are amendable to safe treatment.[8] However, the definition of OMD remains quite variable in the current literature, especially regarding the timing of disease presentation in relation to systemic therapy. Some studies use OMD to refer to patients with limited metastases at the time of diagnosis before receiving any systemic therapies,[9,10] whereas others use it interchangeably with "oligo-recurrence" and define OMD as limited metastases with or without primary tumor control after initiation of systemic therapy.[10–12]

On the other hand, OPD pertains mainly to patients who have previously received systemic therapies or those who are actively undergoing systemic therapy and develop progression in three to five metastatic sites but have otherwise well-controlled or stable systemic disease. The differentiation between OMD and OPD is crucial given the diverging theorized biological basis between the two disease states. In contrast to OMD, OPD is thought to be due to extrinsic pressure from systemic therapy leading to the development of clonal heterogeneity and tumor cell evolution in metastatic sites.[13] Such heterogeneity and evolution under selective pressures can ultimately lead to the development of resistant clones and ultimately uncontrolled proliferation in a few metastatic sites. In essence, OPD is a different clinical entity than OMD, which may necessitate a disparate approach in management.

THE PARADIGM OF LOCAL CONTROL IN STAGE IV DISEASE

With the evolving treatment paradigms for metastatic disease, there has been an increasing interest in the inclusion of local ablative therapies (LATs) to provide durable local control of metastases in stage IV disease. The goal of LAT is to reduce the amount of disease burden and thereby delay the need to progress to the next line of systemic therapy. A study from the University of Colorado reported that 64% of patients with NSCLC treated with first-line chemotherapy presented with local-only extracranial progression, and 53% were considered eligible for LATs.[14] The most common reported sites of OPD were lung, bones, lymph nodes, and brain.[15,16] In theory, LATs may eradicate resistant clones in oligoprogressive sites, especially when used in conjunction with systemic therapy, and thereby further improve survival outcomes. Furthermore, recent studies have suggested that tumor-directed radiation treatment (RT) may stimulate the immune system to cause an immune-mediated abscopal effect in nonirradiated tumors in several cancers, including metastatic NSCLC.[17,18] However, the underlying biological mechanism remains poorly understood, and it is unclear if a similar effect would be observed with molecularly targeted agents and, more importantly, in OPD.

Options for LATs include surgery, radiofrequency ablation (RFA), microwave ablation (MWA), cryoablation, and RT. Historically, RT had a limited role in the setting of metastatic disease, other than for palliation. With the advent of advanced radiation delivery technology, techniques such as stereotactic body radiotherapy (SBRT) are increasingly being employed for local ablation. SBRT is now considered the standard of care (SOC) for patients with inoperable stage I NSCLC.[19] SBRT is an image-guided RT technique that delivers conformal external RT with a higher biologically equivalent dose compared with conventional treatment to extracranial tumors, typically in five or fewer fractions.[20] Fraction doses for SBRT typically range from 6 to 20 Gy, compared with 1.8 to 2.5 Gy per fraction in conventional RT. Most importantly, SBRT allows for delivery of an ablative dose focally to the tumor while sparing adjacent normal tissue. In the same vein, stereotactic radiosurgery (SRS) uses the same precise delivery to target lesions in the brain.

SBRT has several advantages over other LATs. The noninvasive nature of SBRT permits treatment to be given to patients who otherwise are not candidates for surgery or opted for less intrusive therapies. The capability of SBRT to target multiple foci in the same or multiple organs in a single course can reduce the need for patients to undergo multiple procedures or prolonged surgeries. Moreover, SBRT may enhance the immune response of those on a checkpoint inhibitor, in comparison to surgery or other forms of ablation. In the pooled analysis of the pembrolizumab-RT (PEMBRO-RT) (phase II) and M.D. Anderson Cancer Center (MDACC) (phase I/II) trials, the addition of radiotherapy to pembrolizumab, a programmed cell death protein 1 (PD-1) checkpoint inhibitor, was found to improve treatment response and outcomes.[21] Both trials recruited NSCLC immunotherapy-naïve patients with metastatic disease and randomly allocated pembrolizumab with or without RT. The combined analysis of 148 patients (72 patients assigned to pembrolizumab plus radiotherapy) found an out-of-field control rate of 41.7% when radiotherapy was added, compared with 19.7% with immunotherapy alone (odds ratio [OR] 2.96, $P = .0039$).[21] There was also an improvement in median progression-free survival (PFS) (19.2 months with radiotherapy vs 8.7 months without).[21] Despite early data implicating a potential synergistic role of radiation with immunotherapy, dose and fractionation, timing, and the impact of other variables (eg, programmed cell death ligand 1 [PD-L1] status) are still being optimized and determined. These findings have led to the Alliance A082002 (NCT04929041) randomized phase II/III trial which aims to better understand the role of SBRT in PD-L1-negative NSCLC patients with the primary goal of enhancing outcomes by priming the immune system with RT.[22]

LESSONS BORROWED FROM OLIGOMETASTATIC DISEASE

One of the landmark studies supporting the use of LAT in OMD is the (stereotactic ablative radiotherapy for the comprehensive treatment of oligometastases) SABR-COMET trial. This phase II study enrolled 99 patients with one to five metastatic lesions and randomized them to palliative SOC treatment alone or SOC with SBRT to all metastatic lesions.[23,24] With a median follow-up of 51 months, this study demonstrated significant improvements in outcomes when SBRT was added. The trial demonstrated a 5-year overall survival (OS) rate of 42.3% (95% confidence interval [CI], 28% to 56%) with SBRT versus 17.7% (95% CI, 6% to 34%) with palliative treatment ($P = .006$) and PFS rate of 17.3% (95% CI, 8% to 30%) with SBRT and "not reached" (95% CI, 0% to 14%) in the controlled arm ($P = .001$).

The SABR-COMET trial included patients with all tumor types. Nonetheless, other randomized studies of cohorts consisting only of NSCLC patients with OMD reported similar findings. A phase II trial by *Gomez and colleagues* of patients with three or fewer metastases and no progression at three or more months after first-line systemic therapy, assigned patients to either maintenance therapy/observation or LAT (radiation therapy or surgery) to all metastatic sites.[25] At a median follow-up of 38.8 months, they found a median PFS benefit of 9.8 months (14.2 months with LAT vs 4.4 months in the control group; $P = .022$).[26] They also reported an OS benefit with LATs with a median OS of 41.2 months (95% CI, 18.9 months to "not reached"), compared with 17.0 months (95% CI, 10.1–39.8 months) without local treatment ($P = .017$).[26] Similarly, *Iyengar and colleagues* randomized 29 NSCLC patients with up to six sites of extracranial disease to SBRT with maintenance chemotherapy or chemotherapy alone and found improved significant improvement in PFS with SBRT (9.7 months with SBRT vs 3.5 months without; $P = .01$).[27]

Overall, the evidence from these trials has laid down some groundwork in supporting the use of LATs in the setting of metastatic disease. These findings essentially "lowered the threshold" for consideration of LATs in oligoprogressive settings and have become the foundation for future investigations.

THE ROLE OF RADIOTHERAPY IN OLIGOPROGRESSIVE DISEASE

There has been increasing evidence in support of the use of RT in oligoprogressive NSCLC. However, the data from published literature are largely retrospective. **Table 1** summarizes outcomes from published studies on using RT as LAT in patients with oligoprogressive NSCLC. One of the earliest studies by *Shukuya and colleagues* reported on 17 patients with EGFR-positive metastatic NSCLC who developed brain-only OPD with median PFS of 80 days, median extracranial PFS of 171 days, and median OS of 403 days after SRS or whole brain radiotherapy while continuing on TKI therapy.[28] In the current era, most of what we consider oligometastatic or OPD is extracranial alone. Nevertheless, the potential of radiation in local control for oligoprogressive stage IV disease was initially drawn from studies on intracranial progression, as demonstrated by multiple studies including *Shukuya and colleagues*.

The six currently published prospective studies on OPD (five single-arm and one double-arm) included patients with extracranial OPD and found LATs to both intracranial and extracranial sites further improved survival outcomes. The study by *Yu and colleagues*, a review of patient data from a prospective biopsy protocol, identified 184 patients with EGFR-positive NSCLC who experienced disease progression while on TKI. Of the 184 patients, 18 patients received LATs (only three patients underwent RT) and found a median time to progression of 10 months (95% CI, 2–27 months) and median OS of 41 months (95% CI, 26 to "not reached").[12] The study by

Table 1
Summary of studies on radiotherapy in oligoprogressive non-small cell lung cancer

Authors	Study Type	Number of Patients (Received RT, Otherwise Specified)	Systemic Agent	Sites of Oligoprogression Treated with LATs (n)	Median Follow-Up (months)	Outcomes
Hu et al.,[49] 2022	Retrospective	33	TKI (erlotinib/ gefitinib/icotinib)	Lung (14), brain (12), bone (7)	18	Median OS 21.8 mo (14.8–28.8) Median PFS2 (time from oligoprogression to further progression) 6.5 mo (1.4–11.6)
Katz et al.,[50] 2022	Retrospective	8	n/a	lung	34	3-y LFFS 83% (58%–100%) 3-y PFS 33% (12%–95%)
Mok et al.,[51] 2022	Retrospective	55	TKI	Lung (45), bone (15), brain (13), neck lymph node (1), adrenal (1)	13.3	Median OS 25.1 mo (10.0–40.1) Median PFS 6.9 mo (3.1–10.7)
CURB Tsai et al.,[33] 2022 (abstract only)	Phase II prospective, two-arms (SBRT vs palliative standard of care)	55	n/a	n/a	12.8 (51 wk)	Median PFS 22 wk with SBRT (vs 10 wk with palliative; P = .005)
Kroeze et al.,[52] 2021[a]	Retrospective	61	EGFR/ALK inhibitors, immunotherapy, VEGF-antibodies, PARP-inhibitors	Brain (144), lung (18), bone (17), liver (6), adrenal (3), lymph nodes (3), soft tissue (1)	18.7	Median PFS 10.4 mo

(continued on next page)

Table 1
(continued)

Authors	Study Type	Number of Patients (Received RT, Otherwise Specified)	Systemic Agent	Sites of Oligoprogression Treated with LATs (n)	Median Follow-Up (months)	Outcomes
Wang et al.,[53] 2021	Retrospective	24	Anti-PD1/anti-PDL1	Brain (14), lung (10), lymph node (5), adrenal (3), liver (1), cervical vertebra (1)	28.0	Median OS 34 mo (19 to n/a), Median PFS 11 mo (8 to n/a), Median LC 43 mo (77–78.3)
Buglione et al.,[54] 2020	Retrospective	198 (includes 134 patients with oligometastatic disease)	n/a	Brain (204), lung (68), lymph nodes (16), adrenal (12), liver (8), soft tissue (1)	18	Median OS 29.6 mo, Median PFS 10.6 mo, Local PFS "not reached", Out-of-field PFS 10.6 mo
ATOM. Chan et al.,[30] 2020	Phase II prospective, single-arm	16	TKI (gefitinib/erlotinib/afatinib)	Lung (16), bone (4), and lymph nodes (2)	39.1	Median OS 43.3 mo, 1-y PFS rate 68.8%
Friedes et al.,[55] 2020	Retrospective	198	TKI, immunotherapy, chemotherapy	Brain (181), lung (104), others (43)	14.9	Median OS 37.7 mo (31.5–87.9), Median PFS 7.9 mo (6.5–10.0)
Santarpia et al.,[56] 2020	Retrospective	36	Gefitinib	Lung (11), lymph node (9), CNS (9), adrenal (5), bone (2)	n/a	Median PFS 6.3 mo (2–12.5)
Borghetti et al.,[57] 2019[a]	Retrospective	52	TKI (gefitinib, erlotinib, crizotinib)	Brain, bone, lung, others	9.1	Median OS 23 mo

Study	Study type	No. of patients	Treatment	Metastatic sites		Outcomes
Cortellini et al.,[36] 2019	Retrospective	19 (1 received adrenal thermo-ablative therapy)	Osimertinib	lung/mediastinal lymph nodes (10), CNS (6), bone (4), liver (2)	14.5	Median OS 20.2 mo (7.2–20.2) (vs 9.9 mo without LATs; P = .0748) Median PFS 6.4 mo (4.8–10.9) (vs 5.7 mo without LATs; P = .4560)
Rossi et al.,[58] 2019	Retrospective	30	TKI (gefitinib, afatinib)	Bone (11), lung (9), brain (8), lymph nodes (8), liver (1)	46	Median OS 37.3 mo Median PFS2 (time from the first progression to the second progression) 6.7 mo
Schmid et al.,[15] 2019	Retrospective	13[b] (vs 13 without LATs)	Osimertinib	n/a	18	Median OS "not reached" (vs 20.2 mo without LATs; P = .2)
Weiss et al.,[31] 2019	Phase II prospective, single-arm	25	Erlotinib	Lung (15), Bone (7), brain (2), liver (4)	n/a	Median OS 29 mo (21.7–36.3) Median PFS 6 mo (2.5–11.6)
Xu et al.,[59] 2019	Retrospective	206 (32 patients underwent surgery ± RT)	TKI (erlotinib/gefitinib/icotinib)	Brain (124), bone (86), lung (40), adrenal (35), liver (18), chest wall (10), neck lymph nodes (9), intestine (1)	42	Median OS 37.4 mo (35.9–38.9) Median PFS (time from initiation of TKI to stopping TKI) 18.3 mo (17.4–19.2)
Jiang et al.,[40] 2018	Retrospective	24 (8 received RFA, and 3 interventional therapy)	TKI (erlotinib/gefitinib/icotinib)	Liver (69)	n/a	Median OS 28.3 mo Median PFS2 (time to off-TKI progression or switching therapy failure) 13.9 mo

(continued on next page)

Table 1
(continued)

Authors	Study Type	Number of Patients (Received RT, Otherwise Specified)	Systemic Agent	Sites of Oligoprogression Treated with LATs (n)	Median Follow-Up (months)	Outcomes
Merino Lara et al.,[60] 2018	Retrospective	20	TKI (afatinib/erlotinib/gefitinib)	Lung (12), spine (7), liver (3), adrenal (2), non-spine bone (2), lymph node/soft tissue (1)	11.3	Median OS 21.1 mo Median PFS 3.3 mo
Chan et al.,[34] 2017	Retrospective matched-cohort (radiotherapy vs chemotherapy)	25	TKI	Lung (18), brain (5), bone (3), lymph node (2), adrenal (1), and pancreas (1)	24.3	Median OS 28.2 mo (vs 14.7 with chemotherapy; P = .026) Median PFS 7.0 mo (vs 4.1 with chemotherapy; P = .0017)
Qiu et al.,[61] 2017	Retrospective	46 (2 received RFA to lung)	TKI	Brain (24), lung (16), bone (6)	32	Median OS 13.0 mo Median PFS 7.0 mo
Wang et al.,[35] 2017	Retrospective	44	TKI (erlotinib/gefitinib/icotinib)	Bone (19), lung (11), cranial (11), adrenal (5), lymph node (3), liver (1)	25.1	Median OS 26.6 mo (22.2–31) Median PFS (time from initiation of TKI to any disease progression after RT) 21.3 mo (vs 16.0 with no LATs; P = .027) Median TTP (time from initiation of TKI to progression of irradiated lesions after RT) 21.7 mo (vs 16.0 without LATs; P = .010)

Study	Study type	Number	Drug	Metastatic sites	OS	Outcomes
Gan et al.,[62] 2014	Retrospective	14(1 underwent adrenalectomy followed by RT)	Crizotinib	n/a	25.1	Median PFS1 (time to initial progression) 14 mo (5–25) Median PFS2 (time to subsequent progression) 5.5 mo (1–27)
Iyengar et al.,[32] 2014	Phase II prospective, single-arm	24	Erlotinib	Lung (18), mediastinum/hilum (13), adrenal (7), bone (6), liver (4), non-mediastinal lymph nodes (3), kidney (1)	11.6	Median OS 20.4 mo Median PFS 14.7 mo
Yu et al.,[63] 2013	Prospective, single-arm	18(15 underwent surgery/RFA)	TKI (erlotinib/gefitinib)	Lung (15), adrenal (2), lymph node (1)	n/a	Median OS 41 mo (26 to "not reached") Median TTP 10 mo (2–27)
Weickhardt et al.,[64] 2012	Retrospective	25 (1 underwent adrenalectomy)	Crizotinib (for ALK)/erlotinib (for EGFR)	Brain (13), bone (7), lung (7), lymph node (2), adrenal (1), liver (1)	9.4	Median PFS1 9.8 mo (time from initiation of targeted therapy to the first progression) (8.8–13.8) Median PFS2 6.2 mo (time from the first progression to the second progression) (3.7–8.0)

(continued on next page)

Table 1
(continued)

Authors	Study Type	Number of Patients (Received RT, Otherwise Specified)	Systemic Agent	Sites of Oligoprogression Treated with LATs (n)	Median Follow-Up (months)	Outcomes
Salama et al.,[29] 2011	Prospective	61 (included patients with non-lung primaries; 11 NSCLC and 5 SCLC)	n/a	Lung (41), lymph nodes (22), liver (22), bone (15), adrenal (9), soft tissue (3), pancreas (1)	20.9	1-y OS 81.5% (71.1%–91.1%) 2-y OS 56.7% (43.9%–68.9%) 1-y PFS 33.3% (22.8%–46.1%) 2-y PFS 22.0% (12.8%–34.4%)
Shukuya et al.,[28] 2011	Retrospective	17	TKI	CNS	n/a	Median OS 403 d (13.4 mo) Median PFS 80 d (2.7 mo) Median extracranial PFS 171 d (5.7 mo)

Abbreviations: ALK, anaplastic lymphoma kinase; CNS, central nervous system; EGFR, epidermal growth factor receptor; LAT, local ablative therapy; LC, local control; LFFS, local failure-free survival; NSCLC, non-small cell lung cancer; OS, overall survival; PARP, poly ADP ribose polymerase; PD-1, programmed cell death protein 1; PDL1, programmed cell death ligand 1; PFS, progression-free survival; RFA, radiofrequency ablation; RT, radiation treatment; SCLC, small cell lung cancer; SRS, stereotactic radiosurgery; TKI, tyrosine kinase inhibitor; TTP, time to progression, VEGF, vascular endothelial growth factor.
^a Included patients who had oligoprogressive and polyprogressive diseases.
^b Number of patients received radiotherapy vs surgery not available.

Salama and colleagues evaluated patients with multiple histologies, including NSCLC (18%), and demonstrated of the 61 patients with OPD treated with SBRT, the 2-year PFS rate was 22.0% (95% CI, 22.8%–34.4%) and 2-year OS rate was 56.7% (95% CI, 43.9%–68.9%).[29] The other three phase II prospective studies had a combined population of 65 patients, of which a majority received RT to progressive lung metastases, reporting a 1-year PFS rate of 68.8%, median PFS of 6 to 15 months, and median OS of 20 to 43 months.[30–32]

One of the more compelling studies suggesting a role for SBRT in oligoprogressive NSCLC is the CURB trial. The CURB trial is a two-arm prospective trial of NSCLC and patients with breast cancer with fewer than five extracranial metastatic sites.[33] *Tsai and colleagues* randomized these patients 1:1 to either SBRT to all progressive sites or palliative SOC. Per their interim analysis of 102 patients (58 NSCLC and 44 patients with breast cancer), with a median follow-up of 51 weeks, they found a PFS benefit with SBRT (median PFS of 22 weeks in the SBRT arm vs 10 weeks in the palliative SOC arm; P = .005). Interestingly, the observed improvement in PFS was driven entirely by SBRT in NSCLC patients, given no difference in median PFS was observed in the breast cohort (18 weeks with SBRT vs 17 weeks with SOC; P = .5).[33] In the NSCLC cohort, median PFS was 44 weeks with SBRT versus 9 weeks with SOC (P = .004).[33] Last, they also reported that the PFS benefit in the NSCLC cohort remained when age, sex, lines of systemic therapy, and change of systemic therapy were included in the multivariable Cox model.[33]

Our literature search also identified a handful of retrospective studies on LATs in the setting of OPD. Median PFS reported from these studies ranged from 3.3 to 21.3 months from the time of LATs for OPD to further progression and median OS rates of 13 to 41 months. Lung and brain were the most common treated metastatic sites. Four of these retrospective studies compared the survival outcomes after LATs to those who were treated with systemic therapy alone and did not receive LATs. Two of the studies found significant improvement in median OS, PFS, and time to progression after LATs (P < .05),[34,35] whereas the other two comparative studies reported nominal differences in median OS and median PFS, but not of statistical significance.[15,36]

CURRENT EVIDENCE ON SURGERY AND INTERVENTIONAL ABLATION IN OLIGOPROGRESSIVE DISEASE

In addition to RT, surgery and interventional ablation represent other modalities for the treatment of OPD in NSCLC. A summary of published studies is included in **Table 2**. Metastasectomies have long been a treatment option for metastatic lesions in patients who have isolated metastases and are surgical candidates. Surgical resection not only provides an immediate reduction of disease burden but also, unlike RT, allows for sampling of the malignancy tissue for further molecular testing to help guide selection of systemic therapy. One of the earliest studies on complete resection of lung metastases examined 5206 patients with a variety of cancer primaries, found survival rates of 36% at 5 years, 26% at 10 years, and 22% at 15 years, and provided proof of the feasibility of surgery in metastatic settings.[37] The currently available data on the role of surgery in metastatic disease have been primarily on OMD and remain limited for OPD. Our literature search only identified one retrospective study on NSCLC that solely examined the role of surgery (patients receiving other forms of LAT were excluded) in OPD, demonstrating a median PFS of 7 months after metastasectomies in OPD.[38]

Interventional ablation techniques, including RFA, cryoablation, and microwave ablation (MWA), deliver concentrated heat or cold to focally induce cellular damage

Table 2
Summary of studies on surgery or interventional ablation in oligoprogressive non-small cell lung cancer

	Study Type	Number of Patients	Systemic Agent	Sites of Oligoprogression Treated with LATs(n)	Median Follow-Up (months)	Outcomes
Joosten et al.,[38] 2021	Retrospective	28 (all underwent surgery)	Chemotherapy/ immunotherapy/ targeted therapy	Lung, primary tumor (12), adrenal (11), axillary lymph node (3), liver (2)	44	Median OS "not reached" Median PFS 7 mo (6.0–25.0)
Ni et al.,[41] 2019	Retrospective	71 (43 underwent MWA and 28 RFA)	TKI	Lung (45), liver (15), adrenal (9), pleura (7), lymph node (4)	n/a	Median OS 26.4 mo (6–86) Median PFS1 (time from initiation TKI to first progression) 11.8 mo Median PFS2 (time from first progression to second progression after ablation) 10.0 mo (1–82 mo)
Jiang et al.,[40] 2018	Retrospective	24 (8 received RFA, 3 interventional therapy, and 13 RT)	TKI (erlotinib/ gefitinib/icotinib)	Liver (69)	n/a	Median OS 28.3 mo Median PFS2 (time to off-TKI progression or switching therapy failure) 13.9 mo
Yu et al.,[63] 2013	Prospective, single-arm	18 (13 underwent surgery, 2 RFA, and 3 RT)	TKI (erlotinib/ gefitinib)	Lung (15), adrenal (2), lymph node (1),	n/a	Median OS 41 mo (26 to "not reached") Median TTP 10 mo (2–27)

Abbreviations: LAT, local ablative therapy; MWA, microwave ablation; NSCLC, non-small cell lung cancer; OS, overall survival; PFS, progression-free survival; RFA, radiofrequency ablation; RT, radiation treatment; TKI, tyrosine kinase inhibitor; TTP, time to progression.

and consequently, necrosis.[39] Similar to surgery, data on thermal ablation in OPD are scarce. The two studies with a substantial number of patients in their cohort who received interventional ablation to oligoprogressive sites reported a median OS of 26.4 to 28.3 months and median PFS from 10.0 to 13.9 months.[40,41] Overall, data from prospective and randomized studies on these forms of LAT for OPD are lacking.

LIMITATIONS OF CURRENT DATA AND FUTURE DIRECTIONS

High-quality randomized data on the role of local therapies in oligoprogressive NSCLC are limited. As mentioned earlier, contemporary data on the support of LATs in OPD came mostly from retrospective studies. Also, the availability of prospective data is largely from single-arm studies without comparable controls. Data from larger multi-center studies may be needed before LATs becoming the SOC.

Despite our discussion of the possible abscopal effect from SBRT, only three studies from our literature search have examined the effect of LATs on oligoprogressive sites in conjunction with immune checkpoint inhibitors (two studies with RT and one with surgery). In addition, studies on the potential role of LATs have primarily been on NSCLC and there is a dearth of data available on oligoprogressive small cell lung cancer (SCLC). The addition of atezolizumab to chemotherapy as a novel updated SOC for extensive stage SCLC provides some opportunity to investigate the role of LAT in SCLC as well.[42] In the pre-atezolizumab era for extensive stage SCLC, *Slotman and colleagues* demonstrated an OS improvement with the addition of consolidative RT to the residual thoracic disease.[43] The addition of consolidative radiation in extensive-stage SCLC with modern-day chemotherapy and atezolizumab is currently being evaluated by the Raptor Trial (NRG-LU007; NCT04402788).[44] Other limitations include patient selection. Although the current definition of oligometastatic and oligo-progressive is based on the number of disease sites, there may be additional prognostic factors that should be taken into account when properly selecting patients for LAT. Radiation genomics, molecular profiling, biomarker expressions such as PD-L1, volume of disease, and use of novel blood markers such as circulating tumor deoxyribonucleic acid (DNA) are some tests available that should be incorporated into predictive models. The proper selection of patients for either LAT or next-line systemic therapy is important and likely depends on more than just the number of disease sites.

Presently, several large ongoing trials are evaluating the role of LAT in oligoprogressive NSCLC. The Cancer Research UK-funded HALT trial (NCT03256981) started recruitment in 2017.[45] This phase II/III trial randomized patients with advanced mutation-positive NSCLC who developed OPD 2:1 to SBRT (30–52 Gy) to sites of metastatic disease while on TKI versus continuation of TKI alone. The trial aims to recruit 110 patients, with a primary endpoint of PFS and secondary endpoints of OS, toxicity, and quality of life. In addition, there is the STOP trial (NCT02756793), which is a phase II multicenter trial that randomized NSCLC patients with OPD to the SOC therapy or SBRT to all sites of oligoprogressive lesions. SOC may include continuing with current systemic treatment, observation, or switching to next-line treatment, and palliative RT is allowed. The primary endpoint is 5-year PFS and some of the secondary endpoints are OS, quality of life, lesion control rate, and location of sites of further progression after SBRT (in the SBRT arm only). Certainly, results from these trials will further inform our treatment recommendations in the near future.

SUMMARY

The development of molecularly targeted treatments and immune checkpoint inhibitors has changed the therapeutic landscape for stage IV NSCLC. We now have a better understanding of the spectrum of metastatic disease, which has led us to deviate from the one-size-fits-all approach for all stage IV disease. There is an emerging role for RT, specifically SBRT, in the treatment of an OPD pattern in NSCLC. Recent studies suggest a median PFS of 3 to 21 months and a median OS of 13 to 43 months with the integration of LATs into systemic treatments. Despite these encouraging early findings, high-level data remain limited. Without any randomized controlled trial, we could only speculate on the effectiveness of LATs in local control for OPD, which will ultimately need to demonstrate a change in the systemic trajectory of disease and OS to cement a role in routine management.

CLINICS CARE POINTS

- Metastatic cancer represents a spectrum of diseases, including oligometastatic disease and oligoprogressive disease (OPD). OPD represents limited progression while on systemic therapy.
- There is an increasing interest in the use of local ablative therapies, such as stereotactic body radiotherapy, in addressing foci of progressing metastases for patients with OPD.
- Even though some recent retrospective data demonstrated support for the use of local ablative therapies along with systemic therapies in the management of oligoprogressive non-small cell lung cancer, large prospective randomized-controlled trials are required to further validate these findings, ideally demonstrating an improvement in overall survival from these interventions with an acceptable toxicity profile.

DISCLOSURE

The authors have nothing to disclose.

REFERENCES

1. Solomon BJ, Mok T, Kim DW, et al. First-line crizotinib versus chemotherapy in ALK-positive lung cancer. N Engl J Med 2014;371(23):2167–77.
2. Rosell R, Carcereny E, Gervais R, et al. Erlotinib versus standard chemotherapy as first-line treatment for European patients with advanced EGFR mutation-positive non-small-cell lung cancer (EURTAC): a multicentre, open-label, randomised phase 3 trial. Lancet Oncol 2012;13(3):239–46.
3. Shaw AT, Kim DW, Nakagawa K, et al. Crizotinib versus chemotherapy in advanced ALK-positive lung cancer. N Engl J Med 2013;368(25):2385–94.
4. Sequist LV, Yang JCH, Yamamoto N, et al. Phase III study of afatinib or cisplatin plus pemetrexed in patients with metastatic lung adenocarcinoma with EGFR mutations. J Clin Oncol 2013;31(27):3327–34.
5. Pao W, Miller VA, Politi KA, et al. Acquired Resistance of Lung Adenocarcinomas to Gefitinib or Erlotinib Is Associated with a Second Mutation in the EGFR Kinase Domain. Liu ET. PLoS Med 2005;2(3):e73.
6. Kobayashi S, Boggon TJ, Dayaram T, et al. EGFR mutation and resistance of non-small-cell lung cancer to gefitinib. N Engl J Med 2005;352(8):786–92.
7. Hellman S, Weichselbaum RR. Oligometastases. J Clin Oncol 1995;13(1):8–10.
8. Lievens Y, Guckenberger M, Gomez D, et al. Defining oligometastatic disease from a radiation oncology perspective: An ESTRO-ASTRO consensus document. Radiother Oncol 2020;148:157–66.

9. Andratschke N, Alheid H, Allgäuer M, et al. The SBRT database initiative of the German Society for Radiation Oncology (DEGRO): patterns of care and outcome analysis of stereotactic body radiotherapy (SBRT) for liver oligometastases in 474 patients with 623 metastases. BMC Cancer 2018;18(1):283.

10. Fleckenstein J, Petroff A, Schäfers HJ, et al. Long-term outcomes in radically treated synchronous vs. metachronous oligometastatic non-small-cell lung cancer. BMC Cancer 2016;16:348.

11. Hoyer M, Roed H, Sengelov L, et al. Phase-II study on stereotactic radiotherapy of locally advanced pancreatic carcinoma. Radiother Oncol 2005;76(1):48–53.

12. Osti MF, Carnevale A, Valeriani M, et al. Clinical outcomes of single dose stereotactic radiotherapy for lung metastases. Clin Lung Cancer 2013;14(6):699–703.

13. Stanta G, Bonin S. Overview on Clinical Relevance of Intra-Tumor Heterogeneity. Front Med 2018;5:85.

14. Rusthoven KE, Hammerman SF, Kavanagh BD, et al. Is there a role for consolidative stereotactic body radiation therapy following first-line systemic therapy for metastatic lung cancer? A patterns-of-failure analysis. Acta Oncol 2009;48(4):578–83.

15. Schmid S, Klingbiel D, Aeppli S, et al. Patterns of progression on osimertinib in EGFR T790M positive NSCLC: A Swiss cohort study. Lung Cancer 2019;130:149–55.

16. Rheinheimer S, Heussel CP, Mayer P, et al. Oligoprogressive Non-Small-Cell Lung Cancer under Treatment with PD-(L)1 Inhibitors. Cancers 2020;12(4):E1046.

17. Navarro-Martín A, Galiana I, Berenguer Frances M, et al. Preliminary Study of the Effect of Stereotactic Body Radiotherapy (SBRT) on the Immune System in Lung Cancer Patients Unfit for Surgery: Immunophenotyping Analysis. IJMS 2018;19(12):3963.

18. Golden EB, Demaria S, Schiff PB, et al. An abscopal response to radiation and ipilimumab in a patient with metastatic non-small cell lung cancer. Cancer Immunol Res 2013;1(6):365–72.

19. Ettinger DS, Wood DE, Aisner DL, et al. Non–Small Cell Lung Cancer, Version 3.2022, NCCN Clinical Practice Guidelines in Oncology. J Natl Compr Cancer Netw 2022;20(5):497–530.

20. Sahgal A, Roberge D, Schellenberg D, et al. The Canadian Association of Radiation Oncology scope of practice guidelines for lung, liver and spine stereotactic body radiotherapy. Clin Oncol 2012;24(9):629–39.

21. Theelen WSME, Chen D, Verma V, et al. Pembrolizumab with or without radiotherapy for metastatic non-small-cell lung cancer: a pooled analysis of two randomised trials. Lancet Respir Med 2021;9(5):467–75.

22. Schild SE, Wang X, Bestvina CM, et al. Alliance A082002 -a randomized phase II/III trial of modern immunotherapy-based systemic therapy with or without SBRT for PD-L1-negative, advanced non-small cell lung cancer. Clin Lung Cancer 2022;23(5):e317–20.

23. Palma DA, Olson R, Harrow S, et al. Stereotactic Ablative Radiotherapy for the Comprehensive Treatment of Oligometastatic Cancers: Long-Term Results of the SABR-COMET Phase II Randomized Trial. J Clin Oncol 2020;38(25):2830–8.

24. Palma DA, Olson R, Harrow S, et al. Stereotactic ablative radiotherapy versus standard of care palliative treatment in patients with oligometastatic cancers (SABR-COMET): a randomised, phase 2, open-label trial. Lancet 2019;393(10185):2051–8.

25. Gomez DR, Blumenschein GR, Lee JJ, et al. Local consolidative therapy versus maintenance therapy or observation for patients with oligometastatic non-small-cell lung

cancer without progression after first-line systemic therapy: a multicentre, randomised, controlled, phase 2 study. Lancet Oncol 2016;17(12):1672–82.

26. Gomez DR, Tang C, Zhang J, et al. Local Consolidative Therapy Vs. Maintenance Therapy or Observation for Patients With Oligometastatic Non–Small-Cell Lung Cancer: Long-Term Results of a Multi-Institutional, Phase II, Randomized Study. J Clin Orthod 2019;37(18):1558–65.

27. Iyengar P, Wardak Z, Gerber DE, et al. Consolidative Radiotherapy for Limited Metastatic Non–Small-Cell Lung Cancer: A Phase 2 Randomized Clinical Trial. JAMA Oncol 2018;4(1):e173501.

28. Shukuya T, Takahashi T, Naito T, et al. Continuous EGFR-TKI administration following radiotherapy for non-small cell lung cancer patients with isolated CNS failure. Lung Cancer 2011;74(3):457–61.

29. Salama JK, Hasselle MD, Chmura SJ, et al. Stereotactic body radiotherapy for multisite extracranial oligometastases: final report of a dose escalation trial in patients with 1 to 5 sites of metastatic disease. Cancer 2012;118(11):2962–70.

30. Chan OSH, Lam KC, Li JYC, et al. ATOM: A phase II study to assess efficacy of preemptive local ablative therapy to residual oligometastases of NSCLC after EGFR TKI. Lung Cancer 2020;142:41–6.

31. Weiss J, Kavanagh B, Deal A, et al. Phase II study of stereotactic radiosurgery for the treatment of patients with oligoprogression on erlotinib. Cancer Treat Res Commun 2019;19:100126.

32. Iyengar P, Kavanagh BD, Wardak Z, et al. Phase II trial of stereotactic body radiation therapy combined with erlotinib for patients with limited but progressive metastatic non-small-cell lung cancer. J Clin Oncol 2014;32(34):3824–30.

33. Tsai CJ, Yang JT, Guttmann DM, et al. Consolidative Use of Radiotherapy to Block (CURB) Oligoprogression — Interim Analysis of the First Randomized Study of Stereotactic Body Radiotherapy in Patients With Oligoprogressive Metastatic Cancers of the Lung and Breast. Int J Radiat Oncol Biol Phys 2021;111(5):1325–6.

34. Chan OSH, Lee VHF, Mok TSK, et al. The Role of Radiotherapy in Epidermal Growth Factor Receptor Mutation-positive Patients with Oligoprogression: A Matched-cohort Analysis. Clin Oncol 2017;29(9):568–75.

35. Wang Y, Li Y, Xia L, et al. Continued EGFR-TKI with concurrent radiotherapy to improve time to progression (TTP) in patients with locally progressive non-small cell lung cancer (NSCLC) after front-line EGFR-TKI treatment. Clin Transl Oncol 2018;20(3):366–73.

36. Cortellini A, Leonetti A, Catino A, et al. Osimertinib beyond disease progression in T790M EGFR-positive NSCLC patients: a multicenter study of clinicians' attitudes. Clin Transl Oncol 2020;22(6):844–51.

37. Pastorino U, Buyse M, Friedel G, et al. Long-term results of lung metastasectomy: prognostic analyses based on 5206 cases. J Thorac Cardiovasc Surg 1997;113(1):37–49.

38. Joosten PJM, de Langen AJ, van der Noort V, et al. The role of surgery in the treatment of oligoprogression after systemic treatment for advanced non-small cell lung cancer. Lung Cancer 2021;161:141–51.

39. Chu KF, Dupuy DE. Thermal ablation of tumours: biological mechanisms and advances in therapy. Nat Rev Cancer 2014;14(3):199–208.

40. Jiang T, Chu Q, Wang H, et al. EGFR-TKIs plus local therapy demonstrated survival benefit than EGFR-TKIs alone in EGFR-mutant NSCLC patients with oligometastatic or oligoprogressive liver metastases. Int J Cancer 2019;144(10):2605–12.

41. Ni Y, Liu B, Ye X, et al. Local Thermal Ablation with Continuous EGFR Tyrosine Kinase Inhibitors for EGFR-Mutant Non-small Cell Lung Cancers that Developed Extra-Central Nervous System (CNS) Oligoprogressive Disease. Cardiovasc Intervent Radiol 2019;42(5):693–9.
42. Horn L, Mansfield AS, Szczęsna A, et al. First-Line Atezolizumab plus Chemotherapy in Extensive-Stage Small-Cell Lung Cancer. N Engl J Med 2018; 379(23):2220–9.
43. Slotman BJ, van Tinteren H, Praag JO, et al. Use of thoracic radiotherapy for extensive stage small-cell lung cancer: a phase 3 randomised controlled trial. Lancet 2015;385(9962):36–42.
44. Combining Radiotherapy and Immunotherapy in Patients. Available at: https://www.rtog.org/News/Combining-Radiotherapy-and-Immunotherapy-in-Patients. Accessed September 16, 2022.
45. McDonald F, Hanna GG. Oligoprogressive Oncogene-addicted Lung Tumours: Does Stereotactic Body Radiotherapy Have a Role? Introducing the HALT Trial. Clin Oncol 2018;30(1):1–4.
46. Jordan EJ, Kim HR, Arcila ME, et al. Prospective Comprehensive Molecular Characterization of Lung Adenocarcinomas for Efficient Patient Matching to Approved and Emerging Therapies. Cancer Discov 2017;7(6):596–609.
47. Frampton GM, Ali SM, Rosenzweig M, et al. Activation of MET via diverse exon 14 splicing alterations occurs in multiple tumor types and confers clinical sensitivity to MET inhibitors. Cancer Discov 2015;5(8):850–9.
48. Dall'Olio FG, Conci N, Rossi G, et al. Comparison of Sequential Testing and Next Generation Sequencing in advanced Lung Adenocarcinoma patients – A single centre experience. Lung Cancer 2020;149:5–9.
49. Hu C, Wu S, Deng R, et al. Radiotherapy with continued EGFR-TKIs for oligoprogressive disease in EGFR-mutated non-small cell lung cancer: A real-world study. Cancer Med 2023;12(1):266–73.
50. Katz LM, Ng V, Wu SP, et al. Stereotactic Body Radiation Therapy for the Treatment of Locally Recurrent and Oligoprogressive Non-Small Cell Lung Cancer: A Single Institution Experience. Front Oncol 2022;12:870143.
51. Mok FST, Tong M, Loong HH, et al. Local ablative radiotherapy on oligoprogression while continued on epidermal growth factor receptor tyrosine kinase inhibitors in advanced non-small cell lung cancer patients: A longer cohort. Asia Pac J Clin Oncol 2022;18(6):614–24.
52. Kroeze SGC, Schaule J, Fritz C, et al. Metastasis directed stereotactic radiotherapy in NSCLC patients progressing under targeted- or immunotherapy: efficacy and safety reporting from the "TOaSTT" database. Radiat Oncol 2021; 16(1):4.
53. Wang Z, Wei L, Li J, et al. Combing stereotactic body radiotherapy with checkpoint inhibitors after oligoprogression in advanced non-small cell lung cancer. Transl Lung Cancer Res 2021;10(12):4368–79.
54. Buglione M, Jereczek-Fossa BA, Bonù ML, et al. Radiosurgery and fractionated stereotactic radiotherapy in oligometastatic/oligoprogressive non-small cell lung cancer patients: Results of a multi-institutional series of 198 patients treated with "curative" intent. Lung Cancer 2020;141:1–8.
55. Friedes C, Mai N, Fu W, et al. Isolated progression of metastatic lung cancer: Clinical outcomes associated with definitive radiotherapy. Cancer 2020; 126(20):4572–83.

56. Santarpia M, Altavilla G, Borsellino N, et al. High-dose Radiotherapy for Oligo-progressive NSCLC Receiving EGFR Tyrosine Kinase Inhibitors: Real World Data. Vivo 2020;34(4):2009–14.
57. Borghetti P, Bonù ML, Giubbolini R, et al. Concomitant radiotherapy and TKI in metastatic EGFR- or ALK-mutated non-small cell lung cancer: a multicentric analysis on behalf of AIRO lung cancer study group. Radiol Med 2019;124(7):662–70.
58. Rossi S, Finocchiaro G, Noia VD, et al. Survival outcome of tyrosine kinase inhibitors beyond progression in association to radiotherapy in oligoprogressive EGFR-mutant non-small-cell lung cancer. Future Oncol 2019;15(33):3775–82.
59. Xu Q, Liu H, Meng S, et al. First-line continual EGFR-TKI plus local ablative therapy demonstrated survival benefit in EGFR-mutant NSCLC patients with oligo-progressive disease. J Cancer 2019;10(2):522–9.
60. Merino Lara T, Helou J, Poon I, et al. Multisite stereotactic body radiotherapy for metastatic non-small-cell lung cancer: Delaying the need to start or change systemic therapy? Lung Cancer 2018;124:219–26.
61. Qiu B, Liang Y, Li Q, et al. Local Therapy for Oligoprogressive Disease in Patients With Advanced Stage Non-small-cell Lung Cancer Harboring Epidermal Growth Factor Receptor Mutation. Clin Lung Cancer 2017;18(6):e369–73.
62. Gan GN, Weickhardt AJ, Scheier B, et al. Stereotactic radiation therapy can safely and durably control sites of extra-central nervous system oligoprogressive disease in anaplastic lymphoma kinase-positive lung cancer patients receiving crizotinib. Int J Radiat Oncol Biol Phys 2014;88(4):892–8.
63. Yu HA, Sima CS, Huang J, et al. Local therapy with continued EGFR tyrosine kinase inhibitor therapy as a treatment strategy in EGFR-mutant advanced lung cancers that have developed acquired resistance to EGFR tyrosine kinase inhibitors. J Thorac Oncol 2013;8(3):346–51.
64. Weickhardt AJ, Scheier B, Burke JM, et al. Local ablative therapy of oligoprogressive disease prolongs disease control by tyrosine kinase inhibitors in oncogene-addicted non-small-cell lung cancer. J Thorac Oncol 2012;7(12):1807–14.

Advances in Radiotherapy for Breast Cancer

Rituraj Upadhyay, MD[a], Jose G. Bazan, MD, MS[b],*

KEYWORDS

- Radiotherapy • Breast cancer • Hypofractionated • Genomic assay

KEY POINTS

- Breast conservation with lumpectomy followed by adjuvant whole breast or partial breast radiation therapy is the current standard of care for most women with early breast cancer.
- Over the course of two decades, the duration of whole breast radiation has decreased from 5 to 7 weeks (25–33+ fractions) to 5 days (5 fractions) in appropriately selected patients.
- With improvements in molecular classification, biomarkers and genetics, there has been a move towards treatment de-escalation by reducing the irradiation volume and/or omission of radiation.
- Improved planning techniques, such as 3DCRT, inverse planned IMRT, and SBRT, as well as respiratory gating and improved image guidance has reduced radiation exposure to normal tissues.
- Impact of new genomic assays, proton therapy and preoperative radiation therapy, as well as role of ablative RT for patients with metastatic disease continues to evolve.

ADVANCES IN FRACTIONATION SCHEDULES
Evolution of Dose and Fractionation for Adjuvant Whole Breast Irradiation

Radiation[1] therapy (RT) is an integral component of breast conservation. Several seminal randomized trials in the late twentieth century demonstrated that breast radiotherapy following lumpectomy yielded overall survival outcomes equivalent to mastectomy for treatment of early stage invasive breast cancer[2–4] leading to National Institutes of Health consensus statement in 1991 establishing breast conservation treatment. Importantly, all these studies used adjuvant RT delivered with standard fractionation (1.8–2 Gy per fraction) over at least 5 weeks (even longer when a boost dose was delivered to the lumpectomy cavity region). These protracted courses of radiation often proved to be a barrier to successful delivery of adjuvant treatment.

[a] Department of Radiation Oncology, The Ohio State University Medical Center, The Arthur G. James Cancer Hospital D259, 460 W 10th Avenue, Columbus, OH 43210, USA; [b] Department of Radiation Oncology, The Ohio State University Medical Center, The Arthur G. James Cancer Hospital and Solove Research Institute, The Ohio State University Comprehensive Cancer Center, 1145 Olentangy River Road, Columbus, OH 43212, USA
* Corresponding author.
E-mail address: jose.bazan2@osumc.edu

Surg Oncol Clin N Am 32 (2023) 515–536
https://doi.org/10.1016/j.soc.2023.03.002
1055-3207/23/© 2023 Elsevier Inc. All rights reserved.
surgonc.theclinics.com

Hypofractionated RT (HFRT) refers to increasing the daily fraction size with a corresponding reduction in the total delivered dose and number of fractions delivered. Investigators from the United Kingdom exploited the understanding of radiation biology and hypothesized that the fractionation sensitivity for breast adenocarcinomas is close to that of normal breast tissue. Based on the linear-quadratic model, if late normal tissue effects (NTE) α/β ratios exceed the tumor α/β ratio, hypofractionation widens the therapeutic ratio by providing equivalent or lower late toxicity without losing tumor control at a constant tumor biologic effective dose.[5]

Numerous studies have aimed at reducing the treatment duration, without compromising local-regional control and without increasing acute and late toxicities. Pilot studies in the United Kingdom began in 1986[6,7] and then larger, randomized trials including START A, START B, and the Canadian hypofractionation study followed.[8–11] These studies that have recruited more than 7000 patients have established HFRT as the new standard of care for whole breast irradiation (WBI) by demonstrating no difference in local recurrence or survival, with comparable toxicity profiles. Different hypofractionated radiation regimens used in these trials commonly included 40 Gy in 15 fractions and 42.56 Gy in 16 fractions. **Table 1** summarizes the studies evaluating different RT regimens in the postlumpectomy setting.

Shortly thereafter, studies began investigating even shorter WBI regimens with ultrahypofractionation (five fractions). In this realm, the recent UK FAST study, which randomly assigned women with early stage breast cancer (pT1-2N0) to standard WBI or one of two (28.5 Gy or 30 Gy) five-fraction regimens delivered once weekly with no tumor bed boost, found the 28.5-Gy arm to have no difference in moderate or marked NTE as compared with standard WBI, although increased rates of toxicity were seen in the 30-Gy arm at a 10-year follow-up.[12] Subsequently, the FAST-Forward trial compared hypofractionated WBI with two (26 Gy or 27 Gy) five-fraction regimens delivered over 1 week (five consecutive treatment days).[13] At 5 years, the five-fraction treatment regimens were associated with a nonsignificant reduction in local recurrence, and 26-Gy and 27-Gy arms met the noninferiority criteria. In terms of NTEs, 27 Gy in five fractions was associated with worse clinician-reported marked or moderate NTE at 5 years (15.4%) versus 26 Gy in five fractions (11.9%; $P = .020$) and 40 Gy in 15 (9.9%; $P < .001$). These data do suggest that doses greater than or equal to 26 to 30 Gy in five fractions may be in the steep portion of the normal tissue complication probability curve for late cosmetic toxicity, given small changes in dose (1–1.5 Gy) were shown to be associated with worse cosmesis in follow-up. Early NTE are much less responsive to fraction size than late NTE and are more dependent on the total dose.[14] In the FAST-Forward trial, the breast erythema was less intense and occurred about 2 weeks earlier after five-fraction versus 15-fraction schedules.[15] Similarly, acute reactions were also milder in both five-fraction arms of the FAST trial than the 50-Gy arm.[16]

As these studies illustrate, over the course of two decades, the duration of WBI has gone from 5 to 7 weeks (25–33+ fractions) to 5 days (five fractions) in appropriately selected patients. ESTRO consensus guidelines state that moderate hypofractionation can be offered for nearly all patients, regardless of age and clinicopathologic factors, and that ultrahypofractionation can be offered as a standard of care or within a randomized controlled trial or prospective registration cohort.[17]

Evolution of Dose and Fractionation for Regional Nodal Irradiation/Postmastectomy Radiation Therapy

In patients undergoing mastectomy, several randomized trials and the Early Breast Cancer Trialists' Collaborative Group (EBCTCG) meta-analysis have demonstrated that women with axillary node-positive disease benefit from postmastectomy RT (PMRT) to

Table 1
Key studies of hypofractionation versus conventional fractionation after lumpectomy

Trial	Duration of Study	No. of Patients	Follow-up (y)	Radiation Dose	Local Recurrence (%)	Toxicity
Whelan (OCOG)[11]	1993–1996	1234	12	50 Gy/25 F 42.56 Gy/16 F	6.7 6.2	No significant difference in cosmetic outcomes
RMH/GOC[6,7]	1986–1998	1410	9.7	50 Gy/25 F 42.9 Gy/13 F 39 Gy/13 F	7.9 7.1 9.1	28.8% 25.6% 42% (10 y good to excellent cosmesis)
START-A[9]	1999–2002	2236	9.3	50 Gy/25 F 41.6 Gy/13 F 39 Gy/13 F (all over 5 wk)	6.7 5.6 8.1	No difference 50 Gy, 41.6 Gy with moderate or marked normal tissue effects; reduced induration/telangiectasia, edema with 39 Gy vs 50 Gy
START-B[8]	1999–2001	2215	10	50 Gy/25 F 40 Gy/15 F	5.2 3.8 (10 y)	Breast shrinkage, telangiectasia, and edema significantly lower with 40 Gy
HYPO[112]	2009–2014	1854	9	50 Gy/25 F 40 Gy/15 F	3.3 3.0	11.8% 9.0%
FAST[12]	2004–2007	915	9.9	50 Gy/25 F 30 Gy/5 F (once weekly) 28.5 Gy/5 F (once weekly)	3 LRs 4 LRs 4 LRs	Worse marked NTEs with 30 Gy compared with 50 Gy but not 28.5 Gy compared with 50 Gy
FAST-Forward[13]	2011–2014	4096	5.9	40 Gy/15 F 27 Gy/5 F 26 Gy/5 F	2.1 1.7 1.4 (5 y)	Moderate or marked NTEs 40 Gy: 9.9% 26 Gy: 11.9% 27 Gy: 15.4%

Abbreviations: F, number of fractions; LR, local recurrence.

the chest wall and regional lymphatics (supraclavicular, undissected axilla, and internal mammary nodes [IMN]).[18–21] In addition, a randomized clinical trial supported the use of regional nodal irradiation (RNI), which targets the undissected axillary nodes, supraclavicular fossa, and IMN after mastectomy or lumpectomy in patients with limited axillary nodal disease as a means to reduce the risk of distant metastases, the risk of recurrence or death, and the risk of breast cancer mortality.[22,23] Similar to the postlumpectomy setting, PMRT was also delivered with conventional fractionation (1.8–2 Gy/d to total doses of 50–50.4 Gy) in these studies. Some of the early studies evaluating HFRT in the WBI setting also included PMRT/RNI. For example, START-A and B trials included 8.3% and 14.6% patients treated with hypofractionated PMRT, respectively.[8–10]

One concern with HF-PMRT/RNI is radiation-induced brachial plexopathy. Studies done in the two-dimensional (2D) era of breast radiation reported high brachial plexopathy rates of up to 63% and 73% with hypofractionated radiation regimens that delivered a biologic effective dose of greater than 70 to 100 Gy to the brachial plexus.[24,25] As a result, most subsequent PMRT/RNI trials used conventional fractionation schedules. However, as more data emerged regarding the safety of HFRT after breast-conserving surgery (BCS), more prospective studies have re-evaluated the role of HFRT in the PMRT/RNI setting.

Wang and colleagues[26] reported a single institution randomized noninferiority trial of HF PMRT in 810 patients, either T3-4 and/or N2-3, randomized to receive 43.5 Gy in 15 fractions over 3 weeks versus the standard 50 Gy in 25 fractions over 5 weeks. The HF arm was noninferior with a 5-year locoregional recurrence rate of 8.3% compared with 8.1% in the conventional RT group (hazard ratio, 1.10; $P < 0.0001$ for noninferiority).[26] Of note, none of these patients had a breast reconstruction, and they did not target the IMN chain, which is standardly included as part of the radiation target volumes for PMRT/RNI. A recent phase II prospective bi-institutional study by Khan and colleagues[27] evaluated an HF-PMRT dose of 36.63 Gy in 11 fractions to the chest wall and the draining regional lymph nodes, with an optional mastectomy scar boost of 3.33 Gy for four fractions in 69 patients. IMN irradiation was not required but was included in 54% patients, and 61% patients had breast reconstruction. The authors reported a low toxicity rate with acceptable local control (5-year local regional recurrence of 4.6%). There were no grade 3 toxicities, and 24% grade 2 skin toxicities. However, in terms of patients that underwent reconstruction, about 24% of patients had an implant failure or loss, whereas 8% of patients had unplanned surgical correction.

Brachial plexopathy is becoming increasingly rare with modern radiation planning techniques and recent studies report rates of plexopathy close to 1% or less.[6,28] There was only one reported case of brachial plexopathy in the START trials and none in the other two previously mentioned prospective studies. A meta-analysis and systematic review by Liu and colleagues included nearly 4000 postmastectomy patients and concluded that HFRT was not significantly different in either efficacy or toxicity compared with conventional RT.[29] Relative to the intact breast setting, there remains a paucity of randomized data comparing HF PMRT/RNI with conventional fractionation, especially in patients who undergo breast reconstruction. The results from the recently accrued ALLIANCE A221505 trial (RT CHARM, NCT03414970), which is comparing 42.56 Gy in 16 fractions with 50 Gy in 25 fractions in patients undergoing mastectomy with immediate or delayed reconstruction, will provide more answers in the near future.

RADIATION TREATMENT DE-ESCALATION

In addition to the large move toward HFRT schedules for the delivery of adjuvant WBI or PMRT/RNI, improvements in surgical techniques, systemic therapy, and the recognition of various molecular/biologic subtypes of breast cancer, there has been a similar move toward de-escalation of RT in certain clinical scenarios by either reducing the target volume for irradiation and/or omission of radiation altogether. We review these advances in greater detail in this section.

Partial Breast Irradiation

Although hypofractionation after lumpectomy offers to shorten the duration of radiation while maintaining similar efficacy, another way to minimize toxicity (and improve the therapeutic ratio) is to limit the volume of irradiation. It has been observed that most relapses are in the vicinity of tumor bed, especially within 1 cm of the resection margin.[30,31] This has led to a gradual shift in the treatment paradigm from WBI to partial breast radiation (PBI), that is, reducing the radiation fields from the entire breast to a margin around the lumpectomy cavity. With evolving radiation technologies, several PBI techniques have been evaluated including external beam irradiation (three-dimensional [3D] conformal RT [3D-CRT] or intensity-modulated irradiation [IMRT]), intraoperative radiotherapy (IORT), and interstitial or applicator-based brachytherapy. Multiple randomized clinical trials comparing PBI with WBI have been completed with results summarized in **Table 2**.

Overall, the studies comparing brachytherapy or external beam accelerated PBI (APBI) methods with WBI have demonstrated low and essentially equivalent rates of local-regional recurrences with a toxicity profile that favors APBI.[32–36] However, patient selection is of utmost importance for patients receiving APBI. For example, the NSABP B39/RTOG 0413 trial was designed to test the hypothesis that APBI could replace WBI for all patients with breast cancer and therefore enrolled patients with high-risk of local-regional recurrences: younger patients, estrogen receptor (ER)-negative disease, tumors larger than 2 cm, and axillary node-positive disease. This study demonstrated that for the entire population of patients, APBI could not replace WBI because although the difference in Loco-regional recurrence (LRR) was only 0.7% (4.6% vs 3.9%), the hazard ratio for LRR did not meet its prespecified noninferiority criteria.[38] In addition, the recurrence-free interval was significantly worse with APBI than WBI. However, for patients with low-risk invasive disease as defined by the American Society for Radiation Oncology APBI suitable group criteria (size ≤2 cm, ER-positive, ductal histology, node-negative, age ≥50 years old),[39] there was no difference in LRR between APBI and WBI (2.7% vs 2.3%).[38]

However, the results of APBI using IORT methods, either with electrons as in the ELIOT study or low-energy photons in the TARGIT-A study, have demonstrated higher rates of LRR compared with WBI.[40,41] However, these higher but still low risks of in-breast recurrence with IORT must be balanced against the convenience of the treatments in that patients complete surgery and RT on the same day. In addition, there is minimal acute toxicity with IORT and specifically, no radiation dermatitis. In addition, there has been a consistent demonstration of reduced breast cancer mortality in the TARGIT-A IORT group compared with the WBI group. In addition to appropriate patient selection (low-risk invasive disease), these other factors should be considered in patients that have IORT as an option for APBI.

Another important observation is that the fractionation schedule with external-beam APBI seems to have an impact on toxicity and cosmesis. The two largest North American trials of external-beam APBI, RAPID and NSABP B39, both of which delivered APBI to a dose of 38.5 Gy given in 10 fractions of 3.85 Gy, twice per day, have shown conflicting results regarding toxicity and cosmesis. The RAPID study demonstrated a significantly higher rate of late toxicity and significantly higher rate of poor cosmetic outcome rated by patients and providers with twice daily APBI compared with

Table 2
Key randomized studies comparing partial breast irradiation with whole breast irradiation

Trial	Enrollment	No. of Patients	Follow-up	Radiation Dose	LR (%)	Toxicity
Hungary	1998–2004	258	10.2	APBI: 36.4 Gy/7 F (brachy) WBI: 50 Gy/25 F with boost	5.9 5.1	Improved cosmesis with APBI (81% vs 63%)
GEC-ESTRO[36]	2004–2009	1184	6.6	APBI: 32 Gy/8 F (HDR) or 30.3 Gy/7 F (HDR) or 50 Gy (PDR)/interstitial WBI: 50–50.4 Gy/25–28 F with boost	1.4 0.9	Reduced late-grade 2–3 skin toxicity with APBI
U Florence[34]	2005–2013	520	10.7	APBI: 30 Gy/5 F QOD IMRT WBI: 50 Gy/25 F with boost	3.7 2.5	Less acute and chronic toxicity with APBI
NSABP-B39/RTOG 0413[38]	2005–2013	4216	10.2	APBI: 38.5/10 F/BID 3DCRT or 34 Gy/10 F/BID Brachytherapy WBI: 50 Gy/25 F with boost	4.6 3.9	Grade 3 toxicity: 10% APBI vs 7% WBI
RAPID[37]	2006–2011	2135	8.6	APBI: 38.5 Gy/10 F/BID WBI: 50 Gy/25 F or 42.6 Gy/16 F	3.0 2.8	Increased late toxicity with APBI (32% vs 13%) and worse cosmesis with APBI
DBCG[113]	2009–2016	865	7.6	APBI: 40 Gy/15 F WBI: 40 Gy/15F	1.2 0.7	Less breast induration with APBI
IMPORT LOW[33]	2007–2010	2018	6.2	APBI: 40 Gy/15F WBI: 40 Gy/15 F 36 Gy/15 F (with 40 Gy/15 F to the partial breast volume)	0.5 1.1 0.2	Improved breast appearance with PBI and less firmness with PBI and reduced dose WBI relative to standard WBI
ELIOT[40]	2000–2007	1305	12.4	APBI: 21 Gy/1 F (electron IORT) WBI: 50 G/25 F with boost	12.6 2.4	No data collected on long-term adverse events
TARGIT[41]	2000–2012	3451	2.5	APBI: 20 Gy/1 F (kV IORT) WBI: 40–56 Gy ± boost	3.3 1.3	Wound complications similar but less grade 3–4 skin complications with IORT ~15% of IORT patients received WBI

Abbreviations: APBI, accelerated partial breast irradiation; BID, twice daily; F, number of fractions; HDR, high dose rate brachytherapy; IORT, intraoperative radiation therapy; PDR, pulse dose rate brachytherapy; QOD, every other day.

WBI,[37] although these observations were not seen in the NSABP B39 trial.[38,42] However, the University of Florence trial, which delivered 30 Gy in five fractions given once per day on nonconsecutive days, and the UK IMPORT LOW and Danish British Cooperative Group APBI trials, both of which used 40 Gy in 15 fractions given once per day, all show lower rates of acute and late toxicities, particularly breast firmness/induration and better cosmesis with APBI compared with WBI.

In summary, APBI represents a move forward for breast RT, and should be considered as an option in the appropriate patient population, namely those with stage I, ER-positive, lymph node–negative disease in patients 50 years old or older. Although we are likely to never have randomized trials designed to compare the different PBI methods and/or fractionation schedules, it seems that delivering the PBI with once-daily fractionation is convenient for patients and is associated with low rates of toxicity and favorable cosmesis. IORT remains an option to deliver PBI, but patients should understand that the data clearly show a higher risk of in-breast recurrence compared with WBI.

Biomarker-Guided Omission of Radiation Therapy After Breast-Conserving Surgery

One of the evolving questions faced by oncologists is the indications for omitting adjuvant radiation following BCS. The low rates of local recurrence seen in many of these APBI studies brought up the question of omission of RT in appropriately selected patients. Several studies have aimed at identifying women with early breast cancer who did not derive a significant benefit from RT. Initial studies failed to identify any consistent subset of such patients.[43] The EBCTCG meta-analysis further reinforced the value to breast RT postlumpectomy by demonstrating a small, but consistent increase in breast cancer mortality when breast radiotherapy was omitted after BCS.[44] Subsequently, long-term outcomes from two randomized trials (the CALGB 9343 and PRIME II trials) demonstrated increased rates of local recurrence with no impact on survival when radiation was omitted after lumpectomy in women greater than or equal to 70 years and greater than or equal to 65 years, respectively.[45,46] These studies were done in an era where the standard of care for adjuvant irradiation after lumpectomy was WBI, often over 5 to 6.5 weeks. As demonstrated previously, the field has changed to either shorter courses of WBI delivered over 1 to 3 weeks or PBI, delivered over 1 to 5 days. Therefore, incorporating the results of these older studies into modern practice is challenging given that the inconvenience of adjuvant RT is much less. Nonetheless, consideration of omission of RT in elderly women with stage I, ER-positive, lymph node–negative disease that are committed to endocrine therapy remains a standard of care option.

Recent focus on use of biomarkers and genetics for guiding adjuvant systemic therapy decision making has identified Oncotype DX recurrence score (RS) to reliably predict the risk of distant metastasis and chemotherapy benefit in patients with node-negative hormone-sensitive breast cancer receiving endocrine treatment.[47] The recently reported LUMINA study was a single-arm prospective study that evaluated omission of RT in women greater than or equal to 55 years old with grade 1 to 2 tumors that were less than or equal to 2 cm in size, surgical margins greater than or equal to 1 mm, lymph node–negative, and had a low proliferative index (Ki67 ≤13.25%) and found that the 5-year risk of local-regional recurrence in the 727 patients enrolled was extremely low at 2.3%.[48] Although Ki67 may be adequate to identify low-risk tumors, several studies have demonstrated that genomic assays, such as the Oncotype RS, are also prognostic for local-regional recurrence.[49,50] With this information, numerous prospective studies are underway evaluating the use of clinicopathologic factors and assays, such as the Oncotype RS, to better identify low-risk patients in whom adjuvant breast RT may be safely omitted. One such trial, the NRG Oncology BR007 study entitled De-Escalation of Breast Radiation (DEBRA) for hormone-sensitive, HER-2-negative patients with oncotype RS of less than or equal to 18, is evaluating whether omission of radiation can be expanded to a broader group of younger women, aged 50 to 69 years old (NCT04852887).[51] Other similar ongoing trials evaluating RT exclusion in stage I, ER-positive, lymph node–negative tumors include the randomized (adjuvant radiation vs omission) EXPERT trial for patients greater than or equal to 50 years old with stage I, grade 1 to 2, ER-positive disease and a Prosigna (PAM50) assay indicating luminal A subtype with low risk of recurrence (NCT02889874), the single-arm prospective IDEA trial for women between 50 and 69 years with Oncotype DX score less than or equal to 18 (NCT02400190), and the single-arm PRECISION trial for women between 50 and 75 years with T1 tumors and a low-risk by the PAM50 molecular profile (NCT02653755).

Another clinical scenario in which genomic assays are being used to personalize radiation decisions includes patients with ductal carcinoma in situ (DCIS) that have undergone lumpectomy. In patients with DCIS, meta-analysis of the classic randomized trials has demonstrated a greater than 50% relative reduction in in-breast tumor recurrences with radiation but no decrease in breast cancer mortality and no improvement in overall survival.[39] As a result, several studies have used clinicopathologic features to identify a low-risk group of patients with DCIS (grade 1–2; size <2.5 cm; margin width >3 mm) that may have sufficiently low risk of recurrence such that adjuvant RT may be safely omitted.[29,52] Since then, genomic assays have been developed to individualize the risk of recurrence for patients with DCIS to help them make informed decisions regarding adjuvant treatment. The DCIS Score is a prognostic assay that has been validated in several cohorts and DCIS RT is a prognostic and predictive assay that is used for personalization of care.[31,53,54]

Biomarker-Guided Omission of Regional Nodal Irradiation in Node-Positive Breast Cancer

wAs previously mentioned, the preponderance of data supports that patients with low-volume disease in the axilla derive a benefit from RNI/PMRT because most patients in these studies had only one to three positive axillary nodes. However, just as is the case with adjuvant RT in the node-negative setting, there may be subgroups of patients that may derive little benefit from RNI after lumpectomy or PMRT in the setting of mastectomy. Although most patients with lymph node–positive high-risk breast cancer subtypes, such as triple negative (ER-/PR-/HER2-) breast cancer (TNBC) and HER2-positive breast cancer will receive systemic therapy before surgery, most patients with node-positive ER-positive/HER2-negative breast cancer will undergo surgery first. In addition to the Oncotype RS being prognostic for LRR in patients with node-negative disease, several studies have showed that the oncotype RS can also risk stratify patients at highest risk for LRR in the node-positive setting.[55,56] In addition, recent data from the RxPONDER clinical trial demonstrate extremely low rates of LRR in patients with node-positive disease, regardless of receipt of RNI/PMRT with 5-year rates of LRR less than 1% in patients treated with lumpectomy without RNI and less than 2% in patients treated with mastectomy without PMRT.[57] With these data in mind, the Canadian Cancer Trials Group recently initiated TAILOR RT/MA.39 trial, which is randomizing lumpectomy or mastectomy patients with one to three nodal macrometastases or micrometastases, or those who are pT3N0, with Oncotype DX RS less than or equal to 25, to receipt of RNI versus not, with a goal of determining whether RNI/PMRT can be safely omitted in these low-risk patients (NCT03488693).

In patients that have node-positive disease (cN1) and are treated with neoadjuvant systemic therapy, observational data support that those who convert to pathologically lymph node–negative disease (ypN0) have low rates of LRR.[58] However, current practice is to make treatment recommendations based on initial nodal status, which implies that nearly all node-positive patients receive adjuvant RNI/PMRT. The NSABP B51/RTOG 1304 phase 3 trial is using nodal response to chemotherapy as a biomarker to evaluate whether the addition of RNI/PMRT is necessary in patients with cT1-3 cN1 disease at baseline that convert to ypN0 disease at the time of surgery (NCT01872975). Patients treated with lumpectomy will be randomized to breast-only radiation versus breast plus RNI, whereas those treated with mastectomy will be randomized to PMRT versus no PMRT. The primary end point is 5-year invasive breast cancer recurrence-free interval with a superiority margin of 4.6% and a planned sample size of 1636 patients, with results expected in the near future.

TECHNOLOGICAL ADVANCES IN RADIATION THERAPY DELIVERY

Parallel with the move toward hypofractionation, ultrahypofractionation, and omission of RT, there has been a significant revolution in the technology available to plan and deliver RT. The entire field has shifted from a 2D anatomic landmark-based approach to design radiation fields toward 3D computed tomography (CT)-based radiation planning with improved delivery techniques, such as 3DCRT using multileaf collimators to design fields, inverse planned IMRT (iIMRT), volumetric modulated arc radiotherapy (VMAT), and stereotactic body RT (SBRT). Respiratory gating and improved image guidance during treatment delivery including real-time on-board imaging with cone beam CT capabilities further aid radiation oncology to improve targeting and reduce radiation to normal tissue during treatment delivery. However, the field has been slow to fully embrace many of these technologies for patients with breast cancer. Although the reasons for this slow adoption are unclear, some possibilities include that the cancer control outcomes of patients with breast cancer are excellent with traditional techniques that were used in many of the earlier randomized trials and the lack of contouring guidelines for targets in whole/partial breast and RNI/PMRT. In addition, given the large volume of patients receiving adjuvant breast radiotherapy in most practices, the increased workload and time spent to plan and deliver these treatments may have had a negative impact on the uptake of 3D-based planning for breast cancer. With some of these considerations in mind, the thought leaders in the early part of the twentieth century recognized that the first step was creating a resource for contouring targets and organs-at-risk (OARs).

Contouring Atlases

The first breast contouring atlas to be developed was initiated by investigators in the RTOG, now part of NRG Oncology. These investigators recognized the atlas was necessary to develop a systematic consensus of target volume definitions, not only for achieving consistency in breast radiation treatment, but also in the context of prospective clinical trials, to ensure the differences in the comparator arms are not caused by differences in the quality of the breast RT. The RTOG Breast Cancer Atlas was developed in 2009[59] and forms the basis of the contouring definitions across many ongoing and completed clinical trials (NCT01349322, NCT01872975, NCT03414970, NCT03488693, NCT04852887). Since that time, several other atlases have been developed including the European Society for Radiation Oncology (ESTRO) breast atlas and the RADCOMP atlas.[60,61] Although each of these atlases are slightly different and contain their own strengths and weaknesses, these form a major step forward for breast RT. Bazan and Khan recently performed a comprehensive review of target volume delineation and contemporary patterns of recurrence.[62]

Improvements in Radiation Planning Techniques

CT-based planning and field-shaping with Multi-leaf collimators (MLCs) enabled improvements in conformality of radiation dose delivery. The technique of creating multiple field-in-fields to reduce hotspots within the breast has been termed forward-planned IMRT/3DCRT. Randomized studies of forward-planned IMRT compared with 2D techniques demonstrated a significantly lower incidence of acute toxicities (31% vs 48%).[63,64] In addition, significantly fewer patients develop moderate or marked photographic changes in breast appearance with forward-planned IMRT compared with 2D (40% vs 58%).[65]

iIMRT is an advancement in treatment delivery that uses a cost function to optimize beam angles and the fluence of the beam at each angle thereby resulting in dose distributions that optimally conform to the target volume and reduce high-dose radiation to adjacent OARs and has become the standard of care technique in a multitude of disease sites including carcinomas of the prostate and head and neck, where critical OARs are in close proximity to the target.[66,67] iIMRT may have advantages in patients with left-sided breast cancers where radiation dose to the heart is of concern.

In terms of patients receiving APBI, the University of Florence study treated all APBI patients to a dose of 3000 cGy given in five fractions on nonconsecutive days with iIMRT.[34] The low rates of acute toxicity and excellent cosmetic results seen in this trial supports iIMRT for this indication. Since that publication, the group has transitioned from iIMRT to VMAT, a form of rotational iIMRT where continuous arcs are used to deliver radiation.[68] The authors again demonstrate low rates of toxicity with only 32% of patients developing grade 1 acute toxicity and no patients with grade greater than 1 toxicity in the acute or late setting. In the study, 98% of patients had excellent or good cosmesis according to physician assessment.

Although the Florence data do provide solid support for iIMRT or VMAT in patients receiving APBI, the reality is that most patients receiving WBI or APBI are effectively treated with 3DCRT. The situation in which dose to OARs, particularly the heart and ipsilateral lung, becomes challenging is in patients receiving RNI/PMRT. In certain situations, iIMRT may be needed to maintain target volume coverage, including the IMN, and keep dose to the heart and lung at acceptable limits. The RTOG 1304/NSABP B51 study was the first study of RNI/PMRT that used the RTOG Breast atlas to guide the target volume contour definitions and also provided planning objectives for the target volumes and dose constraints for OARs. In 2017, we first published our treatment planning algorithm for RNI/PMRT, which defaults to 3DCRT but then transitions to iIMRT when acceptable 3DCRT plans cannot be created.[69] In this study, we demonstrated that it was feasible to meet the RTOG 1304/NSABP B51 constraints, particularly the most critical constraints of mean heart dose less than or equal to 5 Gy and ipsilateral lung V20 Gy less than or equal to 35%, but iIMRT was associated with a significantly higher rate of deviations from OAR constraints that involved low radiation dose (eg, V5Gy to the ipsilateral lung, V4Gy to the contralateral breast).[69]

In 2019, investigators from the Memorial Sloan Kettering Cancer Center reported results of a prospective phase I study of iIMRT used to deliver PMRT in 104 patients.[70] Although the results met the primary objective of feasibility of meeting dose-volume constraints to targets and OARs, this was primarily because the constraint for mean heart dose OAR was set excessively high (mean heart dose $\leq$20 Gy). As a result, the mean heart dose for all patients on the study was 11.7 Gy (13 Gy for left-sided and 10 Gy for right-sided patients). In addition, the 5-year local-regional failure rate was high at 6.8%.

In 2020, we reported results of toxicities and clinical outcomes of our approach to RNI/PMRT that defaults to 3DCRT but allows for iIMRT adoption when OAR constraints could not be met with 3DCRT.[71] This study included 240 node-positive patients with breast cancer treated with RNI/PMRT from 2013 to 2016, 70% of whom received 3DCRT and the remainder received iIMRT. All target volumes were according the RTOG Breast atlas. The mean heart dose for 3DCRT patients was 1.7 Gy, and for iIMRT patients it was 3.8 Gy, much lower than the 11.7 Gy reported by Ho and colleagues.[70] The 5-year cumulative incidence of local-regional recurrence was low at 2.8% with IMRT and 1.8% with 3DCRT. These data provide reassurance that iIMRT maintains the therapeutic ratio by preserving cancer control outcomes without excess toxicity when 3DCRT fails to meet OAR constraints.[71]

Techniques to Mitigate Cardiac (and Other) Toxicities

The late cardiac effects of radiation remain a major concern for breast cancer survivors given the excellent long-term prognosis of these patients. In 2013, this concern was brought into focus when Darby and colleagues[72] reported that each additional increase in 1 Gy of mean heart dose exposure corresponded to a 7.4% increase in major coronary events in a population-based study involving 2100 women with breast cancer. Several other studies have shown similar findings, reporting that the cumulative risk of cardiac events peaks at 5 to 15 years after treatment.[73,74] Most of these studies are from an era when CT-based planning was not used. A recent systematic review has demonstrated that mean heart doses have declined from 13.3 Gy in the 1970s to 4.7 Gy in the 1990s, to 2.6 Gy between 2014 and 2017.[74–76] With more information about the importance of cardiac exposure, several treatment planning and delivery techniques have helped design radiation fields avoiding exposure to the heart, including the reduction of treatment volumes via PBI and alterations in patient immobilization, including prone positioning as discussed previously and deep inspiration breath hold (DIBH) techniques.

In most patients, DIBH results in an inferior and posterior displacement of the heart such that the heart lies significantly further away from the chest wall resulting in lower dose to the heart.[77,78] A DIBH CT scan is obtained at the time of CT simulation for radiation planning and treatment delivery is performed with the patient holding their breath. The DIBH scan may be obtained via voluntary breath hold technique or an invasive, spirometry-based technique.[79] In a study that compared both types of DIBH techniques, patients and therapists preferred the voluntary DIBH method.[80,81] Although DIBH is most commonly used for patients with left-sided cancers receiving WBI, APBI, or RNI/PMRT, there may also be some advantages for patients with right-sided breast cancer receiving RNI/PMRT in terms of reduction in dose to the ipsilateral lung and liver.[82]

Prone breast radiation techniques are being increasingly used as a consequence of its favorable effects on the dose to the OARs, especially the skin, ipsilateral lung, and the heart.[83–85] The reduced OAR doses result in significantly lower rates of moist desquamation and high rates of good/excellent cosmesis in patients with large, pendulous breasts.[83,85] One common misconception is that prone RT use should be exclusive to patients with large, pendulous breasts. However, as Taylor and colleagues[74] demonstrated, increased radiation dose to the lung is associated with extremely high rates of lung cancer–related mortality in smokers. We have demonstrated a mean total lung dose of 0.62 Gy for patients undergoing prone WBI, which is significantly lower than the 3.9 Gy for patients receiving supine WBI.[86] Therefore, prone positioning is an effective technique that reduces dose to OARs in nearly all patients, regardless of breast size. In addition, RNI is effectively done in the prone position, and also results in lower total lung dose and heart dose compared with supine DIBH.[87,88] Although data are limited, prone RNI with use of DIBH is worthy of further investigation.[89-91]

FUTURE DIRECTIONS
New Genomic Assays

Several newer molecular scoring systems integrate patient- and disease-related clinical features with biomarkers and gene signatures. One novel example is the genomic-adjusted RT dose (GARD) score, which uses the gene expression–based radiosensitivity index and the linear quadratic model to determine the personalized radiosensitivity of the tumor. GARD score has been shown to be an independent predictor of RT-specific outcomes and is able to estimate the probability for relapse- and distant metastasis-free survival.[92] This can prove to be a future segue to consider omission of adjuvant regional nodal radiation in ER-positive/HER2-negative patients with a low risk score for locoregional and distant relapse. GARD score of greater than or equal to 21 has been shown to be associated with local control following whole breast or PMRT in TNBC patients, and an individualized dose range by modeling RT dose effect with GARD has been proposed.[93]

Proton Therapy

The unique physical properties of protons makes their potential use attractive for patients with breast cancer, especially with reducing radiation dose to OARs, such as the heart. However, although dosimetric studies have shown advantages of protons in patients with breast cancer,[94,95] clinical results have been underwhelming and have demonstrated excess toxicity not seen with modern photon-based techniques. For example, Fattahi and colleagues[96] demonstrated an exceedingly high rib fracture rate of 21% in patients with inflammatory breast cancer receiving proton-based PMRT. In addition, Galland-Girodet and coworkers[97] found high rates of fibrosis, telangectasias, and unacceptable cosmesis in patients undergoing proton-based APBI. However, more recent studies using additional treatment fields have shown better results.[98,99] At this time, until results of randomized comparisons of protons to photons demonstrate a significant advantage to proton therapy, the use of protons for breast cancer should be considered investigational especially given that prone RT for APBI/WBI and supine DIBH techniques result in excellent clinical outcomes with minimal dose to OARs. In particular, the RADCOMP consortium RTOG 3510 trial, which is a multicenter study randomizing patients with nonmetastatic breast cancer requiring locoregional RT, including IMNs to receive proton versus photon RT, over standard fractionated, 5 to 7 weeks of treatment is currently enrolling, and aims to assess effectiveness of protons in reducing major cardiovascular events (NCT02603341).

Preoperative Radiation Therapy

With the advent and advancement of APBI techniques, recent studies evaluating preoperative RT targeting the primary tumor have emerged. Preoperative APBI can potentially downstage the tumor and reduce treatment volumes, while avoiding postoperative hypoxia (a factor known to promote radioresistance) and has been shown to be feasible with low postoperative complication rate, limited fibrosis, and good to excellent cosmetic outcomes.[100–102] Nichols and colleagues[102] evaluated preoperative 3D-conformal APBI 38.5 Gy in 10 twice-daily fractions in 27 patients with less than 3 cm, node-negative tumors with BCS greater than 21 days after RT. Furthermore, preoperative RT can facilitate combined oncologic and reconstructive surgery because it may reduce the shrinkage of transferred tissue and affect perfusion or contracture around implants.[103] A recent prospective study conducted by the National Health Service in the United Kingdom evaluated preoperative primary radiation (40 Gy in 15 fractions to the breast ± RNI) and deep inferior epigastric perforator flap reconstruction for patients requiring mastectomy and postmastectomy radiotherapy.[104] Patients underwent skin-sparing mastectomy with reconstruction 2 to 6 weeks after completion of radiation. The authors found that the preoperative RT was feasible and technically safe with similar rates of breast open wounds as in patients receiving postoperative radiation. Future randomized studies may determine whether preoperative APBI or preoperative RT in patients undergoing reconstruction will move forward as a new treatment option.

Radiation Therapy for Metastatic Disease

The role of RT for patients with metastatic breast cancer continues to evolve. Much enthusiasm was garnered for using SBRT to ablate metastases in patients with limited (oligometastatic) metastatic disease. However, the NRG BR002 randomized phase II trial demonstrated no improvement in progression-free survival with SBRT compared with systemic therapy alone (NCT02364557).[105] In particular, the development of new metastases outside of the index lesions was the same in both arms of the study at approximately 40% essentially refuting the hypothesis that oligometastatic breast cancer can be managed as a local disease.

As new trial data continue to emerge, immunotherapy is finding a significant role in the treatment of many solid tumors, although its efficacy in breast cancer seems to be modest, perhaps because of lower immunogenicity and mutational burden of many breast cancers.[106] Given the immunostimulatory effects of radiation, few studies have identified that SBRT may synergize with immunotherapy. A phase I trial evaluated SBRT followed by pembrolizumab in 73 patients, and found the combination to be safe, with an overall survival of 17.8 months in patients with a complete or partial local response compared with 9.1 months in stable disease, and 3.4 months in progressive local disease.[107] This suggests that cytoreduction in the advanced tumor population improved outcomes. A challenge that remains in moving forward with RT and immunotherapy combinations is that there are many different modalities, doses, and fractionation schemes that may affect immunologic changes in the tumor microenvironment differently. Multiple trials assessing the combination of SBRT and immunotherapy are currently ongoing including the P-RAD study that aims to evaluate the optimal immunogenic dose of RT in patients with early stage TNBC or high-risk hormone receptor–positive breast cancer who will be randomized to no, low (9 Gy), or moderate-dose (24 Gy in three fractions) RT followed by treatment with pembrolizumab/chemotherapy (NCT04443348). Another ongoing Australian trial is testing single fraction of 20-Gy SBRT and pembrolizumab for oligometastatic breast cancers (NCT02303366).

Another area of interest is the use of SBRT for patients that have metastatic breast cancer with progression in only a limited number of sites with a hypothesis that SBRT to the progressing lesions can be used as opposed to changing systemic therapy. However, the CURB trial from Memorial Sloan Kettering Cancer Center showed no benefit to this approach in patients with breast cancer. However, two-thirds of the patients with breast cancer had TNBC, a disease in which effective systemic therapies are lacking after progression. Whether the approach to ablate oligoprogressive lesions in subsets of patients with ER-positive/HER2-negative and/or HER2-positive disease, where there are many effective systemic therapies available, may be worthy of future study. The AVATAR study is currently evaluating this question in patients with ER-positive/HER2-negative breast cancer.[108]

Lastly, patients with metastatic breast cancer often benefit from palliative RT. Integration of palliative RT with systemic therapy remains a challenge, particularly for agents that have been developed in the past decade, such as the CDK4/6 inhibitors, and more recently, the antibody drug conjugate molecule fam-trastuzumab deruxtecan-nxki (Enhertu). Case reports of the CDK4/6 inhibitors demonstrated significant toxicities when administered concurrent with palliative RT.[109–111] However, more recent retrospective data suggest it may be safe to administer these agents with palliative RT. However, Enhertu, which is an effective treatment of HER2-positive breast cancer and HER2-negative breast cancer with low HER2 expression, is associated with risk of fatal pneumonitis, and therefore, more studies are needed to determine timing of palliative RT relative to Enhertu, particularly when lung tissue will be exposed to the radiation (eg, in the case with treatment of thoracic vertebral metastases or lung metastases).

SUMMARY

Breast cancer RT has seen significant advancements over the past 20 years with the development of hypofractionated and ultrahypofractionated courses of RT, standardization of target volume definitions, and planning objectives to ensure radiation quality, improved treatment and delivery techniques, use of genomic assays to better inform patient selection for omission of radiation, and a better understanding of the role of RT in patients with metastatic disease. In the next 10 years, we anticipate that the field will see an even better understanding of appropriate candidates for ultrahypofractionated radiation regimens, particularly in patients with nodal disease; improved understanding of patterns of failure and toxicities with modern radiation planning; further clarification of the role of proton therapy; and continued evolution of the role of ablative therapies in metastatic disease.

CLINICS CARE POINTS

- Breast cancer RT has seen significant advancements over the past 20 years with the development of hypofractionated and ultrahypofractionated courses of RT, standardization of target volume definitions, and planning objectives to ensure radiation quality, improved treatment and delivery techniques, use of genomic assays to better inform patient selection for omission of radiation, and a better understanding of the role of RT in patients with metastatic disease.

- In the next 10 years, we anticipate that the field will see an even better understanding of appropriate candidates for ultrahypofractionated radiation regimens, particularly in patients with nodal disease; improved understanding of patterns of failure and toxicities with modern radiation planning; further clarification of the role of proton therapy; and continued evolution of the role of ablative therapies in metastatic disease.

CONFLICTS OF INTEREST

The authors have no relevant conflicts to disclose.

FUNDING

No funding relevant to this work.

REFERENCES

1. Siegel RL, Miller KD, Fuchs HE, et al. Cancer statistics, 2022. CA Cancer J Clin 2022;72:7–33.
2. Fisher B, Anderson S, Bryant J, et al. Twenty-year follow-up of a randomized trial comparing total mastectomy, lumpectomy, and lumpectomy plus irradiation for the treatment of invasive breast cancer. N Engl J Med 2002;347:1233–41.
3. van Dongen JA, Voogd AC, Fentiman IS, et al. Long-term results of a randomized trial comparing breast-conserving therapy with mastectomy: European Organization for Research and Treatment of Cancer 10801 trial. J Natl Cancer Inst 2000;92:1143–50.
4. Veronesi U, Cascinelli N, Mariani L, et al. Twenty-year follow-up of a randomized study comparing breast-conserving surgery with radical mastectomy for early breast cancer. N Engl J Med 2002;347:1227–32.
5. Brand DH, Yarnold JR. The linear-quadratic model and implications for fractionation. Clin Oncol 2019;31:673–7.
6. Owen JR, Ashton A, Bliss JM, et al. Effect of radiotherapy fraction size on tumour control in patients with early-stage breast cancer after local tumour excision: long-term results of a randomised trial. Lancet Oncol 2006;7:467–71.
7. Yarnold J, Ashton A, Bliss J, et al. Fractionation sensitivity and dose response of late adverse effects in the breast after radiotherapy for early breast cancer: long-term results of a randomised trial. Radiother Oncol 2005;75:9–17.
8. Group ST, Bentzen SM, Agrawal RK, et al. The UK Standardisation of Breast Radiotherapy (START) Trial B of radiotherapy hypofractionation for treatment of early breast cancer: a randomised trial. Lancet 2008;371:1098–107.
9. Group ST, Bentzen SM, Agrawal RK, et al. The UK Standardisation of Breast Radiotherapy (START) Trial A of radiotherapy hypofractionation for treatment of early breast cancer: a randomised trial. Lancet Oncol 2008;9:331–41.
10. Haviland JS, Owen JR, Dewar JA, et al. The UK Standardisation of Breast Radiotherapy (START) trials of radiotherapy hypofractionation for treatment of early breast cancer: 10-year follow-up results of two randomised controlled trials. Lancet Oncol 2013;14:1086–94.
11. Whelan TJ, Pignol JP, Levine MN, et al. Long-term results of hypofractionated radiation therapy for breast cancer. N Engl J Med 2010;362:513–20.
12. Brunt AM, Haviland JS, Sydenham M, et al. Ten-year results of FAST: a randomized controlled trial of 5-fraction whole-breast radiotherapy for early breast cancer. J Clin Oncol 2020;38:3261–72.
13. Murray Brunt A, Haviland JS, Wheatley DA, et al. Hypofractionated breast radiotherapy for 1 week versus 3 weeks (FAST-Forward): 5-year efficacy and late normal tissue effects results from a multicentre, non-inferiority, randomised, phase 3 trial. Lancet 2020;395:1613–26.
14. Fowler JF. The linear-quadratic formula and progress in fractionated radiotherapy. Br J Radiol 1989;62:679–94.
15. Brunt AM, Wheatley D, Yarnold J, et al. Acute skin toxicity associated with a 1-week schedule of whole breast radiotherapy compared with a standard 3-week regimen delivered in the UK FAST-Forward Trial. Radiother Oncol 2016;120:114–8.

16. group FT, Agrawal RK, Alhasso A, et al. First results of the randomised UK FAST Trial of radiotherapy hypofractionation for treatment of early breast cancer (CRUKE/04/015). Radiother Oncol 2011;100:93–100.
17. Meattini I, Becherini C, Boersma L, et al. European Society for Radiotherapy and Oncology Advisory Committee in Radiation Oncology Practice consensus recommendations on patient selection and dose and fractionation for external beam radiotherapy in early breast cancer. Lancet Oncol 2022;23:e21–31.
18. Ebctcg, McGale P, Taylor C, et al. Effect of radiotherapy after mastectomy and axillary surgery on 10-year recurrence and 20-year breast cancer mortality: meta-analysis of individual patient data for 8135 women in 22 randomised trials. Lancet 2014;383:2127–35.
19. Overgaard M, Hansen PS, Overgaard J, et al. Postoperative radiotherapy in high-risk premenopausal women with breast cancer who receive adjuvant chemotherapy. Danish Breast Cancer Cooperative Group 82b Trial. N Engl J Med 1997;337:949–55.
20. Overgaard M, Jensen MB, Overgaard J, et al. Postoperative radiotherapy in high-risk postmenopausal breast-cancer patients given adjuvant tamoxifen: Danish Breast Cancer Cooperative Group DBCG 82c randomised trial. Lancet 1999;353:1641–8.
21. Ragaz J, Jackson SM, Le N, et al. Adjuvant radiotherapy and chemotherapy in node-positive premenopausal women with breast cancer. N Engl J Med 1997; 337:956–62.
22. Poortmans PM, Collette S, Kirkove C, et al. Internal mammary and medial supraclavicular irradiation in breast cancer. N Engl J Med 2015;373:317–27.
23. Whelan TJ, Olivotto IA, Levine MN. Regional nodal irradiation in early-stage breast cancer. N Engl J Med 2015;373:1878–9.
24. Johansson S, Svensson H, Denekamp J. Timescale of evolution of late radiation injury after postoperative radiotherapy of breast cancer patients. Int J Radiat Oncol Biol Phys 2000;48:745–50.
25. Stoll BA, Andrews JT. Radiation-induced peripheral neuropathy. Br Med J 1966; 1:834–7.
26. Wang SL, Fang H, Song YW, et al. Hypofractionated versus conventional fractionated postmastectomy radiotherapy for patients with high-risk breast cancer: a randomised, non-inferiority, open-label, phase 3 trial. Lancet Oncol 2019;20: 352–60.
27. Khan AJ, Poppe MM, Goyal S, et al. Hypofractionated postmastectomy radiation therapy is safe and effective: first results from a prospective phase II trial. J Clin Oncol 2017;35:2037–43.
28. Galecki J, Hicer-Grzenkowicz J, Grudzien-Kowalska M, et al. Radiation-induced brachial plexopathy and hypofractionated regimens in adjuvant irradiation of patients with breast cancer: a review. Acta Oncol 2006;45:280–4.
29. Liu L, Yang Y, Guo Q, et al. Comparing hypofractionated to conventional fractionated radiotherapy in postmastectomy breast cancer: a meta-analysis and systematic review. Radiat Oncol 2020 Jan 17;15(1):17.
30. Shah C, Bremer T, Cox C, et al. The Clinical Utility of DCISionRT((R)) on Radiation Therapy Decision Making in Patients with Ductal Carcinoma In Situ Following Breast-Conserving Surgery. Ann Surg Oncol 2021;28:5974–84.
31. Fisher ER, Anderson S, Redmond C, et al. Ipsilateral breast tumor recurrence and survival following lumpectomy and irradiation: pathological findings from NSABP protocol B-06. Semin Surg Oncol 1992;8:161–6.

32. Vicini FA, Kestin LL, Goldstein NS. Defining the clinical target volume for patients with early-stage breast cancer treated with lumpectomy and accelerated partial breast irradiation: a pathologic analysis. Int J Radiat Oncol Biol Phys 2004;60:722–30.

33. Coles CE, Griffin CL, Kirby AM, et al. Partial-breast radiotherapy after breast conservation surgery for patients with early breast cancer (UK IMPORT LOW trial): 5-year results from a multicentre, randomised, controlled, phase 3, non-inferiority trial. Lancet 2017;390:1048–60.

34. Meattini I, Marrazzo L, Saieva C, et al. Accelerated partial-breast irradiation compared with whole-breast irradiation for early breast cancer: long-term results of the randomized phase III APBI-IMRT-Florence Trial. J Clin Oncol 2020; 38:4175–83.

35. Polgar C, Fodor J, Major T, et al. Breast-conserving therapy with partial or whole breast irradiation: ten-year results of the Budapest randomized trial. Radiother Oncol 2013;108:197–202.

36. Strnad V, Ott OJ, Hildebrandt G, et al. 5-year results of accelerated partial breast irradiation using sole interstitial multicatheter brachytherapy versus whole-breast irradiation with boost after breast-conserving surgery for low-risk invasive and in-situ carcinoma of the female breast: a randomised, phase 3, non-inferiority trial. Lancet 2016;387:229–38.

37. Whelan TJ, Julian JA, Berrang TS, et al. External beam accelerated partial breast irradiation versus whole breast irradiation after breast conserving surgery in women with ductal carcinoma in situ and node-negative breast cancer (RAPID): a randomised controlled trial. Lancet 2019;394:2165–72.

38. Vicini FA, Cecchini RS, White JR, et al. Long-term primary results of accelerated partial breast irradiation after breast-conserving surgery for early-stage breast cancer: a randomised, phase 3, equivalence trial. Lancet 2019;394:2155–64.

39. Correa C, Harris EE, Leonardi MC, et al. Accelerated partial breast irradiation: executive summary for the update of an ASTRO Evidence-Based Consensus Statement. Pract Radiat Oncol 2017;7:73–9.

40. Orecchia R, Veronesi U, Maisonneuve P, et al. Intraoperative irradiation for early breast cancer (ELIOT): long-term recurrence and survival outcomes from a single-centre, randomised, phase 3 equivalence trial. Lancet Oncol 2021;22: 597–608.

41. Vaidya JS, Wenz F, Bulsara M, et al. Risk-adapted targeted intraoperative radiotherapy versus whole-breast radiotherapy for breast cancer: 5-year results for local control and overall survival from the TARGIT-A randomised trial. Lancet 2014;383:603–13.

42. White JR, Winter K, Cecchini RS, et al. Cosmetic outcome from post lumpectomy whole breast irradiation (WBI) versus partial breast irradiation (PBI) on the NRG Oncology/NSABP B39-RTOG 0413 phase III clinical trial. Int J Radiat Oncol Biol Phys 2019;105:S3–4.

43. Veronesi U, Marubini E, Mariani L, et al. Radiotherapy after breast-conserving surgery in small breast carcinoma: long-term results of a randomized trial. Ann Oncol 2001;12:997–1003.

44. Early Breast Cancer Trialists' Collaborative G, Darby S, McGale P, et al. Effect of radiotherapy after breast-conserving surgery on 10-year recurrence and 15-year breast cancer death: meta-analysis of individual patient data for 10,801 women in 17 randomised trials. Lancet 2011;378:1707–16.

45. Hughes KS, Schnaper LA, Bellon JR, et al. Lumpectomy plus tamoxifen with or without irradiation in women age 70 years or older with early breast cancer: long-term follow-up of CALGB 9343. J Clin Oncol 2013;31:2382–7.

46. Kunkler IH, Williams LJ, Jack WJ, et al. Breast-conserving surgery with or without irradiation in women aged 65 years or older with early breast cancer (PRIME II): a randomised controlled trial. Lancet Oncol 2015;16:266–73.

47. Sparano JA, Gray RJ, Makower DF, et al. Adjuvant chemotherapy guided by a 21-gene expression assay in breast cancer. N Engl J Med 2018;379:111–21.

48. Whelan TJ, Smith S, Nielsen TO, et al. LUMINA: a prospective trial omitting radiotherapy (RT) following breast conserving surgery (BCS) in T1N0 luminal A breast cancer (BC). J Clin Oncol 2022;40:LBA501.

49. Mamounas EP, Tang G, Fisher B, et al. Association between the 21-gene recurrence score assay and risk of locoregional recurrence in node-negative, estrogen receptor-positive breast cancer: results from NSABP B-14 and NSABP B-20. J Clin Oncol 2010;28:1677–83.

50. Solin LJ, Gray R, Goldstein LJ, et al. Prognostic value of biologic subtype and the 21-gene recurrence score relative to local recurrence after breast conservation treatment with radiation for early stage breast carcinoma: results from the Eastern Cooperative Oncology Group E2197 study. Breast Cancer Res Treat 2012;134:683–92.

51. White JR, Anderson SJ, Harris EE, et al. NRG-BR007: a phase III trial evaluating de-escalation of breast radiation (DEBRA) following breast-conserving surgery (BCS) of stage 1, hormone receptor1, HER2-, RS ≤ 18 breast cancer. J Clin Oncol 2022;40(16_suppl). TPS613-TPS613.

52. McCormick B, Winter KA, Woodward W, et al. Randomized phase III trial evaluating radiation following surgical excision for good-risk ductal carcinoma in situ: long-term report from NRG Oncology/RTOG 9804. J Clin Oncol 2021; 39:3574–82.

53. Warnberg F, Karlsson P, Holmberg E, et al. Prognostic risk assessment and prediction of radiotherapy benefit for women with ductal carcinoma in situ (DCIS) of the breast, in a randomized clinical trial (SweDCIS). Cancers 2021;13:6103.

54. Weinmann S, Leo MC, Francisco M, et al. Validation of a ductal carcinoma in situ biomarker profile for risk of recurrence after breast-conserving surgery with and without radiotherapy. Clin Cancer Res 2020;26:4054–63.

55. Mamounas EP, Liu Q, Paik S, et al. 21-Gene recurrence score and locoregional recurrence in node-positive/ER-positive breast cancer treated with chemoendocrine therapy. J Natl Cancer Inst 2017;109:djw259.

56. Woodward WA, Barlow WE, Jagsi R, et al. Association between 21-gene assay recurrence score and locoregional recurrence rates in patients with node-positive breast cancer. JAMA Oncol 2020;6:505–11.

57. Jagsi R, Barlow W, Woodward WA, et al. Radiotherapy use and locoregional recurrence rates on SWOG 1007, a US cooperative group trial enrolling patients with favorable-risk node-positive breast cancer. Int J Radiat Oncol Biol Phys 2022;114:S43.

58. Mamounas EP, Anderson SJ, Dignam JJ, et al. Predictors of locoregional recurrence after neoadjuvant chemotherapy: results from combined analysis of National Surgical Adjuvant Breast and Bowel Project B-18 and B-27. J Clin Oncol 2012;30:3960–6.

59. White J, Tai A, Arthur D, et al. (2009) Breast Cancer Atlas for Radiation Therapy Planning: Consensus Definitions Collaborators. Breast Cancer Atlas for Radiation Therapy Planning, 73, 944–951. https://www.rtog.org.

60. MacDonald S CL, Fagundes M, Feigenber S, et al. Breast Contouring RAD-COMP Consortium 2016. http://www.crtog.org/UploadFiles/2016-12/94/N131266924114721.pdf.
61. Offersen BV, Boersma LJ, Kirkove C, et al. ESTRO consensus guideline on target volume delineation for elective radiation therapy of early stage breast cancer, version 1.1. Radiother Oncol 2016;118:205–8.
62. Bazan JG, Khan AJ. Target volume delineation and patterns of recurrence in the modern era. Semin Radiat Oncol 2022;32:254–69.
63. Pignol JP, Olivotto I, Rakovitch E, et al. A multicenter randomized trial of breast intensity-modulated radiation therapy to reduce acute radiation dermatitis. J Clin Oncol 2008;26:2085–92.
64. Vicini FA, Sharpe M, Kestin L, et al. Optimizing breast cancer treatment efficacy with intensity-modulated radiotherapy. Int J Radiat Oncol Biol Phys 2002;54:1336–44.
65. Donovan E, Bleakley N, Denholm E, et al. Randomised trial of standard 2D radiotherapy (RT) versus intensity modulated radiotherapy (IMRT) in patients prescribed breast radiotherapy. Radiother Oncol 2007;82:254–64.
66. Gupta T, Agarwal J, Jain S, et al. Three-dimensional conformal radiotherapy (3D-CRT) versus intensity modulated radiation therapy (IMRT) in squamous cell carcinoma of the head and neck: a randomized controlled trial. Radiother Oncol 2012;104:343–8.
67. Sheets NC, Goldin GH, Meyer AM, et al. Intensity-modulated radiation therapy, proton therapy, or conformal radiation therapy and morbidity and disease control in localized prostate cancer. JAMA 2012;307:1611–20.
68. Marrazzo L, Meattini I, Simontacchi G, et al. Updates on the APBI-IMRT-Florence Trial (NCT02104895) Technique: from the intensity modulated radiation therapy trial to the volumetric modulated arc therapy clinical practice. Pract Radiat Oncol 2022;13(1):e28–34.
69. Bazan J, DiCostanzo D, Kuhn K, et al. Likelihood of unacceptable normal tissue doses in breast cancer patients undergoing regional nodal irradiation in routine clinical practice. Pract Radiat Oncol 2017;7:154–60.
70. Ho AY, Ballangrud A, Li G, et al. Long-term pulmonary outcomes of a feasibility study of inverse-planned, multibeam intensity modulated radiation therapy in node-positive breast cancer patients receiving regional nodal irradiation. Int J Radiat Oncol Biol Phys 2019;103:1100–8.
71. Bazan JG, Healy E, Beyer S, et al. Clinical effectiveness of an adaptive treatment planning algorithm for intensity modulated radiation therapy versus 3D conformal radiation therapy for node-positive breast cancer patients undergoing regional nodal irradiation/postmastectomy radiation therapy. Int J Radiat Oncol Biol Phys 2020;108(5):1159–71.
72. Darby SC, Ewertz M, McGale P, et al. Risk of ischemic heart disease in women after radiotherapy for breast cancer. N Engl J Med 2013;368:987–98.
73. Saiki H, Petersen IA, Scott CG, et al. Risk of heart failure with preserved ejection fraction in older women after contemporary radiotherapy for breast cancer. Circulation 2017;135:1388–96.
74. Taylor C, Correa C, Duane FK, et al. Estimating the risks of breast cancer radiotherapy: evidence from modern radiation doses to the lungs and heart and from previous randomized trials. J Clin Oncol 2017;35:1641–9.
75. Lin H, Dong L, Jimenez RB. Emerging technologies in mitigating the risks of cardiac toxicity from breast radiotherapy. Semin Radiat Oncol 2022;32:270–81.

76. Taylor CW, Nisbet A, McGale P, et al. Cardiac exposures in breast cancer radiotherapy: 1950s-1990s. Int J Radiat Oncol Biol Phys 2007;69:1484–95.
77. Nissen HD, Appelt AL. Improved heart, lung and target dose with deep inspiration breath hold in a large clinical series of breast cancer patients. Radiother Oncol 2013;106:28–32.
78. Sixel KE, Aznar MC, Ung YC. Deep inspiration breath hold to reduce irradiated heart volume in breast cancer patients. Int J Radiat Oncol Biol Phys 2001;49: 199–204.
79. Bergom C, Currey A, Desai N, et al. Deep inspiration breath hold: techniques and advantages for cardiac sparing during breast cancer irradiation. Front Oncol 2018;8:87.
80. Bartlett FR, Colgan RM, Carr K, et al. The UK HeartSpare Study: randomised evaluation of voluntary deep-inspiratory breath-hold in women undergoing breast radiotherapy. Radiother Oncol 2013;108:242–7.
81. Bartlett FR, Donovan EM, McNair HA, et al. The UK HeartSpare Study (Stage II): multicentre evaluation of a voluntary breath-hold technique in patients receiving breast radiotherapy. Clin Oncol 2017;29:e51–6.
82. Peters GW, Gao SJ, Knowlton C, et al. Benefit of deep inspiratory breath hold for right breast cancer when regional lymph nodes are irradiated. Pract Radiat Oncol 2022;12:e7–12.
83. Bergom C, Kelly T, Morrow N, et al. Prone whole-breast irradiation using three-dimensional conformal radiotherapy in women undergoing breast conservation for early disease yields high rates of excellent to good cosmetic outcomes in patients with large and/or pendulous breasts. Int J Radiat Oncol Biol Phys 2012;83: 821–8.
84. Formenti SC, DeWyngaert JK, Jozsef G, et al. Prone vs supine positioning for breast cancer radiotherapy. JAMA 2012;308:861–3.
85. Vesprini D, Davidson M, Bosnic S, et al. Effect of supine vs prone breast radiotherapy on acute toxic effects of the skin among women with large breast size: a randomized clinical trial. JAMA Oncol 2022;8:994–1000.
86. Healy EH, Pratt DN, DiCostanzo D, et al. Evaluation of lung and heart dose in patients treated with radiation for breast cancer. Cancer Res 2018; 78(4_Supplement):P2-11-07.
87. Deseyne P, Speleers B, De Neve W, et al. Whole breast and regional nodal irradiation in prone versus supine position in left sided breast cancer. Radiat Oncol 2017;12:89.
88. Shin SM, No HS, Vega RM, et al. Breast, chest wall, and nodal irradiation with prone set-up: results of a hypofractionated trial with a median follow-up of 35 months. Pract Radiat Oncol 2016;6:e81–8.
89. Mulliez T, Van de Velde J, Veldeman L, et al. Deep inspiration breath hold in the prone position retracts the heart from the breast and internal mammary lymph node region. Radiother Oncol 2015;117:473–6.
90. Mulliez T, Veldeman L, Speleers B, et al. Heart dose reduction by prone deep inspiration breath hold in left-sided breast irradiation. Radiother Oncol 2015; 114:79–84.
91. Mulliez T, Veldeman L, Vercauteren T, et al. Reproducibility of deep inspiration breath hold for prone left-sided whole breast irradiation. Radiat Oncol 2015; 10:9.
92. Scott JG, Berglund A, Schell MJ, et al. A genome-based model for adjusting radiotherapy dose (GARD): a retrospective, cohort-based study. Lancet Oncol 2017;18:202–11.

93. Ahmed KA, Liveringhouse CL, Mills MN, et al. Utilizing the genomically adjusted radiation dose (GARD) to personalize adjuvant radiotherapy in triple negative breast cancer management. EBioMedicine 2019;47:163–9.

94. Lin LL, Vennarini S, Dimofte A, et al. Proton beam versus photon beam dose to the heart and left anterior descending artery for left-sided breast cancer. Acta Oncol 2015;54:1032–9.

95. Milligan MG, Zieminski S, Johnson A, et al. Target coverage and cardiopulmonary sparing with the updated ESTRO-ACROP contouring guidelines for postmastectomy radiation therapy after breast reconstruction: a treatment planning study using VMAT and proton PBS techniques. Acta Oncol 2021;60: 1440–51.

96. Fattahi S, Mullikin TC, Aziz KA, et al. Proton therapy for the treatment of inflammatory breast cancer. Radiother Oncol 2022;171:77–83.

97. Galland-Girodet S, Pashtan I, MacDonald SM, et al. Long-term cosmetic outcomes and toxicities of proton beam therapy compared with photon-based 3-dimensional conformal accelerated partial-breast irradiation: a phase 1 trial. Int J Radiat Oncol Biol Phys 2014;90:493–500.

98. Bush DA, Do S, Lum S, et al. Partial breast radiation therapy with proton beam: 5-year results with cosmetic outcomes. Int J Radiat Oncol Biol Phys 2014;90: 501–5.

99. Mutter RW, Jethwa KR, Gonuguntla K, et al. 3 fraction pencil-beam scanning proton accelerated partial breast irradiation: early provider and patient reported outcomes of a novel regimen. Radiat Oncol 2019;14:211.

100. Bosma SCJ, Leij F, Vreeswijk S, et al. Five-year results of the Preoperative Accelerated Partial Breast Irradiation (PAPBI) Trial. Int J Radiat Oncol Biol Phys 2020; 106:958–67.

101. Horton JK, Blitzblau RC, Yoo S, et al. Preoperative single-fraction partial breast radiation therapy: a novel phase 1, dose-escalation protocol with radiation response biomarkers. Int J Radiat Oncol Biol Phys 2015;92:846–55.

102. Nichols E, Kesmodel SB, Bellavance E, et al. Preoperative accelerated partial breast irradiation for early-stage breast cancer: preliminary results of a prospective, phase 2 trial. Int J Radiat Oncol Biol Phys 2017;97:747–53.

103. Lightowlers SV, Boersma LJ, Fourquet A, et al. Preoperative breast radiation therapy: indications and perspectives. Eur J Cancer 2017;82:184–92.

104. Thiruchelvam PTR, Leff DR, Godden AR, et al. Primary radiotherapy and deep inferior epigastric perforator flap reconstruction for patients with breast cancer (PRADA): a multicentre, prospective, non-randomised, feasibility study. Lancet Oncol 2022;23:682–90.

105. Chmura SJ, Winter KA, Woodward WA, et al. NRG-BR002: a phase IIR/III trial of standard of care systemic therapy with or without stereotactic body radiotherapy (SBRT) and/or surgical resection (SR) for newly oligometastatic breast cancer (NCT02364557). J Clin Oncol 2022;40(16_suppl):1007–1007.

106. Schmid P, Rugo HS, Adams S, et al. Atezolizumab plus nab-paclitaxel as first-line treatment for unresectable, locally advanced or metastatic triple-negative breast cancer (IMpassion130): updated efficacy results from a randomised, double-blind, placebo-controlled, phase 3 trial. Lancet Oncol 2020;21:44–59.

107. Luke JJ, Lemons JM, Karrison TG, et al. Safety and clinical activity of pembrolizumab and multisite stereotactic body radiotherapy in patients with advanced solid tumors. J Clin Oncol 2018;36:1611–8.

108. Alomran R, White M, Bruce M, et al. Stereotactic radiotherapy for oligoprogressive ER-positive breast cancer (AVATAR). BMC Cancer 2021;21:303.

109. Hans S, Cottu P, Kirova YM. Preliminary results of the association of palbociclib and radiotherapy in metastatic breast cancer patients. Radiother Oncol 2018; 126:181.
110. Kawamoto T, Shikama N, Sasai K. Severe acute radiation-induced enterocolitis after combined palbociclib and palliative radiotherapy treatment. Radiother Oncol 2019;131:240–1.
111. Meattini I, Desideri I, Scotti V, et al. Ribociclib plus letrozole and concomitant palliative radiotherapy for metastatic breast cancer. Breast 2018;42:1–2.
112. Offersen BV, Alsner J, Nielsen HM, et al. Hypofractionated versus standard fractionated radiotherapy in patients with early breast cancer or ductal carcinoma in situ in a randomized phase III trial: the DBCG HYPO Trial. J Clin Oncol 2020;38:3615–25.
113. Offersen BV, Alsner J, Nielsen HM, et al. Partial breast irradiation versus whole breast irradiation for early breast cancer patients in a randomized phase III trial: the Danish Breast Cancer Group Partial Breast Irradiation Trial. J Clin Oncol 2022;40(36):4189–97.

Intraoperative Radiation Therapy for Gastrointestinal Malignancies

Alex R. Ritter, MD[a], Eric D. Miller, MD, PhD[a],*

KEYWORDS

- Intraoperative radiation therapy • Gastrointestinal malignancies • Pancreatic cancer
- Rectal cancer • Local control • Recurrence • Unresectable

KEY POINTS

- Intraoperative radiation therapy involves the delivery of a large dose of radiation during surgery directly to the tumor or tumor bed, allowing dose escalation to the treatment target while minimizing radiation dose to adjacent structures.
- Intraoperative radiation therapy has been evaluated for use in a variety of gastrointestinal malignancies, primarily pancreatic and rectal cancers, and is typically implemented in patients with unresectable disease or those at high risk of local recurrence.
- Predominantly retrospective data indicate intraoperative radiation therapy improves local control without significant toxicity, with some studies suggesting potential survival benefit in carefully selected patients.

INTRODUCTION

Gastrointestinal malignancies account for approximately 27% of all new cancer cases and 37% of cancer-related deaths worldwide.[1] Advancements in systemic therapy over time have resulted in improved distant disease control for these malignancies, increasing the importance of local control (LC) for overall oncologic outcomes. External beam radiotherapy (EBRT) is a primary treatment modality for local disease control, but the radiosensitivity of many gastrointestinal structures limits the dose of EBRT that can be safely delivered.

Intraoperative radiotherapy (IORT), in contrast, involves the precise delivery of radiotherapy (RT) directly to the tumor or tumor bed at the time of surgery, which offers

[a] Department of Radiation Oncology, The Ohio State University Comprehensive Cancer Center, Arthur G. James Cancer Hospital and Richard J. Solove Research Institute, 460 West 10th Avenue, Columbus, OH 43210, USA
* Corresponding author. Department of Radiation Oncology, Arthur G. James Cancer Hospital and Richard J. Solove Research Institute, 460 West 10th Avenue, Room A209, Columbus, OH 43210.
E-mail address: eric.miller@osumc.edu

Surg Oncol Clin N Am 32 (2023) 537–552
https://doi.org/10.1016/j.soc.2023.02.005
1055-3207/23/© 2023 Elsevier Inc. All rights reserved.

numerous advantages over EBRT.[2] For example, the ability to directly visualize the treatment target allows for precise localization of RT delivery. In addition, the rapid dose fall-off of IORT facilitates dose escalation to the target while minimizing further dose to adjacent radiosensitive structures, thereby, improving the therapeutic ratio. Because IORT is delivered in a single dose at the time of surgery, it also offers increased convenience to patients compared with weeks of daily treatment associated with EBRT.

IORT can be delivered via multiple modalities, including use of electrons, high-dose rate (HDR) brachytherapy, and kilovoltage (KV) x-rays, each with strengths and limitations. IORT using electrons most commonly involves placement of an applicator at the site of desired treatment followed by docking of a mobile linear accelerator and delivery of treatment. In addition to being the most well-studied modality in the literature, the use of IORT with electrons has the advantage of relatively short set-up and treatment time, but the inflexibility of the applicators can make delivery to narrow, constrained sites challenging. HDR IORT is delivered by placing temporary applicators at the treatment site and connecting them to a machine that inserts radioactive material into the applicators, which are then removed at the completion of treatment. In comparison to electron IORT, HDR IORT typically uses flexible applicators that allow for treatment to more anatomically challenging locations, but its disadvantages include prolonged planning and treatment time and decreased depth of penetration. KV IORT delivers kilovoltage x-rays at the time of surgery with very limited depth of penetration and is most frequently used in breast cancer. The vast majority of studies included in this review focus primarily on the use of electron IORT. Herein, we review the role of IORT in gastrointestinal malignancies with a primary focus on rectal and pancreatic cancer.

Esophago-Gastric

The majority of studies of IORT in esophago-gastric cancer have been in gastric cancer, not esophageal cancer, in part due to technical limitations. As such, this section will predominantly focus on gastric cancer. Although less prevalent in the United States, gastric cancer contributes significant disease burden worldwide, ranking sixth for incidence and fourth for mortality of all malignancies globally.[1] Surgery is the mainstay of treatment of resectable, non-metastatic cases, and perioperative chemotherapy has become standard-of-care for locoregionally advanced cases. Since this time, the role of EBRT in the management of gastric cancer has diminished and is typically indicated for instances of non-R0 resection and for those with unresectable disease. Although initially a predominant pattern of failure, rates of locoregional recurrence have declined significantly in the era of modern surgical techniques and systemic therapy.[3] Therefore, most research regarding IORT for gastric cancer comes from trials that accrued patients before the current standard-of-care, and as such, caution should be warranted when interpreting these data.

A study-level meta-analysis performed by Yu and colleagues evaluating the use of IORT for resectable gastric cancer demonstrated no improvement in overall survival (OS) but statistically significant benefit to locoregional control (HR = 0.40, P <.001) with the addition of IORT.[4] When evaluating patients with stage III disease, IORT was associated with significantly improved OS (HR = 0.60, P =.011). Another meta-analysis performed by Gao and colleagues evaluating 11 studies (nine gastric, two esophageal) with IORT used for resectable disease similarly demonstrated improved locoregional control but no improvement in OS with the use of IORT, as well as no significant increase in complication rate.[5]

Pancreas

Pancreas cancer remains, arguably, the most lethal cancer with an estimated 62,210 cases and nearly 50,000 deaths in the United States in 2022.[6] Surgical resection remains the only curative treatment modality for localized pancreas cancer, however, the majority of patients present with metastatic disease or have involvement of critical structures making resection difficult or impossible.[7] In patients who present with either borderline resectable or locally advanced disease, neoadjuvant chemotherapy serves as the mainstay of treatment both to facilitate a margin-negative resection and for early treatment of potential micrometastatic disease.[8,9] In patients with an inadequate response to initial systemic therapy, RT can be considered with or without concurrent systemic therapy to increase response rates.[10] Radiation as part of neoadjuvant therapy has been demonstrated to improve OS, disease-free survival (DFS), locoregional failure-free interval, and R0 resection rates in patients with resectable and borderline resectable pancreas cancer compared with immediate surgery.[11,12] In patients with locally advanced disease, the addition of RT to systemic therapy has shown improved LC compared with continued systemic therapy alone.[13] However, outcomes in pancreas cancer remain suboptimal, and, despite multimodality treatment, the rate of conversion from unresectable disease to a margin-negative resection remains low with both unresectable disease and margin positivity associated with a poor prognosis.[14] Although distant failure remains a challenge, local failure and primary tumor control in patients not eligible for resection are of paramount importance. Locally destructive disease has been suggested to be the direct cause of death in up to 30% of pancreas cancer patients based on autopsy series.[15]

Recent data suggest that delivering higher doses of RT in patients with locally advanced disease results in improved outcomes.[16,17] However, one limitation to delivering higher RT doses is the tolerance of adjacent structures including the luminal gastrointestinal tract. The anatomic location of pancreas cancer makes this site readily amenable to treatment with high-energy electrons using an applicator and an intraoperative linear accelerator as shown in **Fig. 1**. An excellent overview of IORT for patients with borderline-resectable and unresectable pancreatic cancer including the technical aspects of the procedure has been published by Calvo and colleagues[18,19]

Intraoperative Radiation Therapy in Resectable Disease

The anatomic location of pancreatic cancer with frequent retroperitoneal soft tissue involvement presents a challenge to achieving wide resection margins.[20] In cases of

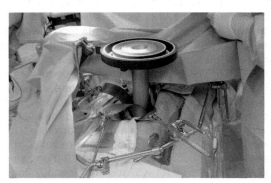

Fig. 1. Photo of intraoperative electron beam applicator secured in place to treat the postoperative bed of a patient following resection of pancreatic cancer with concerns for a positive retroperitoneal surgical margin.

involved or close surgical margins, IORT is an efficient method of delivering a focal RT boost to the post-operative bed while minimizing the dose to adjacent radiosensitive organs. A small prospective randomized clinical trial of IORT in 24 patients with resectable pancreatic cancer was performed at the National Cancer Institute.[21] Patients were randomized to either receive IORT (20 Gy) to the resection bed or standard treatment consisting of resection alone for patients with disease confined to the pancreatic capsule or post-operative EBRT for patients with extrapancreatic extension or nodal disease. Enrolled patients had locally advanced disease, traditionally considered unresectable, but extensive surgical resection was allowed which resulted in a perioperative mortality rate of 27%. The median OS of patients treated with IORT was 18 months compared with 12 months for the control group. The local recurrence rate was 33% in the IORT group versus 100% in the control group.

Larger series investigating the utility of an IORT boost primarily include single or multi-institution retrospective series. Valentini and colleagues reported a joint analysis of five European institutions evaluating the role of IORT with either pre-operative or post-operative EBRT in 270 patients.[22] Surgery was performed in 91.5% of cases with 47% of patients undergoing an R1 or R2 resection. Preoperative EBRT was delivered in 23.9% of cases. At a median follow-up of 96 months, the 5-year LC was 23.3% with a median LC of 15 months. The median OS was 19 months with a 5-year OS of 17.7%. Improved LC and OS were observed in patients treated with preoperative EBRT compared with patients receiving post-operative EBRT or IORT alone. Ogawa and colleagues reported the results of a multi-institutional retrospective analysis of 210 patients treated with IORT (n = 62) with or without EBRT (n = 148).[23] R1 resections were performed in 30% of patients. Two-year LC in all patients was 83.7% with a median OS of 19.1 months. Calvo and colleagues reported on a cohort of 60 patients treated with chemoradiation and surgery with (n = 29) or without (n = 31) IORT.[24] Most patients (n = 41) received post-operative chemoradiation, and adjuvant chemotherapy was delivered in approximately 60% of patients. R1 resections were performed in 41% of the IORT group and 45% of the non-IORT group (P =.77). At a median follow-up of 15.9 months, 5-year OS and locoregional control were 20% and 58%, respectively. On multivariate analysis, margin resection status (HR = 3.0, P =.05) and not receiving IORT (HR = 6.75, P =.01) were associated with higher locoregional recurrence. Patients treated with IORT had a similar rate of perioperative complications and perioperative mortality as those not treated with IORT.

The Massachusetts General Hospital (MGH) recently reported a more modern series of patients with borderline resectable or locally advanced pancreas cancer treated with neoadjuvant therapy and IORT.[25] Most patients received neoadjuvant FOLFIRINOX (83%) followed by consolidative photon-based RT (95%) or treatment with stereotactic body radiation therapy (SBRT) or protons (5%). Of 158 patients, 86 received neoadjuvant FOLFIRINOX-based therapy and underwent combined surgical resection with IORT (10 Gy). The median progression-free survival and OS were 21.5 and 46.7 months, respectively, with local progression occurring in 12.7% of patients. A recent publication from Sekigami and colleagues and the MGH group reported on the utility of IORT to mitigate the effects of a microscopically positive tumor margin following neoadjuvant FOLFIRINOX followed by chemoradiation and then resection.[26] No significant difference was observed in DFS (R0 – 29 months vs R1 – 20 months, P =.114) or OS (R0 – 48 months vs R1 – 37 months, P =.307) in patients with an R0 versus an R1 resection if IORT was delivered. For patients with an R1 resection, receiving IORT showed a trend for significance for improved OS (37 months vs 21 months, P =.064). A recent meta-analysis consisting of 15 studies with 834 patients compared outcomes of patients with resectable pancreatic cancer who underwent surgery with or without IORT.[27] The pooled analysis showed favorable OS (median survival rate = 1.20, 95% confidence interval 1.06–1.37, P =.005) and reduced local recurrence (relative risk = 0.70, 95% confidence interval 0.51–0.97, P =.03) in patients treated with surgery plus IORT. Select studies investigating IORT for patients with resected pancreatic cancer are summarized in **Table 1**.

Intraoperative Radiation Therapy in Unresectable Disease

IORT is an effective boost strategy for patients with unresectable disease given the ability to remove adjacent radiosensitive organs from the target volume. Following promising results from early single-institution studies, the utility of IORT for unresectable pancreatic cancer was evaluated in the cooperative group setting in Radiation Therapy Oncology Group (RTOG) 8505.[29] In this study, patients received a dose of 20 Gy intraoperatively followed by 5-fluorouracil (5-FU)-based chemoradiation to a dose of 50.4 Gy. The median survival was 9 months with major post-operative complications occurring in 12% of patients. Mohiuddin and colleagues reported on 49 patients with unresectable pancreatic cancer treated with IORT (15–20 Gy) followed by EBRT to a dose of 40 to 55 Gy in 1.8 to 2.0 Gy fractions with concurrent 5-FU followed by maintenance 5-FU.[30] The median survival was 16 months with a 2-year survival rate of 22% and freedom from local progression of disease achieved in 71% of patients. Treatment was well-tolerated with early and late grade 3/4 toxicity in 14% and 19% of patients, respectively.

The Japanese Radiation Oncology Study Group reported 144 patients with localized unresectable pancreatic cancer treated with IORT (median of 25 Gy) with (n = 113) or without (n = 31) EBRT (median of 45 Gy).[31] Systemic therapy with the majority of patients receiving either gemcitabine or 5-FU was administered concurrently with RT and then after completion of RT until progression. Two-year LC in all patients was 44.6% and was improved in patients treated with IORT plus EBRT versus IORT alone (50.9% vs 17.5%, P =.0004). The median OS for all patients was 10.5 months with a 2-year OS of 14.7%. Late grade 3 gastrointestinal toxicity was reported in 1.4% of patients. Chen and colleagues reported on the outcomes of 247 patients with unresectable pancreatic cancer treated with IORT at the China National Cancer Center.[32] The majority of patients were treated with IORT alone with a median dose of 15 Gy. Less than 40% of patients received treatment with adjuvant EBRT or systemic therapy. The median OS was 9.0 months for all patients with a 2-year actuarial survival rate of 14%. Of note, on multivariate analysis, receipt of post-operative chemoradiation followed by systemic therapy was significantly associated with improved OS with a median OS of 16.2 months in this subset of patients.

MGH reported their long-term outcomes in 194 patients with unresectable pancreatic cancer treated with IORT.[33] In their series, 97% of patients received EBRT before IORT with the majority receiving concurrent systemic therapy and a lower percentage of patients receiving adjuvant systemic therapy. The median OS of all patients was 12.0 months with a 2-year survival rate of 16%. In the more contemporary MGH experience where patients received neoadjuvant FOLFIRINOX before consolidation RT, 46 patients had unresectable primary tumors and were treated with IORT alone to doses of 15 to 20 Gy.[25] Local progression occurred in 15% of patients with an encouraging median progression-free survival of 14.7 months and an impressive median OS of 23 months. Treatment was shown to be safe with one death in the IORT alone group due to spontaneous bacterial peritonitis. Select studies investigating IORT for patients with unresectable pancreatic cancer are summarized in **Table 2**.

Table 1
Select studies of intraoperative radiation therapy for patients with resectable pancreatic cancer

Study	Patient Number	IORT Dose Range (Gy)	EBRT Dose Range (Gy)	Systemic Therapy	Local Control	Median Overall Survival
Valentini et al,[22] 2009	270 (169 IORT + EBRT, 95 IORT alone)	7.5–25	18–61	11.8% concurrent with EBRT	Median local control 15 mo	19 mo
Showalter et al,[28] 2009	37 (23 IORT + EBRT)	10–20	45–50.4	70% adjuvant	23% locoregional recurrence	19.2 mo
Ogawa et al,[23] 2010	210 (62 IORT + EBRT, 148 IORT alone)	20–30	20–60	19% concurrent with EBRT; 46% adjuvant	2-y local control 83.7%	19.1 mo
Calvo et al,[24] 2013	29	10–15	45–50.4	100% concurrent with EBRT; 62% adjuvant	5-y locoregional control 92.2%	5-y 20% for all patients (including no IORT)
Harrison et al,[25] 2020	86 (all treated with EBRT + IORT)	10.2 (mean)	50.4–58.8 or SBRT	100% received neoadjuvant treatment	12.7% local recurrence rate	46.7 mo

Abbreviations: EBRT, external beam radiation therapy; Gy, gray; IORT, intraoperative radiation therapy; SBRT, stereotactic body radiation therapy.

Table 2
Select studies of intraoperative radiation therapy for patients with unresectable pancreatic cancer

Study	Patient Number	IORT Dose Range (Gy)	EBRT Dose Range (Gy)	Systemic Therapy	Local Control	Median Overall Survival
Tepper et al,[29] 1991	51	15–20	50.4	100% concurrent with EBRT; no adjuvant	Not evaluated	9.0 mo
Mohiuddin et al,[30] 1995	49	15–20	40–55	100% concurrent with EBRT; 100% adjuvant	31% local recurrence rate	16.0 mo
Ogawa et al,[31] 2011	144 (113 IORT + EBRT, 31 IORT alone)	12–35	14–50.8	69% concurrent with EBRT; 45% adjuvant	2-y local control rate 44.6%	10.5 mo
Chen et al,[32] 2016	247 (90 IORT + EBRT, 157 IORT alone)	10–20	36–40	32% concurrent with EBRT; 35% adjuvant	2-y local PFS rate of 40.1%	9.0 mo
Harrison et al,[25] 2020	46 (all treated with EBRT + IORT)	15 (mean)	50.4–58.8 or SBRT	100% received neoadjuvant treatment	15% local recurrence rate	23.0 mo

Abbreviations: EBRT, external beam radiation therapy; Gy, gray; IORT, intraoperative radiation therapy; PFS, progression-free survival; SBRT, stereotactic body radiation therapy.

Bile Duct and Gallbladder Cancer

Gallbladder cancer and extrahepatic cholangiocarcinoma are rare malignancies with approximately 12,000 new cases diagnosed in 2022.[6] Surgical resection remains the mainstay for eligible patients; however, the majority of patients with this diagnosis present with locally advanced disease making surgical removal challenging.[34] In addition, biliary tract cancer has traditionally been thought to be resistant to conventional systemic therapy and RT, possibly secondary to stromal desmoplasia, making dose escalation of RT an attractive treatment option for this malignancy.[35] Given its rarity, limited prospective studies are available for bile duct cancer, and fewer studies have investigated the role of IORT. Select series are highlighted here.

In gallbladder cancer, Todoroki and colleagues reported on 85 patients with stage IV disease who underwent tumor resection with intraoperative, external, or intracavitary RT used as a supplement in 47 patients.[36] The addition of RT significantly improved LC (59.1% vs 36.1%, $P = .0467$) and 5-year OS (8.9% vs 2.9%, $P = .0023$) with a particular benefit seen in those who underwent an R1 resection. In a second small series from Lindell and colleagues of 20 patients who underwent extended resection with or without IORT for gallbladder cancer, the actuarial 5-year OS was 47% in the RT group versus 13% in the surgery alone group, which was not statistically significant but limited by the small number of patients included.[37] Treatment was well-tolerated with a post-operative complication rate of only 15%.

Similar small series have been published for extrahepatic cholangiocarcinoma. The Mayo Clinic experience includes 13 patients with unresectable extrahepatic cholangiocarcinoma treated with biliary stenting along with EBRT and IORT (15–20 Gy).[38] Local progression in the IORT field was evident in 31% of patients, and the median OS for the entire group was 16.5 months with six patients achieving survival ranging from 21 to 61 months from diagnosis. Kaiser and colleagues reported on the addition of IORT to surgery alone in patients with unresectable hilar cholangiocarcinoma.[39] Nine patients were treated with palliative IORT (group 1) whereas surgery alone was performed in a case-matched group of nine patients (group 2). Group 1 was also compared with a larger group of 36 patients with unresectable disease treated without IORT (group 3). The median OS for the IORT group was 23.3 months compared with the case-matched surgery-alone group at 9.4 months, $P = .0359$, and the unmatched surgery-alone group (group 3) at 5.7 months, $P = .0367$. Toxicity from IORT was minimal with no post-operative complications reported. Based on these limited data, IORT is a well-tolerated treatment that can be considered for patients with unresectable bile duct cancer as an effective means of improving LC that may impact OS.

Colorectal Cancer

Colorectal cancer (CRC) is the fourth most common cancer and the second most common cause of cancer death in the United States.[6] Historically, management of locally-advanced rectal cancer (LARC) consisted of surgery alone, which resulted in significant local recurrence rates of approximately 25%.[40] With the adoption of neoadjuvant therapy before total mesorectal excision as standard-of-care for locally-advanced rectal cancer, rates of locoregional failure have declined significantly to <10%.[41] However, certain risk factors such as increasing T-stage, regional lymph node involvement, poor response to neoadjuvant therapy, involved circumferential resection margin, and close or positive surgical margins portend a higher risk for locoregional recurrence.[42,43] R0 resection is unable to be achieved in approximately 15% of patients with T4 rectal cancer undergoing surgery even after neoadjuvant chemoradiation.[44] Given the poor outcomes associated with incomplete resection and recurrent disease, IORT has been evaluated in the setting of unresectable rectal cancers and those with a high risk of local recurrence.

Locally-Advanced Rectal Cancer

Various studies evaluating IORT in the setting of LARC have been reported, although few randomized studies comparing IORT to standard treatment exist. Dubois and colleagues randomized 142 patients with LARC undergoing surgical resection following preoperative EBRT to surgical resection alone versus surgical resection with IORT.[45] No improvement in 5-year LC (91.8% vs 92.8%, P = .6018) or 5-year OS (69.8% vs 74.8%, P = .2578) was seen with the addition of IORT, although nearly 90% of patients had T3 tumors, meaning the potential benefit of IORT may have been diminished due to high rates of complete resection. IORT was not associated with an increased risk of post-operative complications. Masaki and colleagues published the final results of their trial that randomized 79 patients with LARC to standard surgical treatment, including bilateral lateral lymph node dissection (LLND) and limited pelvic autonomic nerve preservation (PANP), versus surgery (including bilateral LLND and complete PANP) with IORT to the bilateral preserved pelvic nerve plexuses.[46] This trial also failed to show benefit in terms of LC or OS with the addition of IORT and was terminated prematurely due to significantly worsened distant metastasis-free survival in the IORT group. Post-operative complication rates were similar between groups, and both short-term and long-term urinary functions were improved in the IORT group.

Nevertheless, non-randomized comparisons have suggested LC benefit with the usage of IORT in this patient population, particularly in patients with positive surgical margins, as demonstrated in two prospective pooled analyses.[47,48] Kusters and colleagues reported outcomes of 605 patients undergoing IORT as part of multimodality therapy for their LARC.[47] The five-year local recurrence rate among all patients was 12.0% and was 45.1% in those who underwent incomplete resection, which are favorable results compared with historical controls not receiving IORT. Holman and colleagues reported outcomes for 417 patients treated with multimodality therapy including IORT for their T4b rectal cancers at either Mayo Clinic Rochester or Catharina Hospital Eindhoven in The Netherlands.[48] As discussed by the authors in their manuscript, compared with patients with non-R0 resections reported in a separate, non-IORT series from Mayo, patients in this study with non-R0 resections receiving IORT had higher 5-year OS (56% vs 24%) and lower 5-year local recurrence (19% vs 76%), acknowledging the limitations of this comparison.

Locally-Recurrent Rectal Cancer

Although less likely with modern treatment paradigms, locoregional recurrence of rectal cancer following surgery does still occur. Managing locally-recurrent rectal cancer (LRRC) is particularly challenging in patients who have received prior pelvic radiation, as further re-irradiation is limited in terms of dose and volume due to the prior dose received by the adjacent healthy tissues. Additionally, recurrent tumors following pelvic radiation are generally more radioresistant and have more limited surgical options due to prior surgery.[49] For patients with isolated LRRC, treatment often consists of preoperative chemoradiation (or re-irradiation in the case of previously radiated patients) followed by surgical resection if feasible. The ability to deliver additional radiation to the site of disease with IORT while limiting dose to the adjacent critical structures makes it a particularly attractive therapy in the LRRC setting.

Previous non-randomized comparison studies have demonstrated improved LC with the addition of IORT to the treatment regimen for patients with LRRC with no extra-pelvic disease.[50,51] Holman and colleagues published their pooled analysis of

Table 3
Select studies of intraoperative radiation therapy for patients with locally advanced and locally-recurrent rectal cancer

Study	Patient Number	Disease Type	IORT Dose Range (Gy)	Perioperative EBRT Dose Range (Gy)	Systemic Therapy	Local Control	5-y Survival
Roeder et al,[56] 2012	97	LRRC	10–20	15–54 (56% received)	89% concurrent with EBRT; 34% adjuvant	5-y = 54%	30%
Sole et al,[57] 2014	335	LARC	10–15	45–50.4 (100% received)	100% concurrent with EBRT	10-y = 92%	75%
Hyngstrom et al,[58] 2014	30 (LARC) and 70 (LRRC)	LARC and LRRC	10–15	39–59 (LARC) 30–50.4 (LRRC) (82% total received)	37% concurrent with EBRT	5-y = 94% (LARC) 5-y = 56% (LRRC)	61% (LARC) 56% (LRRC)
Zhang[59] 2014	45	LARC (pT3)	15–25	None	100% received adjuvant	5-y = 84%	84%
Zhang et al,[60] 2014	71	LARC (pT4 or pN+)	10–20	45–50.4 Gy (100% received adjuvant)	100% concurrent with adjuvant EBRT	5-y = 90%	75%
Holman et al,[48] 2016	417	LARC	10–15+	45–54 (97% preop; 6% adjuvant)	78% concurrent with EBRT; 17% adjuvant	5-y = 81%	56%
Holman et al,[52] 2018	565	LRRC	10–30	5–54 (90% received)	75% concurrent with EBRT; 8.7% adjuvant	5-y = 54.7%	33%

Abbreviations: EBRT, external beam radiation therapy; Gy, gray; IORT, intraoperative radiation therapy; LARC, locally-advanced rectal cancer; LRRC, locally-recurrent rectal cancer.

565 patients undergoing IORT-containing multimodality treatment of LRRC at two major treatment centers.[52] In this study, 90% of patients received preoperative EBRT before surgery for their recurrent disease (either re-irradiation or full-course radiation). Typical IORT dose ranged from 10 to 20 Gy. The five-year local re-recurrence rate was 43.5% and 5-year OS was 33%. In total, 44% of patients achieved R0 resection, with significantly higher rates in those who had undergone preoperative EBRT. The radicality of resection and preoperative (chemo)radiotherapy were the strongest prognostic factors and were associated with significant improvements in local recurrence rate, metastasis-free survival, and OS.

Multiple meta-analyses evaluating IORT outcomes for LARC and LRRC have been published recently. Mirnezmi and colleagues published a meta-analysis including 3003 patients from 29 studies from 1965 to 2011, reporting outcomes after IORT for advanced or recurrent colorectal cancer.[53] The IORT dose was typically 10 to 15 Gy for R1 resections and 15 to 20 Gy for R2 resections. The IORT was associated with significantly improved 5-year LC, 5-year DFS, and 5-year OS. There was no overall difference in total, urologic, or anastomotic complications; however, IORT patients did have higher rates of wound complications. Fahy and colleagues published a meta-analysis including 833 patients from seven papers from 2000 to 2020 evaluating outcomes of IORT received as part of multimodal treatment of LARC/LRRC.[54] There was a trend toward improvement in locoregional recurrence with the addition of IORT compared with surgery/EBRT alone (14.7% vs 21.4%; $P = .11$) but no survival difference. The IORT was not associated with higher rates of wound infection, pelvic abscess, anastomotic leak, or need for repeat surgical intervention compared with the surgery/EBRT cohort. Liu and colleagues performed a meta-analysis including 1460 patients from 15 studies evaluating outcomes from IORT included as part of the treatment regimen for rectal cancer.[55] In this analysis, IORT showed significantly improved 5-year LC, with no significant difference in 5-year OS, 5-year DFS, or complication rate. Select studies investigating IORT for patients with LARC and LRRC are summarized in **Table 3**.

Taken together, IORT can be utilized for both LARC and LRRC to achieve dose escalation without significant increased toxicity to adjacent critical structures. Although randomized data supporting its use are lacking, numerous nonrandomized studies evaluating IORT demonstrate benefits with regard to improved LC, particularly in patients unable to achieve an R0 resection. Future studies are needed to investigate how IORT may fit in the modern paradigm of total neoadjuvant therapy for LARC.

SUMMARY

Gastrointestinal malignancies cause significant suffering globally, accounting for more than one-third of all cancer-related deaths. Given improvements in systemic therapy, optimizing LC remains vitally important in the management of these malignancies, but the radiosensitive nature of surrounding gastrointestinal structures limits the doses of EBRT that can be safely given. IORT offers a promising strategy for dose escalation and improvement in therapeutic ratio in patients with unresectable disease or those at high risk of local recurrence and has been explored across a variety of gastrointestinal malignancies. Our summary of the literature regarding this topic demonstrates that IORT is frequently associated with improvements in LC, at times suggesting potential survival benefit, and is generally associated with low rates of complications or significant toxicity. Additional studies, particularly prospective trials, are needed to clarify specific indications for IORT in gastrointestinal cancers.

CLINICS CARE POINTS

- Intraoperative radiation therapy is a valuable part of multimodality cancer therapy with the ability to improve the therapeutic ratio by delivering radiation at the time of surgery directly to the tumor or post-operative bed, allowing intensified treatment while sparing dose to adjacent radiosensitive structures.
- Intraoperative radiation therapy has been evaluated in the management of gastrointestinal malignancies, particularly in rectal and pancreatic cancers, though data are largely retrospective in nature.
- Intraoperative radiation therapy has been associated with improved local control, and at times, improvements in survival, without a significant increase in toxicity.
- Further prospective studies are needed to further define the role of intraoperative radiation therapy in the management of gastrointestinal cancers.

DISCLOSURE

EDM has served as a consultant for Varian Medical Systems. This publication was supported in part by the NIH, United States (grant P30 CA16058).

REFERENCES

1. Sung H, Ferlay J, Siegel RL, et al. Global Cancer Statistics 2020: GLOBOCAN Estimates of Incidence and Mortality Worldwide for 36 Cancers in 185 Countries. CA Cancer J Clin 2021;71:209–49.
2. Willett CG, Czito BG, Tyler DS. Intraoperative radiation therapy. J Clin Oncol 2007; 25:971–7.
3. Lee J, Lim DH, Kim S, et al. Phase III trial comparing capecitabine plus cisplatin versus capecitabine plus cisplatin with concurrent capecitabine radiotherapy in completely resected gastric cancer with D2 lymph node dissection: the ARTIST trial. J Clin Oncol 2012;30:268–73.
4. Yu WW, Guo YM, Zhang Q, et al. Benefits from adjuvant intraoperative radiotherapy treatment for gastric cancer: A meta-analysis. Mol Clin Oncol 2015;3:185–9.
5. Gao P, Tsai C, Yang Y, et al. Intraoperative radiotherapy in gastric and esophageal cancer: meta-analysis of long-term outcomes and complications. Minerva Med 2017;108:74–83.
6. Siegel RL, Miller KD, Fuchs HE, et al. Cancer statistics, 2022. CA Cancer J Clin 2022;72:7–33.
7. Patel SH, Katz MHG, Ahmad SA. The Landmark Series: Preoperative Therapy for Pancreatic Cancer. Ann Surg Oncol 2021;28:4104–29.
8. Suker M, Beumer BR, Sadot E, et al. FOLFIRINOX for locally advanced pancreatic cancer: a systematic review and patient-level meta-analysis. Lancet Oncol 2016;17:801–10.
9. Janssen QP, O'Reilly EM, van Eijck CHJ, et al. Neoadjuvant Treatment in Patients With Resectable and Borderline Resectable Pancreatic Cancer. Front Oncol 2020;10:41.
10. Murphy JE, Wo JY, Ryan DP, et al. Total Neoadjuvant Therapy With FOLFIRINOX Followed by Individualized Chemoradiotherapy for Borderline Resectable Pancreatic Adenocarcinoma: A Phase 2 Clinical Trial. JAMA Oncol 2018;4:963–9.

11. Versteijne E, Suker M, Groothuis K, et al. Preoperative Chemoradiotherapy Versus Immediate Surgery for Resectable and Borderline Resectable Pancreatic Cancer: Results of the Dutch Randomized Phase III PREOPANC Trial. J Clin Oncol 2020;38:1763–73.

12. Versteijne E, van Dam JL, Suker M, et al. Neoadjuvant Chemoradiotherapy Versus Upfront Surgery for Resectable and Borderline Resectable Pancreatic Cancer: Long-Term Results of the Dutch Randomized PREOPANC Trial. J Clin Oncol 2022;40:1220–30.

13. Hammel P, Huguet F, van Laethem JL, et al. Effect of Chemoradiotherapy vs Chemotherapy on Survival in Patients With Locally Advanced Pancreatic Cancer Controlled After 4 Months of Gemcitabine With or Without Erlotinib: The LAP07 Randomized Clinical Trial. JAMA 2016;315:1844–53.

14. Konstantinidis IT, Warshaw AL, Allen JN, et al. Pancreatic ductal adenocarcinoma: is there a survival difference for R1 resections versus locally advanced unresectable tumors? What is a "true" R0 resection? Ann Surg 2013;257:731–6.

15. Iacobuzio-Donahue CA, Fu B, Yachida S, et al. DPC4 gene status of the primary carcinoma correlates with patterns of failure in patients with pancreatic cancer. J Clin Oncol 2009;27:1806–13.

16. Krishnan S, Chadha AS, Suh Y, et al. Focal Radiation Therapy Dose Escalation Improves Overall Survival in Locally Advanced Pancreatic Cancer Patients Receiving Induction Chemotherapy and Consolidative Chemoradiation. Int J Radiat Oncol Biol Phys 2016;94:755–65.

17. Reyngold M, O'Reilly EM, Varghese AM, et al. Association of Ablative Radiation Therapy With Survival Among Patients With Inoperable Pancreatic Cancer. JAMA Oncol 2021;7:735–8.

18. Calvo FA, Asencio JM, Roeder F, et al. ESTRO IORT Task Force/ACROP recommendations for intraoperative radiation therapy in borderline-resected pancreatic cancer. Clin Transl Radiat Oncol 2020;23:91–9.

19. Calvo FA, Krengli M, Asencio JM, et al. ESTRO IORT Task Force/ACROP recommendations for intraoperative radiation therapy in unresected pancreatic cancer. Radiother Oncol 2020;148:57–64.

20. Willett CG, Lewandrowski K, Warshaw AL, et al. Resection margins in carcinoma of the head of the pancreas. Implications for radiation therapy. Ann Surg 1993; 217:144–8.

21. Sindelar WF, Kinsella TJ. Studies of intraoperative radiotherapy in carcinoma of the pancreas. Ann Oncol 1999;10(Suppl 4):226–30.

22. Valentini V, Calvo F, Reni M, et al. Intra-operative radiotherapy (IORT) in pancreatic cancer: joint analysis of the ISIORT-Europe experience. Radiother Oncol 2009;91:54–9.

23. Ogawa K, Karasawa K, Ito Y, et al. Intraoperative radiotherapy for resected pancreatic cancer: a multi-institutional retrospective analysis of 210 patients. Int J Radiat Oncol Biol Phys 2010;77:734–42.

24. Calvo FA, Sole CV, Atahualpa F, et al. Chemoradiation for resected pancreatic adenocarcinoma with or without intraoperative radiation therapy boost: Long-term outcomes. Pancreatology 2013;13:576–82.

25. Harrison JM, Wo JY, Ferrone CR, et al. Intraoperative Radiation Therapy (IORT) for Borderline Resectable and Locally Advanced Pancreatic Ductal Adenocarcinoma (BR/LA PDAC) in the Era of Modern Neoadjuvant Treatment: Short-Term and Long-Term Outcomes. Ann Surg Oncol 2020;27:1400–6.

26. Sekigami Y, Michelakos T, Fernandez-Del Castillo C, et al. Intraoperative Radiation Mitigates the Effect of Microscopically Positive Tumor Margins on Survival

Among Pancreatic Adenocarcinoma Patients Treated with Neoadjuvant FOLFIR-INOX and Chemoradiation. Ann Surg Oncol 2021;28:4592–601.

27. Jin L, Shi N, Ruan S, et al. The role of intraoperative radiation therapy in resectable pancreatic cancer: a systematic review and meta-analysis. Radiat Oncol 2020;15:76.

28. Showalter TN, Rao AS, Rani Anne P, et al. Does intraoperative radiation therapy improve local tumor control in patients undergoing pancreaticoduodenectomy for pancreatic adenocarcinoma? A propensity score analysis. Ann Surg Oncol 2009; 16:2116–22.

29. Tepper JE, Noyes D, Krall JM, et al. Intraoperative radiation therapy of pancreatic carcinoma: a report of RTOG-8505. Radiation Therapy Oncology Group. Int J Radiat Oncol Biol Phys 1991;21:1145–9.

30. Mohiuddin M, Regine WF, Stevens J, et al. Combined intraoperative radiation and perioperative chemotherapy for unresectable cancers of the pancreas. J Clin Oncol 1995;13:2764–8.

31. Ogawa K, Karasawa K, Ito Y, et al. Intraoperative radiotherapy for unresectable pancreatic cancer: a multi-institutional retrospective analysis of 144 patients. Int J Radiat Oncol Biol Phys 2011;80:111–8.

32. Chen Y, Che X, Zhang J, et al. Long-term results of intraoperative electron beam radiation therapy for nonmetastatic locally advanced pancreatic cancer: Retrospective cohort study, 7-year experience with 247 patients at the National Cancer Center in China. Medicine (Baltim) 2016;95:e4861.

33. Cai S, Hong TS, Goldberg SI, et al. Updated long-term outcomes and prognostic factors for patients with unresectable locally advanced pancreatic cancer treated with intraoperative radiotherapy at the Massachusetts General Hospital, 1978 to 2010. Cancer 2013;119:4196–204.

34. Jarnagin WR, Fong Y, DeMatteo RP, et al. Staging, resectability, and outcome in 225 patients with hilar cholangiocarcinoma. Ann Surg 2001;234:507–17 [discussion: 517-509].

35. Sirica AE, Gores GJ. Desmoplastic stroma and cholangiocarcinoma: clinical implications and therapeutic targeting. Hepatology 2014;59:2397–402.

36. Todoroki T, Kawamoto T, Otsuka M, et al. Benefits of combining radiotherapy with aggressive resection for stage IV gallbladder cancer. Hepato-Gastroenterology 1999;46:1585–91.

37. Lindell G, Holmin T, Ewers SB, et al. Extended operation with or without intraoperative (IORT) and external (EBRT) radiotherapy for gallbladder carcinoma. Hepato-Gastroenterology 2003;50:310–4.

38. Monson JR, Donohue JH, Gunderson LL, et al. Intraoperative radiotherapy for unresectable cholangiocarcinoma–the Mayo Clinic experience. Surg Oncol 1992;1: 283–90.

39. Kaiser GM, Fruhauf NR, Lang H, et al. Impact of intraoperative radiotherapy (IORT) on survival of patients with unresectable hilar cholangiocarcinoma. Hepato-Gastroenterology 2008;55:1951–4.

40. Fisher B, Wolmark N, Rockette H, et al. Postoperative adjuvant chemotherapy or radiation therapy for rectal cancer: results from NSABP protocol R-01. J Natl Cancer Inst 1988;80:21–9.

41. Conroy T, Bosset JF, Etienne PL, et al. Neoadjuvant chemotherapy with FOLFIR-INOX and preoperative chemoradiotherapy for patients with locally advanced rectal cancer (UNICANCER-PRODIGE 23): a multicentre, randomised, open-label, phase 3 trial. Lancet Oncol 2021;22:702–15.

42. Masaki T, Matsuoka H, Kishiki T, et al. Site-specific risk factors for local recurrence after rectal cancer surgery. Surg Oncol 2021;37:101540.
43. Maas M, Nelemans PJ, Valentini V, et al. Long-term outcome in patients with a pathological complete response after chemoradiation for rectal cancer: a pooled analysis of individual patient data. Lancet Oncol 2010;11:835–44.
44. Braendengen M, Tveit KM, Berglund A, et al. Randomized phase III study comparing preoperative radiotherapy with chemoradiotherapy in nonresectable rectal cancer. J Clin Oncol 2008;26:3687–94.
45. Dubois JB, Bussieres E, Richaud P, et al. Intra-operative radiotherapy of rectal cancer: results of the French multi-institutional randomized study. Radiother Oncol 2011;98:298–303.
46. Masaki T, Matsuoka H, Kishiki T, et al. Intraoperative radiotherapy for resectable advanced lower rectal cancer-final results of a randomized controlled trial (UMIN000021353). Langenbeck's Arch Surg 2020;405:247–54.
47. Kusters M, Valentini V, Calvo FA, et al. Results of European pooled analysis of IORT-containing multimodality treatment for locally advanced rectal cancer: adjuvant chemotherapy prevents local recurrence rather than distant metastases. Ann Oncol 2010;21:1279–84.
48. Holman FA, Haddock MG, Gunderson LL, et al. Results of intraoperative electron beam radiotherapy containing multimodality treatment for locally unresectable T4 rectal cancer: a pooled analysis of the Mayo Clinic Rochester and Catharina Hospital Eindhoven. J Gastrointest Oncol 2016;7:903–16.
49. Haddock MG, Miller RC, Nelson H, et al. Combined modality therapy including intraoperative electron irradiation for locally recurrent colorectal cancer. Int J Radiat Oncol Biol Phys 2011;79:143–50.
50. Suzuki K, Gunderson LL, Devine RM, et al. Intraoperative irradiation after palliative surgery for locally recurrent rectal cancer. Cancer 1995;75:939–52.
51. Valentini V, Morganti AG, De Franco A, et al. Chemoradiation with or without intraoperative radiation therapy in patients with locally recurrent rectal carcinoma: prognostic factors and long term outcome. Cancer 1999;86:2612–24.
52. Holman FA, Bosman SJ, Haddock MG, et al. Results of a pooled analysis of IOERT containing multimodality treatment for locally recurrent rectal cancer: Results of 565 patients of two major treatment centres. Eur J Surg Oncol 2017;43:107–17.
53. Mirnezami R, Chang GJ, Das P, et al. Intraoperative radiotherapy in colorectal cancer: systematic review and meta-analysis of techniques, long-term outcomes, and complications. Surg Oncol 2013;22:22–35.
54. Fahy MR, Kelly ME, Power Foley M, et al. The role of intraoperative radiotherapy in advanced rectal cancer: a meta-analysis. Colorectal Dis 2021;23:1998–2006.
55. Liu B, Ge L, Wang J, et al. Efficacy and safety of intraoperative radiotherapy in rectal cancer: A systematic review and meta-analysis. World J Gastrointest Oncol 2021;13:69–86.
56. Roeder F, Goetz JM, Habl G, et al. Intraoperative Electron Radiation Therapy (IOERT) in the management of locally recurrent rectal cancer. BMC Cancer 2012;12:592.
57. Sole CV, Calvo FA, Serrano J, et al. Post-chemoradiation intraoperative electron-beam radiation therapy boost in resected locally advanced rectal cancer: long-term results focused on topographic pattern of locoregional relapse. Radiother Oncol 2014;112:52–8.

58. Hyngstrom JR, Tzeng CW, Beddar S, et al. Intraoperative radiation therapy for locally advanced primary and recurrent colorectal cancer: ten-year institutional experience. J Surg Oncol 2014;109:652–8.
59. Zhang Q, Tey J, Yang Z, et al. Intraoperative radiotherapy in the combination of adjuvant chemotherapy for the treatment of pT3N0M0 rectal cancer after radical surgery. Am J Clin Oncol 2014;37:8–12.
60. Zhang Q, Tey J, Yang Z, et al. Adjuvant chemoradiation plus intraoperative radiotherapy versus adjuvant chemoradiation alone in patients with locally advanced rectal cancer. Am J Clin Oncol 2015;38:11–6.

Biology-Guided Radiation Therapy

An Evolving Treatment Paradigm

Colton Ladbury, MD, Nicholas Eustace, MD, PhD, Arya Amini, MD,
Savita Dandapani, MD, PhD, Terence Williams, MD, PhD*

KEYWORDS

- PET • Radiotherapy • BgRT • Biology-guided radiotherapy • lung cancer
- lymphoma • gastrointestinal cancer • molecular imaging

KEY POINTS

- PET is a valuable imaging modality that can prognosticate outcomes and predict response to therapy, including radiation.
- PET can be used as a strategy for adapting, escalating, or de-escalating radiotherapy.
- Optimal PET metrics and thresholds need to be further clarified.
- Real-time biology-guided radiation therapy PET-guided linear accelerator technology is forthcoming as a potential promising augmentation to radiotherapy options.

INTRODUCTION

In radiation oncology, imaging guides patient selection, treatment volume delineation, and accurate treatment delivery. Therefore, improvements in radiotherapy delivery are intrinsically linked to advances in imaging technology. The advent of 3D-radiotherapy was made possible by computed tomography (CT)-based radiation treatment planning, and more recently, novel magnetic resonance-guided radiation treatment has provided increasing soft tissue resolution to enable more precise anatomic targeting.[1,2] Advances in functional imaging modalities such as PET have demonstrated promise for further informing radiotherapy delivery by providing risk stratification and a means of gauging treatment response via correlation with biological activity. Indeed, early studies assessing the incorporation of PET into radiation treatment planning suggested improved radiation planning (eg, incorporation of CT-subclinical disease) and outcomes when combining PET with radiation.[3–5] This has led to the concept of biology-guided radiotherapy (BgRT), an emerging external beam

Department of Radiation Oncology, City of Hope National Medical Center, 1500 East Duarte Road, Duarte, CA 91010, USA
* Corresponding author.
E-mail address: terwilliams@coh.org

Surg Oncol Clin N Am 32 (2023) 553–568
https://doi.org/10.1016/j.soc.2023.02.006
1055-3207/23/© 2023 Elsevier Inc. All rights reserved.

surgonc.theclinics.com

radiotherapy treatment paradigm that uses biological/molecular imaging to inform radiation treatment.

A primary way of BgRT functions is by using imaging as a biomarker that is both prognostic and predictive of response to therapy. PET imaging is the most common modality, with the associated radiotracer being used to characterize relevant treatment metrics such as tumor burden/distribution, hypoxia, angiogenesis, metabolism, and proliferation.[6] Functional imaging like PET can provide relevant information at several points in the radiation delivery process: before and following treatment as a prognostic indicator, as an indicator of response to therapy, during radiation to inform treatment planning and adaptation.

Radiation therapy is at the cusp of integrating advanced functional imaging and treatment delivery systems and is poised to use biological information afforded by molecular imaging during BgRT to deliver more effective therapies. This potentially will enable treatment of multiple disease sites simultaneously, improve motion management, decrease treatment margins, and optimize targeting of biologically active tumor. This review highlights prior applications of PET imaging to prognosticate patients and guide radiation treatment, which will be relevant as integrated BgRT develops. A summary of included studies is summarized in **Table 1**.

PET Imaging for Response Assessment and Posttreatment Prognostication

Lung
In the ACRIN 6668/RTOG 0235 trial, the prognostic value of post-chemoradiation fluorodeoxyglucose (FDG)-PET was evaluated in patients with stage III non-small cell lung cancer (NSCLC).[7] In this study, 14 weeks after completion of chemoradiation, an FDG-PET was obtained to evaluate treatment response using two metrics: Standardized Uptake Value $(SUV)_{max}$ (the highest single-voxel SUV) and SUV_{peak} (mean SUV in a circular region of interest with diameter between 0.75 and 1.5 cm encompassing the SUV_{max}). Of 250 enrolled patients, 173 were evaluable for posttreatment analyses, whereas 226 had pretreatment imaging available. Neither pretreatment SUV_{max} nor SUV_{peak} correlated with survival. However, posttreatment SUV_{max} (Hazard Ratio [HR]: 1.125, $P < .001$) and SUV_{peak} (HR: 1.098, $P < .001$) as continuous variables did significantly correlate with overall survival. Further, although the prespecified binary SUV_{max} value of greater than 3.5 was not a significant predictor of overall survival, an exploratory analysis using a threshold of greater than 5 did significantly correlate with survival using both SUV_{max} (HR: 1.596, $P = .038$) and SUV_{peak} (HR: 2.148, $P = .002$).

Lymphoma
The introduction of PET has revolutionized assessment of treatment response in lymphoma, which had previously been assessed with the Cotswold criteria in the CT era.[8] The incorporation of PET was first published in 1999 by the National Cancer Institute Working Group,[9] with guidelines revised in 2007 by the International Working Group.[10] These lymphoma response criteria have since been succeeded by the Lugano classification criteria, which comprise the basis of modern lymphoma treatment response assessment.[11] The Lugano classification recognizes the importance of both CT and PET changes, primarily using a five-point scoring scale (Deauville criteria) that is based on metabolic activity relative to the liver and mediastinum to assess treatment response. By incorporating information from PET, the "complete response unconfirmed" category was removed because PET facilitated differentiation of patients with a "complete response" (CR) from patients with a "partial response" (PR), with PET-negative patients classified as CR even with residual CT findings. This framework improves the accuracy of disease assessment in patients with high-grade non-

Table 1
Summary of selected studies using PET to inform radiation therapy

Study, Year Published	Study Name	Study Type	Patient Number	Disease	Clinical Question	Takeaway
Role of PET for response assessment and posttreatment prognostication						
Machtay et al,[7] 2013	ACRIN 6668/RTOG 0235	Prospective	173	NSCLC	Can prognosis be based on pre- and post-CRT SUVpeak and SUVmax?	Post-CRT but not pre-CRT SUVmax and SUVpeak correlated with OS. A binary classification based on an SUV of 5 but not 3.5 was prognostic
Itti et al,[14] 2013	-	Retrospective	114	Non-Hodgkin lymphoma	How do PET metrics compare with Deauville scale?	SUVmax out-prognosticates the Deauville scale and has better interobserver reproducibility
Hasenclever et al,[15] 2014	-	Retrospective	898	Non-Hodgkin lymphoma	What is the prognostic role of SUVpeak/average liver uptake?	With threshold of 1.3, SUVpeak/average liver uptake can identify favorable responses with high sensitivity
Role of PET for guiding radiation therapy						
van Diessen J et al,[16] 2019 & Cooke et al[17] 2020	PET-boost	Prospective (phase II)	352	NSCLC	Can PET be used for definition of radiation boost (boost to entire PTV vs only area with a SUVmax ≥50% within the PTV)?	No significant difference in toxicity, LC, or OS

(continued on next page)

Table 1
(continued)

Study, Year Published	Study Name	Study Type	Patient Number	Disease	Clinical Question	Takeaway
Nestle et al,[18] 2020	PET-PLAN	Prospective (phase III)	205	NSCLC	Can PET be used for definition of radiation treatment volumes (all FDG-avid disease plus elective nodes vs only FDG-avid sites)?	Improved locoregional progression with PET-guided only treatment
Greally et al,[19] 2019	-	Retrospective	111	Esophageal	Should chemotherapy component of chemoradiation (CRT) be changed based on post-induction chemotherapy disease response?	No difference in progression-free survival (PFS) or overall survival (OS) when changing chemotherapy in nonresponders
Goodman et al,[20] 2021	CALGB 80803	Prospective (phase II)	225	Esophageal	Should chemotherapy component of CRT be changed based on post-induction chemotherapy disease response?	No difference in pCR when changing chemotherapy in nonresponders. Higher pCR rate in responders treated with FOLFOX
Cotter et al,[21] 2006	-	Retrospective	41	Anal	How does PET/CT compare with CT in delineating the primary for radiation treatment planning?	PET is better able to aid in identification of the primary and positive lymph nodes compared to CT
Nguyen et al,[22] 2008	-	Retrospective	50	Anal	How does PET/CT compare with CT in delineating the primary for radiation treatment planning?	PET is better able to aid in identification of the primary and positive lymph nodes compared with CT

Study	Name	Type and number	Cancer type	Question	Result
Friedman et al,[24] 2014	AHOS0031	Prospective (phase III) 1712	Hodgkin Lymphoma	Can radiation be omitted in rapid early responders to chemotherapy (IFRT vs observation)?	No difference in EFS when omitting radiation in rapid early responders
Radford et al,[25] 2015	UK NCRI RAPID	Prospective (phase III) 602	Hodgkin Lymphoma	Can radiation be omitted in patients with CR following three cycles of chemotherapy (IFRT vs observation)?	No difference in PFS with RT omission
Borchmann et al,[26] 2021	GHSG HD17	Prospective (phase III) 1100	Hodgkin Lymphoma	Can radiation be omitted in patients with CR following four cycles of chemotherapy (IFRT vs observation)?	No difference in OS, PFS with RT omission
Keller et al,[27] 2018	AHOD0431	Prospective (phase III) 278	Hodgkin Lymphoma	Can radiation be omitted in patients with CR following 3 cycles of chemotherapy (IFRT vs observation)?	No difference in OS, EFS with RT omission
Pfreundschuh et al,[28] 2017	OPTIMAL>60 DSHNHL	Prospective (phase III) 187	Non-Hodgkin Lymphoma	Can radiation be omitted in elderly patients with bulky disease and CR to chemotherapy?	RT omission leads to comparable PFS to historical controls

(continued on next page)

Table 1
(continued)

Study, Year Published	Study Name	Study Type	Patient Number	Disease	Clinical Question	Takeaway
Role of PET for adaptive radiation therapy						
Kong et al,[32] 2017		Prospective (phase II)	42	NSCLC	Can radiation dose and volumes based on mid-treatment PET be adapted based on initial response?	Dose escalation was feasible with a PET-adaptive approach with acceptable toxicity, though associated local control (LC) and OS were still comparable with historical controls
Kong et al,[34] 2021	NRG-RTOG 1106/ ACRIN 6697	Prospective (phase II)	127	NSCLC	Can radiation dose and volumes based on mid-treatment PET be adapted based on initial response (standard treatment vs adaptive dose escalation)?	Adaptive dose escalation did not improve OS or loco-regional progression though exploratory analysis showed that in-field local primary tumor control and loco-regional tumor control were improved. Pulmonary toxicity was increased
Yuan et al,[35] 2020	CRTOG 1601	Prospective (phase III)	243	NSCLC	Can radiation dose and volumes based on mid-treatment PET be adapted based on initial response (standard treatment vs adaptive dose escalation)?	OS and PFS were improved with an adaptive approach without increased serious adverse events

Hodgkin lymphoma (NHL) and has since been validated in multiple studies including patients from the International Extranodal Lymphoma Study Group study.[12,13]

Despite the adoption of the Lugano classification, it must be emphasized that other PET metrics might still provide further information. In an international confirmatory study of the prognostic value of early PET in NHL, although the Deauville scale was found to be prognostic, the change in SUV_{max} led to better performance and interobserver reproducibility.[14] Other approaches include adaptations of the Deauville scale such as the quotient between SUV_{peak} of residual tumors and average uptake of the liver as measured with standardized volumes of interest, with a value of less than 1.3 excluding abnormal response with high sensitivity.[15] Therefore, although modern criteria are a major step in the right direction and synergizes with the concept of BgRT (as treatment is directed to areas of increased metabolism), more work will be required to further optimize its use.

Pre-Radiation PET Imaging for Guiding Radiation Therapy

Lung
PET imaging before and during radiation has been used to direct radiation treatment dose and fractionation. Recently, in the phase II PET-boost trial, patients were randomized to receive ≥72 Gy in 24 fractions (≥3 Gy/fraction) with an integrated boost to the planning target volume (PTV) of the entire primary tumor delineated on the CT scan (Arm A) or only to the regions with a SUV_{max} ≥50% within the PTV of the primary tumor on the pretreatment FDG-PET scan (Arm B).[16] The actual boost dose was calculated for each patient based on meeting organ-at-risk constraints. Of note, this trial was associated with significant acute and late grade ≥3 (41% and 42%, respectively) and grade 5 (5% and 11%, respectively) toxicity. There was no significant difference in OS and LC, with 3-year OS of 37% and 33% and 1-year LC of 97% and 91% in Arms A and B, respectively.[17]

Another trial in stage III NSCLC examined the ability of PET to guide treatment volumes. In PET-PLAN, a randomized phase III trial, patients underwent an FDG-PET and CT for planning and were randomized to radiation treatment with volumes inclusive of all sites of FDG-avid disease plus elective nodal irradiation (Group A) or target volumes inclusive of only FDG-avid sites (Group B), the latter allowing target volume reduction.[18] Dose was prescribed to 60 to 74 Gy as possible while respecting nearby structures. By tailoring dose only to sites of FDG-avid disease, mean dose in Group B was significantly higher (67.3 Gy vs 65.3, $P = .007$). One-year locoregional progression was decreased in Group B (14% vs 27%, $P = .039$), and there was no significant difference in toxicity between groups. Therefore, this trial has become a prime example of using PET to fully guide radiation therapy volumes.

Esophageal
There have also been attempts at using PET to guide chemoradiation in esophageal squamous cell carcinoma (SCC). In a retrospective analysis, Greally and colleagues investigated whether it is beneficial to change chemotherapy for the chemoradiation component of treatment if the post-induction therapy PET scan showed poor response to induction chemotherapy.[19] Responders were defined as a 35% or more decrease in SUV_{max}. A total of 37% of patients were classified as nonresponders, and of those patients, 61% had their systemic therapy changed during radiation. This strategy improved neither median PFS (6.4 months vs 8.3 months, $P = .556$) nor OS (14.1 vs 17.2 months, $P = .81$).

Interestingly, a similar approach has since been reported for esophageal and esophagogastric adenocarcinoma in the phase II CALGB 80803 trial.[20] In this study, patients underwent a baseline PET and were subsequently randomized to induction chemotherapy with either modified oxaliplatin, leucovorin, and fluorouracil (FOLFOX) or carboplatin-paclitaxel (CP). PET was repeated after induction chemotherapy, and nonresponders (again defined as a <35% decrease in SUV_{max}) were switched to the alternative chemotherapy regimen during the radiation portion of their treatment. Among nonresponders, pathologic CR (pCR) rate in patients who switched to FOLFOX and CP was 18% and 20%, respectively. In comparison, responders who received FOLFOX and CP had a pCR of 40.3% and 14.1%, respectively. The investigators concluded that using PET imaging as an early response assessment biomarker could be used to improve pCR rates in PET nonresponders.

Anal

PET has also proven useful in delineating anal cancer disease extent, which is critical to defining radiation treatment volumes. In a retrospective review by Cotter and colleagues, FDG-PET/CT was compared with CT alone in 41 patients.[21] PET imaging detected the primary tumor in 91% of patients compared with 59% with CT alone. It also identified 12% more patients with positive pelvic nodes and 17% of patients with positive inguinal nodes that were not detected by either CT or physical examination. In a similar study of 50 patients by Nguyen and colleagues, PET detected 98% of primary tumors compared with 58% with CT. PET upstaged 17% of patients nodal disease and led to changes in radiation plans in 19% of patients.[22] Accurate delineation of the primary and nodal disease is critical to dose selection and treatment volume determination based on updated standards defined by RTOG 0529, so the value of PET for radiation planning cannot be stressed enough.[23] An example of the utility PET provides for delineating the primary tumor is shown in **Fig. 1**A, B.

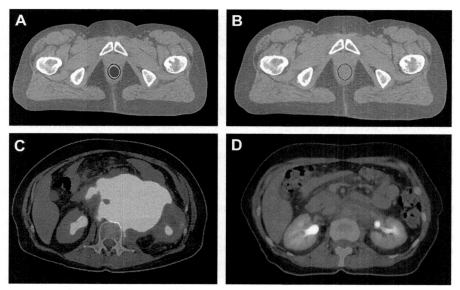

Fig. 1. Use of PET/CT (*A*) versus CT alone (*B*) for delineation of primary tumor (purple contour) in anal cancer. Pre-chemotherapy (*C*) and post-chemotherapy PET/CT (*D*) of an elderly patient with bulky DLBCL eligible for radiation omission due to complete response at the posttreatment PET/CT. DLBCL, diffuse large B-cell.

Lymphoma

In addition to providing information on treatment response in lymphoma, pre-radiation PET also has been used to guide treatment, largely as a means of treatment de-escalation. In Hodgkin lymphoma (HL), the AHOS0031 study examined omission of radiation in patients with rapid early response (RER) to chemotherapy, defined as having a CR on PET or CR following two cycles of doxorubicin, bleomycin, vincristine, etoposide, cyclophosphamide, and prednisone Adriamycin, Bleomycin, Vinblastine, Dacarbazine (ABVD).[24] Patients with RER were randomized to 21 Gy involved-field radiation therapy (IFRT) versus observation. In patients with PET-confirmed RER, 4-year event-free survival was 87% in both arms, demonstrating the ability of PET to help guide treatment de-escalation.

Similarly, in the UK NCRI RAPID study, patients with stage I or IIA HL with CR by PET following three cycles of ABVD were randomized to IFRT versus observation.[25] Three-year PFS was not significantly different, with 95% in the RT arm versus 91% in the observation arm. Several other studies have also used PET to support RT omission in early-stage HL, including HD17 GHSG[26] and COG AHOD0431 trials.[27]

PET has also been used to guide treatment in NHL, where indications for radiotherapy have decreased to select cases of bulky disease or PR in the rituximab era. In the OPTIMAL>60 DSHNHL trial, elderly patients with CR and bulky disease received no further treatment, whereas patients with PR received 39.6 Gy.[28] When compared with the RICOVER-60 trial,[29] which had previously established the role of RT for bulky disease, results were non-inferior. Again, in this study, PET permitted potential treatment de-escalation for lymphoma. An example of the utility PET provides for identifying candidates for radiation omission in patients under the OPTIMAL greater than 60 DSHNHL paradigm is shown in **Fig. 1**C, D.

Adaptive Approaches to Biology-Guided Radiation Therapy

Lung

Following disappointing results from the radiation dose-escalation study RTOG 0617, a popular area of study for adaptive radiotherapy is in locally advanced NSCLC in order to further attempts to improve outcomes with treatment escalation.[30,31] In one such study by Kong and colleagues, as part of a phase II trial, patients were treated with a mid-treatment CT and PET-based adaptation to facilitate dose escalation to gross disease to up to 86 Gy in 30 fractions, with actual dose determined based on limiting risk of radiation-induced lung toxicity to less than 17.2% based on normal tissue complication probability modeling.[32] This was accomplished by performing a PET/CT after an equivalent 2 Gy dose of 40 to 50 Gy was delivered, at which point radiation was replanned with an updated GTV based on PET using a tumor-aorta auto-segmentation method.[33] Ultimately in the trial of 42 patients, median dose was 83 Gy. By using this approach, dose escalation was feasible without the excessive toxicity observed in RTOG 0617, with only a 7% Grade ≥ 3 toxicity rate. However, outcomes were still comparable to those achieved in RTOG 0617 with 2-year local control of 62% and median OS of 25 months. The approach was also tested in RTOG 1106/ACRIN 6697, this time as part of a randomized phase II trial. A total of 127 patients were randomized to either standard 60 Gy/30 fractions or treatment to approximately 40 Gy/20 fractions followed by PET-based adaptive replanning to a maximum of 80.4 Gy in the last 10 fractions.[34] There was no improvement in 2-year freedom from loco-regional progression (59.5% vs 54.6%, $P = .66$) or 3-year OS (49.1% vs 47.5%, $P = .80$). However, an exploratory analysis demonstrated improvements in 2-year in-field local primary tumor control (58.5% vs 75.6%) and local-regional tumor control (55.6% vs 66.3%). As opposed to RTOG 0617, rates of cardiac toxicity were low (<3%), though grade 3+ pulmonary toxicity was increased in the PET-adaptive arm (23.8% vs 14.3%).

Better oncologic results were achieved with the CRTOG 1601 trial, which was a phase III trial where patients were randomized to receive standard dosing (60 Gy/30 fractions), or PET-adapted dose escalation, where a repeat PET/CT was obtained after 36 to 40 Gy was delivered.[35] An adaptive boost (22–32 Gy) was then planned based on the updated imaging, to a minimum dose of 66 Gy or more in the last 10 fractions. In the initial presentation of these data, the PET-adaptive boost has led to improvements in median OS (44.6 months vs 28.0 months, $P = .001$) and PFS (15.1 months vs 11.6 months, $P = .001$) with no significant difference in serious adverse events.

Challenges

Despite the established role PET has in BgRT, several barriers remain to achieving optimal integration. A major question is determining how best to interpret PET scan data and then apply the data to guide treatments and predict outcomes. Several PET metrics are commonly used in the clinic.[36] SUV_{max} and SUV_{peak} are frequently used due to often correlating well with outcomes, being straightforward to calculate, and have abundant representation in the literature. Other relatively simple metrics include SUV_{mean} metabolic tumor volume (MTV; defined as the total volume of metabolically active tumor) and total lesion glycolysis (TLG; defined as MTV $\times$ SUV_{mean}). More complicated metrics being tested include radiomic analysis, such as texture features and contrast agent kinetics. Although all these metrics might be prognostic and/or predictive, some metrics may lend themselves better to certain clinical scenarios, whereas others are currently too complicated for broad adoption in the everyday oncology clinic until more streamlined analysis algorithms are developed. Identification of clinically relevant PET metric cutoff values for definition of prognostic groups is also relevant, which can be a challenge. This is evidenced by the ACRIN 6668/RTOG 0235 study, where the protocol specified SUV_{max} threshold of 3.5 was not prognostic, whereas an exploratory value of 5.0 was.[7] In contrast, lymphoma tends to use patient-specific thresholds defined by the liver or mediastinal blood pool, but these definitions require some degree of interpretation and, as illustrated by the study by Hasenclever and colleagues,[15] further refinement of how such thresholds should be defined is needed. As imaging data sets grow, it will be more feasible to empirically identify candidate thresholds that might be independently validated in additional data sets or prospective trials.

Other challenges to integration of PET with treatment delivery relate to the actual acquisition and nature of the resulting images. SUV is by its nature a semiquantitative metric that depends on factors including body weight, timing of SUV evaluation, competing transport effects, reconstruction methods, and scanner characteristics.[37] This leads to intra-patient, inter-patient, and inter-institution variability in SUV measurements, which can make multi-institutional studies and generalizations difficult. Next, there is the issue of nonspecific SUV uptake, which can influence multiple PET metrics and thresholds if not accounted for. The sources of nonspecific uptake include inflammation, infection, and physiologic uptake from normal organs.[38]

FUTURE DIRECTIONS AND REAL-TIME BIOLOGY-GUIDED RADIATION THERAPY

As detailed above, PET has demonstrated utility as a prognostic and predictive functional imaging modality, with the potential to inform adaptive treatment approaches and monitor disease response over the course of treatment. The advent of PET and some of its applications is demonstrating the feasibility of BgRT in clinical practice. The next step is to expand on incorporation into existing treatment protocols as well as improving PET imaging itself.

In recent years, "real-time" BgRT PET-guided linear accelerator technology (RefleXion X1) has been developed and is awaiting final US Food and Drug Administration approval. This technology has the potential to improve BgRT in several ways. One such example is by potentially obviating the need for motion management. As part of the treatment, the tumor's emitted PET profile or biological signature acts as a fiducial, which increases the confidence in lesion localization during treatment.[39] When combined with a tomographic delivery algorithm with sub-second latency, treatment can be administered rapidly by targeting the emitted PET profile without the need for breath holding or other motion management technology. The goal of this technology is to manage motion across multiple targets throughout the body, thereby facilitating radiation treatment of disseminated or metastatic tumors as a debulking modality, which has previously been challenging due to technologic limitations relating to throughput and accurate targeting. An overview of the real-time BgRT RefleXion X1 workflow is shown in **Fig. 2**. Of course, the adoption of real-time BgRT will not be without challenges. One such challenge arises due to the intrinsic nature of the technology of BgRT; for PET scans to guide radiation and monitor response of the course of a fractionated radiation treatment, radiotracer must be present in the patient. However, the half-life of FDG is approximately 2 hours,[40] meaning a new injection would be required for each fraction of radiation. This means more injections, added costs, radiation dose, and thereby burden on and/or risk to patients. Thus, the onus will be on real-time BgRT technology to generate enough clinical benefit to counteract these encumbrances and hazards. One possible way to remedy the issue of cost and frequent injections is to use alternative radiotracers with longer half-lives that can be imaged over the course of multiple radiation fractions.

Other challenges relate to the stability of the PET signal throughout the course of radiation, and the threshold of PET signal needed to accurately target the lesion. Toward the former issue, a prospective pilot study by Tian and colleagues assessed FDG-PET metrics in 14 patients with early-stage NSCLC being treated with stereotactic body radiation therapy (SBRT) to a dose of 50 Gy in 5 fractions. These patients underwent serial PETs obtained within 2 weeks before treatment start, between fractions 1 and 2 and between fractions 3 and 4.[41] The initial work demonstrated no significant change in PET metrics over the course of treatment aside from the ratio between MTV and

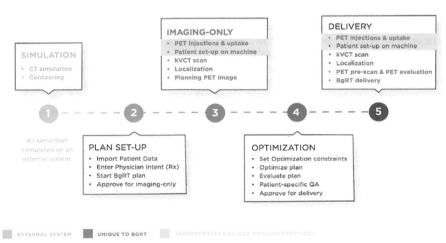

Fig. 2. Overview of the real-time BgRT clinical workflow and associated PET tracer-related steps. kvCT, kilovoltage computed tomography; QA, quality assurance.

Table 2 Summary of clinically available PET tracers			
Tracer	**Base**	**Half-Life**	**Application**
FDG	^{18}F	110 min	Glucose metabolism
Fluoride			Bone metabolism
FMISO			Hypoxia
FAZA			Hypoxia
PyL			Prostate-specific membrane antigen
Fluciclovine			Amino acid transport
FES			Estrogen binding
PSMA	^{68}Ga	68 min	Prostate-specific membrane antigen
FAP			Stromal activity
Choline	^{11}C	20 min	Phospholipid activity
MIBG	^{124}I	4.2 d	Neuronal activity
CD8	^{64}Cu	12.7 h	Immune activity

Abbreviations: CD8, cluster of differentiation 8; FAZA, F18-Fluoroazomycin arabinoside; MIBG, metaiodobenzylguanidine.

gross tumor volume (GTV), suggesting relative feasibility of using FDG signal as a fiducial.[41] Interestingly, with additional follow-up, an increase in SUV_{max} between the second and third PET scans correlated with distant failure in patients with recurrent/metastatic disease ($P = .025$).[42]

The most commonly used PET radiotracer in the aforementioned studies is FDG, but FDG has limitations related to the lack of specificity to tumor and short half-life, which both are potential obstacles to successful incorporation with BgRT. More recent radiotracers have been developed that may help address one or both of those problems, either through increased specificity or longer half-life that enables imaging of a single injection at multiple timepoints over the course of treatment. These include PyL, prostate-specific membrane antigen (PSMA), fluoro-estradiol (FES), and fibroblast activation protein (FAP). The ability to image non-tumor cell-related biological features is an attractive feature of this technology and includes innovative molecular imaging tools such as fluoromisonidazole (FMISO) and CD8 ImmunoPET.[43] These novel tracers offer additional exciting opportunities for implementation of BgRT in future studies by providing new applications and means of identifying tumors (or tumor-related features) to target over the course of RT. A summary of clinically available PET tracers can be found in **Table 2**.

Certainly, many questions remain regarding the use of FDG-based real-time BgRT. For example, is targeting mostly the pre-radiation PET-avid portions of the tumor the best targeting strategy, or should the non-FDG-avid portions of the CT-based tumor volume also be included? Does persistent mid-treatment FDG-avidity correlate with poor prognosis and radioresistance warranting dose escalation to these portions of the tumor? How do we differentiate FDG activity secondary to active cancer versus noncancer causes of uptake (eg, infection, inflammation, treatment-related inflammation, and other etiologies)? These questions and the above-mentioned challenges toward optimal implementation of real-time BgRT will be the subject of much research over the coming years.

SUMMARY

PET imaging has been extensively used as a treatment planning tool in radiation treatment planning but also to provide prognostic and predictive information for patients receiving radiation therapy. In addition, FDG-PET has a demonstrated role in adaptive planning and monitoring of tumor response over the course of treatment. Although there are several areas where further research is needed to clarify how PET can be best incorporated into clinical workflows, the advent of real-time PET-guided BgRT via incorporation of a dual molecular imaging-linear accelerator system is imminent. As further developments in PET imaging occur and are incorporated into radiotherapy, we should be cognizant to perform the necessary rigorous studies to establish the validity of novel ways of incorporating PET imaging and data metrics into the clinical practice of radiation oncology. Taken together, BgRT is an exciting and evolving field and could potentially significantly advance the field of radiation oncology through more personalized treatment.

CLINICS CARE POINTS

- In addition to general prognostication, PET has been used to monitor, escalate (eg, for lung cancer), or de-escalate (eg, for lymphoma) radiotherapy.
- Despite its established role in radiotherapy, the optimal use of PET needs to be further elucidated; efforts to standardize SUV metrics and thresholds, as well as imaging protocols, are warranted and ongoing.
- Although fluorodeoxyglucose represents the most widely used radiotracer, several emerging options might be able to improve sensitivity, specificity, and positive/negative predictive values depending on the clinical application.
- Real-time biology-guided radiation therapy PET-guided linear accelerator technology is a novel technology that incorporates PET into radiotherapy, allowing for improved motion management, smaller margins, simultaneous treatment of multiple targets, and using PET emissions to guide external beam radiation treatment.

DISCLOSURE

C. Ladbury has research grant funding from RefleXion Medical, United States. T. Williams has funding from the National Institutes of Health, United States and American Cancer Society, United States. The authors have nothing further to disclose.

REFERENCES

1. Mazzara GP, Velthuizen RP, Pearlman JL, et al. Brain tumor target volume determination for radiation treatment planning through automated MRI segmentation. Int J Radiat Oncol Biol Phys 2004;59(1):300–12.
2. Lagendijk JJ, Raaymakers BW, van Vulpen M. The magnetic resonance imaging-linac system. Semin Radiat Oncol 2014;24(3):207–9.
3. Turgeon GA, Iravani A, Akhurst T, et al. What (18)F-FDG PET Response-Assessment Method Best Predicts Survival After Curative-Intent Chemoradiation in Non-Small Cell Lung Cancer: EORTC, PERCIST, Peter Mac Criteria, or Deauville Criteria? J Nucl Med 2019;60(3):328–34.
4. Kalff V, Hicks RJ, MacManus MP, et al. Clinical impact of (18)F fluorodeoxyglucose positron emission tomography in patients with non-small-cell lung cancer: a prospective study. J Clin Oncol 2001;19(1):111–8.
5. Mac Manus MP, Wong K, Hicks RJ, et al. Early mortality after radical radiotherapy for non-small-cell lung cancer: comparison of PET-staged and conventionally

staged cohorts treated at a large tertiary referral center. Int J Radiat Oncol Biol Phys 2002;52(2):351–61.

6. Stewart RD, Li XA. BGRT: Biologically guided radiation therapy-The future is fast approaching. Med Phys 2007;34(10):3739–51.

7. Machtay M, Duan F, Siegel BA, et al. Prediction of Survival by F18 Fluorodeoxy-glucose Positron Emission Tomography in Patients With Locally Advanced Non–Small-Cell Lung Cancer Undergoing Definitive Chemoradiation Therapy: Results of the ACRIN 6668/RTOG 0235 Trial. J Clin Oncol 2013;31(30):3823–30.

8. Lister T, Crowther D, Sutcliffe S, et al. Report of a committee convened to discuss the evaluation and staging of patients with Hodgkin's disease: Cotswolds meeting. J Clin Oncol 1989;7(11):1630–6.

9. Cheson BD, Horning SJ, Coiffier B, et al. Report of an international workshop to standardize response criteria for non-Hodgkin's lymphomas. J Clin Oncol 1999; 17(4):1244.

10. Cheson BD, Pfistner B, Juweid ME, et al. Revised response criteria for malignant lymphoma. J Clin Oncol 2007;25(5):579–86.

11. Cheson BD, Fisher RI, Barrington SF, et al. Recommendations for Initial Evalua-tion, Staging, and Response Assessment of Hodgkin and Non-Hodgkin Lym-phoma: The Lugano Classification. J Clin Oncol 2014;32(27):3059–67.

12. Juweid ME, Wiseman GA, Vose JM, et al. Response assessment of aggressive non-Hodgkin's lymphoma by integrated International Workshop Criteria and fluorine-18-fluorodeoxyglucose positron emission tomography. J Clin Oncol 2005;23(21):4652–61.

13. Ceriani L, Martelli M, Gospodarowicz MK, et al. Positron emission tomography/computed tomography assessment after immunochemotherapy and irradiation using the Lugano classification criteria in the IELSG-26 study of primary medias-tinal B-cell lymphoma. Int J Radiat Oncol Biol Phys 2017;97(1):42–9.

14. Itti E, Meignan M, Berriolo-Riedinger A, et al. An international confirmatory study of the prognostic value of early PET/CT in diffuse large B-cell lymphoma: compar-ison between Deauville criteria and ΔSUVmax. Eur J Nucl Med Mol Imag 2013; 40(9):1312–20.

15. Hasenclever D, Kurch L, Mauz-Körholz C, et al. qPET – a quantitative extension of the Deauville scale to assess response in interim FDG-PET scans in lymphoma. Eur J Nucl Med Mol Imag 2014;41(7):1301–8.

16. van Diessen J, De Ruysscher D, Sonke JJ, et al. The acute and late toxicity results of a randomized phase II dose-escalation trial in non-small cell lung cancer (PET-boost trial). Radiother Oncol 2019;131:166–73.

17. Cooke S, De Ruysscher D, Reymen B, et al. The PET-boost trial: isotoxic homo-geneous or FDG-directed dose escalation in stage II-III NSCLC. Radiother Oncol 2020;152:S345–6.

18. Nestle U, Schimek-Jasch T, Kremp S, et al. Imaging-based target volume reduc-tion in chemoradiotherapy for locally advanced non-small-cell lung cancer (PET-Plan): a multicentre, open-label, randomised, controlled trial. Lancet Oncol 2020; 21(4):581–92.

19. Greally M, Chou JF, Molena D, et al. Positron-Emission Tomography Scan–Directed Chemoradiation for Esophageal Squamous Cell Carcinoma: No Benefit for a Change in Chemotherapy in Positron-Emission Tomography Nonre-sponders. J Thorac Oncol 2019;14(3):540–6.

20. Goodman KA, Ou F-S, Hall NC, et al. Randomized Phase II Study of PET Response–Adapted Combined Modality Therapy for Esophageal Cancer: Mature Results of the CALGB 80803 (Alliance) Trial. J Clin Oncol 2021;39(25):2803–15.

21. Cotter SE, Grigsby PW, Siegel BA, et al. FDG-PET/CT in the evaluation of anal carcinoma. Int J Radiat Oncol Biol Phys 2006;65(3):720–5.

22. Nguyen BT, Joon DL, Khoo V, et al. Assessing the impact of FDG-PET in the management of anal cancer. Radiother Oncol 2008;87(3):376–82.

23. Kachnic LA, Winter K, Myerson RJ, et al. RTOG 0529: a phase 2 evaluation of dose-painted intensity modulated radiation therapy in combination with 5-fluorouracil and mitomycin-C for the reduction of acute morbidity in carcinoma of the anal canal. Int J Radiat Oncol Biol Phys 2013;86(1):27–33.

24. Friedman DL, Chen L, Wolden S, et al. Dose-Intensive Response-Based Chemotherapy and Radiation Therapy for Children and Adolescents With Newly Diagnosed Intermediate-Risk Hodgkin Lymphoma: A Report From the Children's Oncology Group Study AHOD0031. J Clin Oncol 2014;32(32):3651–8.

25. Radford J, Illidge T, Counsell N, et al. Results of a Trial of PET-Directed Therapy for Early-Stage Hodgkin's Lymphoma. N Engl J Med 2015;372(17):1598–607.

26. Borchmann P, Plütschow A, Kobe C, et al. PET-guided omission of radiotherapy in early-stage unfavourable Hodgkin lymphoma (GHSG HD17): a multicentre, open-label, randomised, phase 3 trial. Lancet Oncol 2021;22(2):223–34.

27. Keller FG, Castellino SM, Chen L, et al. Results of the AHOD0431 trial of response adapted therapy and a salvage strategy for limited stage, classical Hodgkin lymphoma: A report from the Children's Oncology Group. Cancer 2018;124(15): 3210–9.

28. Pfreundschuh M, Christofyllakis K, Altmann B, et al. Radiotherapy to bulky disease PET-negative after immunochemotherapy in elderly DLBCL patients: Results of a planned interim analysis of the first 187 patients with bulky disease treated in the OPTIMAL>60 study of the DSHNHL. J Clin Oncol 2017;35(15_suppl):7506.

29. Held G, Murawski N, Ziepert M, et al. Role of Radiotherapy to Bulky Disease in Elderly Patients With Aggressive B-Cell Lymphoma. J Clin Oncol 2014;32(11): 1112–8.

30. Bradley JD, Hu C, Komaki RR, et al. Long-Term Results of NRG Oncology RTOG 0617: Standard- Versus High-Dose Chemoradiotherapy With or Without Cetuximab for Unresectable Stage III Non–Small-Cell Lung Cancer. J Clin Oncol 2020;38(7):706–14.

31. Bradley JD, Paulus R, Komaki R, et al. Standard-dose versus high-dose conformal radiotherapy with concurrent and consolidation carboplatin plus paclitaxel with or without cetuximab for patients with stage IIIA or IIIB non-small-cell lung cancer (RTOG 0617): a randomised, two-by-two factorial p. Lancet Oncol 2015;16(2):187–99.

32. Kong F-M, Ten Haken RK, Schipper M, et al. Effect of Midtreatment PET/CT-Adapted Radiation Therapy With Concurrent Chemotherapy in Patients With Locally Advanced Non–Small-Cell Lung Cancer. JAMA Oncol 2017;3(10):1358.

33. Mahasittiwat P, Yuan S, Xie C, et al. Metabolic Tumor Volume on PET Reduced More than Gross Tumor Volume on CT during Radiotherapy in Patients with Non-Small Cell Lung Cancer Treated with 3DCRT or SBRT. J Radiat Oncol 2013;2(2):191–202.

34. Kong F-MS, Hu C, Ten Haken R, et al. NRG-RTOG 1106/ACRIN 6697: A phase IIR trial of standard versus adaptive (mid-treatment PET-based) chemoradiotherapy for stage III NSCLC—Results and comparison to NRG-RTOG 0617 (non-personalized RT dose escalation). J Clin Oncol 2021;39(15_suppl):8548.

35. Yuan S, Yu Q, Wang S, et al. Individualized Adaptive Radiotherapy versus Standard Radiotherapy with Chemotherapy for Patients with Locally Advanced Non-

Small Cell Lung Cancer: A Multicenter Randomized Phase III Clinical Trial CRTOG1601. Int J Radiat Oncol Biol Phys 2020;108(3):S105.

36. Zaidi H, Karakatsanis N. Towards enhanced PET quantification in clinical oncology. Br J Radiol 2017;91(1081):20170508.

37. Thie JA. Understanding the standardized uptake value, its methods, and implications for usage. J Nucl Med 2004;45(9):1431–4.

38. Rosenbaum SJ, Lind T, Antoch G, et al. False-Positive FDG PET Uptake—the Role of PET/CT. Eur Radiol 2006;16(5):1054–65.

39. Oderinde OM, Shirvani SM, Olcott PD, et al. The technical design and concept of a PET/CT linac for biology-guided radiotherapy. Clinical and Translational Radiation Oncology 2021;29:106–12.

40. Yu S. Review of F-FDG Synthesis and Quality Control. Biomed Imaging Interv J 2006;2(4):e57.

41. Tian S, Sethi I, Yang X, et al. Characterization of Inter-Fraction 18-FDG PET Variability During Lung SBRT: Results of a Prospective Pilot Study. Int J Radiat Oncol Biol Phys 2019;105(1):E536.

42. Tian S, Switchenko J, Yang X, et al. Increased 18F-FDG Metabolic Activity during Lung SBRT Predicts Risk of Disease Progression: Results from a Prospective Study of Serial Inter-Fraction PET/CTs. Int J Radiat Oncol Biol Phys 2020;108(3):S59–60.

43. Ballinger J, Gnanasegaran G. F-FDG and Non-FDG PET Radiopharmaceuticals. In: Bomanji JB, Gnanasegaran G, Fanti S, Macapinlac HA, editors. PET/CT imaging, 18. New York City: Springer; 2022. p. 27–31.

Advances in Radiotherapy for Brain Metastases

Jennifer K. Matsui, PhD[a], Haley K. Perlow, MD[b], Rituraj Upadhyay, MD[b], Aliah McCalla, BS[c], Raju R. Raval, MD, DPhil[b], Evan M. Thomas, MD, PhD[b], Dukagjin M. Blakaj, MD, PhD[b], Sasha J. Beyer, MD, PhD[b], Joshua D. Palmer, MD[b,*]

KEYWORDS

- Brain metastases • Radiotherapy • Hippocampal avoidance
- Stereotactic radiosurgery • Radiation necrosis

KEY POINTS

- Hippocampal avoidance-whole-brain radiation therapy plus memantine may reduce neurocognitive decline for patients prescribed whole-brain radiotherapy.
- Stereotactic radiosurgery (SRS) is recommended for patients with limited brain metastases; however, patients with up to 15 brain metastases may benefit from SRS.
- Preoperative SRS has emerged as a safe and effective treatment option for patients with large and/or symptomatic brain metastases and may decrease rates of meningeal disease and radiation necrosis. Fractionation may reduce the risk of local failure.
- Treatment strategies for managing radiation necrosis include steroids, surgical resection, laser interstitial thermal therapy, Vitamin E and pentoxifylline, Boswellia serrata, and bevacizumab.
- Novel imaging techniques for distinguishing radiation necrosis from local recurrence include fluciclovine positron emission tomography and perfusion MRI.

INTRODUCTION

Brain metastases are the most common central nervous system (CNS) tumor in the adult population and are projected to increase in incidence as survival outcomes improve for primary malignancies.[1] Currently, the primary treatment options for brain metastases include surgery, whole-brain radiation therapy (WBRT), and stereotactic radiosurgery (SRS). Historically, WBRT was considered the radiation treatment standard for brain metastases[2] but patients that receive WBRT commonly experience long-term neurotoxicity.[3] As patients with brain metastases live longer, there has been a shift toward improving quality of life and neurocognitive function for patients

[a] College of Medicine, The Ohio State University, Columbus, OH 43201, USA; [b] Department of Radiation Oncology, The Ohio State University Wexner Medical Center, Columbus, OH 43201, USA; [c] College of Medicine, Central Michigan University, Mount Pleasant, MI 48858, USA
* Corresponding author.
E-mail address: joshua.palmer@osumc.edu

Surg Oncol Clin N Am 32 (2023) 569–586
https://doi.org/10.1016/j.soc.2023.02.007
1055-3207/23/© 2023 Elsevier Inc. All rights reserved.
surgonc.theclinics.com

receiving radiation therapy. This review article will focus on various advancements in radiation treatment of brain metastases. More specifically, hippocampal avoidance-WBRT (HA-WBRT), preoperative versus postoperative SRS, and single-fraction versus multifraction SRS will be discussed. Novel strategies for treating radiation necrosis will also be evaluated. Finally, ongoing clinical trials that are currently recruiting patients are highlighted.

ADVANCES IN WHOLE-BRAIN RADIOTHERAPY

For decades, radiotherapy has been a cornerstone treatment modality for patients with brain metastases. Historically, WBRT has been utilized to treat intracranial disease regardless of disease burden. Patchell conducted seminal studies demonstrating (1) the addition of surgery to WBRT improves overall survival (OS) and functional independence[4] and (2) adjuvant WBRT reduces recurrence and neurologic death but does not significantly affect OS.[5] Subsequent WBRT studies aimed to assess associated neurocognitive and quality of life decline in addition to survival outcomes. The QUARTZ trial reported patients with lung cancer brain metastases receiving WBRT plus optimal supportive care (OSC) compared with OSC alone had significantly more episodes of drowsiness, alopecia, nausea, and dry/itchy scalp, although there was no significant difference in serious adverse events.[6] Furthermore, there was no significant difference in OS, overall quality of life, or steroid use between the 2 groups. The results from this study suggest WBRT may not benefit a subset of patients with brain metastases (eg, poor performance status, older patients, uncontrolled primary non-small cell lung cancer), although a subgroup analysis showed that patients with 5 or greater metastases had an improved survival, suggesting that SRS may be more appropriate for patients with fewer lesions. Given the reports of cognitive decline and decreased quality of life associated with WBRT, strategies to mitigate these adverse effects have been explored.

Hippocampal Avoidance

HA-WBRT may be an option to improve cognition in this patient population.[7,8] The hippocampus, a critical structure for memory consolidation, is rarely involved in the setting of brain metastases.[9,10] RTOG 0933 compared patients receiving HA-WBRT with standard WBRT and found HA-WBRT results in greater cognitive preservation.[11] Neuroprotective agents such as memantine, an N-methyl-D-aspartate receptor antagonist, have been explored in the setting of brain irradiation after promising preclinical studies.[12–14] RTOG 0614 sought to determine if there is a cognitive function benefit when prescribing memantine during WBRT.[15] Although the authors noted less cognitive decline at 24 weeks (the primary endpoint) in patients that received memantine, this finding did not reach statistical significance, potentially due to patient loss (only 29% of eligible patients completed the assessment but an 80% completion rate was assumed). Notably, memantine was associated with better cognitive function preservation and was well tolerated. Given the promising preclinical and clinical results suggesting memantine is associated with better cognitive function preservation and HA-WBRT preserves memory and quality of life, the NRG-CC001 investigated the role of WBRT versus HA-WBRT with memantine in both arms.[16] The randomized phase III trial found no significant difference in OS or intracranial progression-free survival (PFS), and the time to neurocognitive function failure was significantly longer in the HA-WBRT plus memantine arm. HA-prophylactic cranial irradiation (PCI) for patients with lung cancer has also been explored to preserve cognitive function. The PREMER phase III study measured delayed free recall at 3 months comparing patients who received standard PCI or HA-PCI.[17] The authors found hippocampal avoidance preserved cognitive function with no observed survival or quality of life differences.

Simultaneous Integrated Boost

Although HA-WBRT limits cognitive decline associated with WBRT for brain metastases, investigators have sought to improve long-term local control rates. Some hypothesized that delivering a radiosurgery boost to gross disease in a simultaneous fashion (as opposed to sequential) may reduce tumor cell proliferation and repopulation.[18,19] RTOG 9508 evaluated WBRT with or without an SRS boost for patients with 1 to 3 brain metastases, and found that an SRS boost improved local control.[20] Modern data have evaluated the efficacy of a simultaneous integrated boost (SIB) with HA-WBRT compared with SRS. One single-institution phase II trial in adult patients with brain metastases consisted of 20 Gy in 10 fractions to the whole brain with an SIB of 40 Gy in 10 fractions to metastatic lesions.[21] The authors found SIB-WBRT significantly improved cognitive outcomes compared with traditional WBRT (evaluated with the Hopkins Verbal Learning Test-Revised delayed recall) while achieving intracranial control rates similar to patients who received WBRT plus SRS. Another study by Popp and colleagues compared HA-WBRT plus SIB to conventional WBRT in patients with multiple brain metastases and found the addition of SIB was associated with improved local control, longer intracranial PFS, and reduced neurologic death rate.[22] The HIP-PORAD randomized phase II trial (NCT02147028) is currently evaluating neurocognitive function outcomes of HA-WBRT plus SIB.[23]

Future Directions

In addition to hippocampal sparing (HA), researchers are exploring other memory sparing structures that may improve cognitive outcomes.[24] The amygdala, fornix, and mammary bodies are critical components of the limbic system that are responsible for functions such as decision-making, processing memories, and memory recall.[25] Studies have found structures such as the fornix are exquisitely sensitive to irradiation, and future studies evaluating the cognitive function benefit of avoiding these structures is warranted.[26]

ADVANCES IN STEREOTACTIC RADIOSURGERY

Although WBRT has historically been used to treat brain metastases, SRS utilization is increasingly utilized, particularly in patients with limited brain metastases.[27] Compared with WBRT, SRS delivers a precise local treatment that achieves good local control while mitigating neurocognitive decline.[28] A seminal study conducted in Japan compared SRS plus WBRT to SRS alone.[29] In this randomized control trial, the addition of WBRT to SRS did not improve survival for patients with 1 to 4 brain metastases, although intracranial recurrence occurred more frequently in patients who did not receive WBRT. A subsequent randomized trial compared SRS plus WBRT with SRS alone and utilized formal neurocognitive testing.[30] An important finding was memory preservation was greater in patients treated with SRS alone (measured by the Hopkins Verbal Learning Test-Revised total recall). Interestingly, the median survival was higher in the SRS subgroup (15.2 vs 5.7 months; $P = .003$), possibly due to more prompt initiation of systemic therapy or a greater systemic disease burden in the SRS plus WBRT arm. One-year local recurrence rates were significantly lower in the SRS alone arm. Collectively, the study provided level 1 evidence supporting the utilization of SRS alone for patient with 1 to 3 brain metastases. In 2016, Brown and colleagues conducted a randomized trial that assessed the cognitive effect of WBRT in addition to SRS and found SRS alone among patients with 1 to 3 brain metastases experienced less cognitive deterioration at 3 months.[31]

Although numerous studies have evaluated survival, disease control, quality of life, and neurocognitive function outcomes for patients with 1 to 3 brain metastases treated with SRS, fewer studies have focused on patients with 4 or more brain metastases. A recent retrospective study by Hughes and colleagues pooled data from 8 academic centers and compared outcomes of patients with 5 to 15 brain metastases treated with upfront SRS.[32] The authors found the number of intracranial metastases (5–15 vs 2–4) did not affect survival outcomes, suggesting that patients with up to 15 metastases may benefit from SRS. However, the recently published American Society for Radiation Oncology task force guidelines suggest that the current quality of evidence for treating patients with good performance status with 5 to 10 intact brain metastases is low.[33] Additional prospective evidence for treating patients with more than 3 brain metastases is warranted.[34] To address this significant gap in the literature, the Canadian Clinical Trials Group and Alliance for Clinical Trials in Oncology are conducting a phase III trial comparing SRS with WBRT for patients with 5 to 15 brain metastases (CCTG CE.7, NCT03550391).[35]

Preoperative versus Postoperative Stereotactic Radiosurgery

Postoperative radiosurgery has notable disadvantages: risk of tumor spillage during the time of surgical resection, larger treatment volumes, potential for decreased compliance in the case of postoperative surgical complications, and treatment planning uncertainty related to irregular tumor resection cavities.[36–38] More specifically, tumor spillage during resection can result in meningeal disease (MD) spread, which is a condition associated with poor survival rates and limited treatment options.[39] Preoperative SRS theoretically has the ability to sterilize cancerous cells via irradiation, preventing viable tumor spillage while also reducing treatment volumes and thereby minimizing healthy brain tissue doses. In particular, patients with factors associated with MD (eg, primary breast cancer, piecemeal resection, posterior fossa location) may significantly benefit from preoperative SRS.[40] Furthermore, preoperative SRS target volume delineation of brain metastases is relatively straightforward, whereas contouring surgical cavities may be challenging due to postoperative changes.[41]

Multiple recent publications have examined preoperative SRS as a treatment alternative for this patient population.[42–44] One early study evaluated 47 patients with brain metastases treated with preoperative SRS.[45] Patients were treated with a dose reduction strategy, where a median dose of 14 Gy was prescribed to the 80% isodose line. The authors reported local control at 1 and 2 years were 85.6% and 71.8%, respectively. Less than 15% of patients in the study were ultimately treated with WBRT, and there were no reports of MD and few incidences of radionecrosis. Subsequently, the group compared preoperative and postoperative SRS.[42] In this study, the median dose was relatively lower for preoperative SRS (14.5 Gy vs 18 Gy) with no differences observed in local or distant control. MD and radionecrosis rates were both significantly lower in the preoperative SRS arm. In 2018, Patel and colleagues evaluated the safety and efficacy of preoperative SRS in an additional cohort of patients treated at the University of Texas Southwestern Medical Center.[46] MD was noted in 2 of the 12 patients, possibly due to posterior fossa location. The authors concluded their findings support preoperative SRS as a safe and effective treatment option for select patients with cerebral metastases. In 2021, Prabhu and colleagues evaluated outcomes from the Preoperative Radiosurgery for Brain Metastases, a large multicenter cohort.[47] The median OS rate was 16.9 months and local recurrence rates were low (15% and 17.9% at 1 and 2 years, respectively). Subtotal resection was found to be a strong independent predictor of local recurrence. Additionally, there were low rates of MD and radiation necrosis when compared with historical controls. These findings suggest preoperative SRS may be a reasonable treatment of patients with large or symptomatic brain metastases when compared with postoperative SRS but randomized data are necessary.

Palmer and colleagues conducted a multi-institutional retrospective analysis of patients with brain metastases who received fractionated stereotactic radiation therapy (FSRT; 24 Gy –25 Gy in 3–5 fractions).[48] Within the cohort of 53 patients with 55 lesions, there were no local failures, 3 Grade 2+ radiation necrosis events, and 1 report of MD. This compared favorably with postoperative SRS studies that had higher incidences of MD and radiation necrosis, as well as historical preoperative SRS studies that had a higher rate of local failure due to single fraction treatments.[47,49–52] A more detailed discussion of single-fraction versus multifraction stereotactic radiotherapy for brain metastases is found in a later section.

Dosimetric analyses comparing postoperative SRS with preoperative SRS plans and showed that preoperative SRS plans have significantly reduced volume of irradiated healthy brain tissue.[53–56] One study found the volume of healthy brain irradiated with 28 Gy or greater was 6.79 cc in the preoperative plans and 10.79 in the postoperative plans ($P = .005$).[54] Beard and Rahimian also compared patients treated with postoperative SRS for brain metastases less than 4 cm in maximum dimension with a 2-mm PTV expansion to preoperative plans using the intact tumor as the PTV.[55] In their study, mean integral brain doses were significantly decreased in the preoperative plans (1.3 Gy vs 2.36 Gy), although integral doses to organs at risk did not differ significantly between the 2 groups. These data may explain the decreased incidence of radiation necrosis in patients who receive preoperative SRS. Another explanation may be avoidance of a proinflammatory cytokine reaction that increases the risk of radiation necrosis.[57]

It is important to note that preoperative treatment may not be suitable for all situations because patients may be unstable, or the lesion may need to be removed for a pathologic diagnosis. However, imaging techniques are constantly advancing, making it possible to distinguish brain metastases from other intracranial processes.[4] This makes it unlikely that the greater than 10% of lesions resected in the seminal Patchell study and found to be a primary malignancy would be replicated in modern clinical practice.[58] In the study by Prabhu and colleagues, only one patient out of 118 had a nonmetastatic intracranial disease and was inadvertently treated with preoperative SRS.[59] Another potential disadvantage is preoperative SRS may increase the risk of wound complications but studies have not found a clear association.[60]

Single-fraction Versus Multifraction Treatment

The most common late toxicity observed with SRS treatment of brain metastases is the development of radionecrosis that can result in neurologic deficits in a significant number of patients.[61–63] Studies have found when normal brain tissue is exposed to 12 Gy ($V_{12-Gy} > 10$ cm^3) during SRS, up to 60% of patients develop necrosis.[62,64] FSRT has been utilized as an alternative to single-fraction SRS in an attempt to mitigate the risk of radiation-related toxicity while also improving local failure rates.[65] Milano and colleagues pooled data from 51 reports to identify dosimetric and clinical predictors of radiation-induced toxicity for patients with either brain metastases or arteriovenous malformations treated with single-fraction or multifraction SRS.[66] The authors found radiation-related brain toxicity is related to tissue volumes that include target volumes; for tissue volumes of 5, 10, and more than 15 cm^3, the risk of symptomatic radionecrosis were approximately 10%, 15%, and 20%, respectively. The study found, if the treatment volumes were larger, FSRT is associated with reduced toxicity risk. In 2006, a phase II trial prospectively evaluated efficacy and toxicities associated with FSRT for irresectable brain metastases (1–4 metastases, median GTV 6 cc) not amenable to single-fraction radiosurgery (eg, gross tumor volume >3 ccs; location in brainstem, basal ganglia).[67] [(p)] In their study, complete response was relatively high (66.7% after a median follow-up of 7 months). Local tumor control at 6 and 12 months was 89% and 76%, respectively. The authors noted increased rates of edema or necrosis if a volume greater than 23 cc of normal brain tissue was exposed to more than 4 Gy per fraction. OS was comparable to historical studies.[5,68–72] These data suggest that FSRT (5 × 7 Gy) seems to be safe and effective for brain metastases with larger tumor volumes or located in critical anatomic sites but caution should be taken when irradiating more than 20 cc of normal brain volume. In 2014, Minniti et al evaluated outcomes of FSRT in patients with 1 to 3 brain metastases.[73] The 1-year and 2-year local control rates were 88% and 72%, respectively, and melanoma histology was an independent predictive factor of increased local failure (HR 6.1, 95% CI 1.5–24, $P = .02$). Radiation necrosis was diagnosed in 7% of the 171 lesions. Severe neurologic complications related to radiation necrosis (grade 3 or higher) was observed in only 4% of patients. In comparison, studies have found patients treated with single-fraction SRS (doses of 16 Gy–22 Gy) develop radionecrosis in up to 68% of the treated lesions.[62,63] The authors commented that FSRT may be ideal in the case where the volume of normal brain receiving a dose of 12 Gy is greater than 10 cc.

In 2019, Lehrer and colleagues performed a meta-analysis comparing single-fraction and multifraction SRS, comparing local control and radionecrosis rates in patients with large brain metastases.[74] In this study, large brain metastases (4–14 cc) treated with definitive multifraction SRS resulted in a 20% improvement in 1-year local control and a 68% relative reduction in radionecrosis. The authors surmised the radiobiological advantage of multifraction SRS contributes to the decrease in radionecrosis.[65,75] Furthermore, the breaks between treatments in fractionated regimens allows for higher biologically effective dose (BED) compared with single-fraction SRS and that the higher BED should improve local control rates. The results of this study support previous retrospective and prospective studies that have found multifraction SRS results in lower rates of radiation necrosis while maintaining or improving local control compared with single-fraction SRS for large brain metastases.[44,50,65,76]

TREATMENT STRATEGIES FOR MANAGING RADIATION NECROSIS
Steroids

For symptomatic patients (eg, headaches, nausea, cognitive impairment), oral corticosteroids are the preferred first-line treatment. Corticosteroids decrease edema through a reduction in inflammatory signals and cytokine production.[77] Notably, long-term steroid use can result in undesired toxicities such as Cushing syndrome, immunosuppression, hyperglycemia, and myopathy. Therefore, a gradual taper is typically recommended.

Surgical Resection

Surgical resection of necrotic tissue causing mass effect may provide patients symptomatic relief. Additional advantages include histologic confirmation and the potential for facilitating steroid weaning. Clinical judgment must be utilized to determine which patients are suitable candidates; some studies have found patients with preoperative

Karnofsky Performance Status (KPS) scores of 70 or less had increased risk of post-operative morbidity.[78]

Laser Interstitial Thermal Therapy

Laser interstitial thermal therapy (LITT) has emerged as a promising treatment of brain necrosis.[79] The procedure is minimally invasive and involves thermal ablation using a stereotactically placed laser probe. To date, LITT has demonstrated utility for recurrent metastatic disease or radiation-related necrosis. In a prospective study, Ahluwalia and colleagues demonstrated LITT stabilized KPS scores, quality of life, and cognition in patients with either biopsy-proven radiation necrosis or recurrent tumor.[80]

Boswellia Serrata

Following irradiation, patients with brain tumors often experience cerebral edema and are treated with steroids (eg, dexamethasone). Steroids have many adverse side effects; thus, replacement therapies are actively sought. Boswellia serrata is a medication that has demonstrated potent anti-inflammatory properties[81] and has been evaluated for the treatment of radiation-related cerebral edema. In a prospective study by Kirste and colleagues, Boswellia serrata significantly reduced edema compared with placebo treatment (>75% reduction in 60% of patients receiving Boswellia and 26% in patients receiving placebo).[82]

Bevacizumab

Currently, researchers believe radiation-induced necrosis is a result of endothelial cell dysfunction and the release of vasoactive compounds (eg, vascular endothelial growth factor [VEGF]).[83–85] Blocking VEGF can reduce the intracranial leakage of plasma and plasma water, thereby reducing edema. Bevacizumab, a VEGF-inhibitor, has been explored as a therapeutic option for symptomatic radiation necrosis. Levin and colleagues conducted a randomized controlled trial and found bevacizumab decreased volumes of necrosis, providing class I evidence supporting the use to bevacizumab for CNS radiation necrosis.[86]

Vitamin E and Pentoxifylline

Vitamin E is a free radical scavenger that may prevent localized cell damage caused by radiotherapy.[87] Pentoxyifylline is a methylxanthine derivative that increases blood circulation, and preclinical studies have demonstrated the ability to modify late-radiation induced injury.[88,89] In a study by Lefaix and colleagues, the combination of vitamin E and pentoxyifylline resulted in a greater than 50% reduction in skin fibrosis in an animal model.[90] Currently, the combination therapy is utilized to treat radiation-induced fibrosis.[91] A recent study has suggested vitamin E and pentoxyifylline is safe for the treatment of radiation necrosis,[92] and a phase II study (NCT01508221) is assessing whether the combination prevents radiation necrosis after radiosurgery.

Imaging to Diagnose Radiation Necrosis

Despite imaging advances, tumor recurrence and radiation necrosis have similar appearances on MRI, CT, and positron emission tomography (PET) imaging.[93,94] Fluciclovine (anti-1-amino-3-18F-fluorocyclobutane-1-carboxylic acid) is a synthetic amino acid that has been shown to have increased uptake in brain gliomas[95] and has been utilized to differentiate high-grade and low-grade gliomas.[96] In 2020, Parent and colleagues investigated the sensitivity and specificity of fluciclovine PET for distinguishing radiation necrosis from tumor recurrence and found that fluciclovine PET can accurately differentiate the two diagnoses.[97] NCT04410133 is a phase III study evaluating the diagnostic performance of fluciclovine PET for detecting radiation necrosis versus local recurrence after radiation.

Perfusion (dynamic susceptibility-weighted contrast-enhanced) MRI can measure vascularity and permeability of brain tissue and has been utilized for grading, predicting RT response, and histologic differentiation of gliomas.[98–101] More recently, perfusion MRI has emerged as a useful tool for distinguishing necrosis and tumor recurrence after SRS in patients with brain metastases.[102,103] A study by Mitsuya and colleagues used MR perfusion imaging to calculate the relative cerebral blood volume (rCBV) ratio of 28 lesions that were followed-up with gadolinium-enhanced MR images at 1 to 2-month intervals.[103] The authors reported a rCBV ratio of greater than 2.1 had the best sensitivity (100%) and specificity (95.2%) for identifying recurrent brain metastases.

CLINICAL TRIALS
Whole-Brain Radiation Therapy

Various phase II and III studies are evaluating HA-WBRT outcomes in addition to other WBRT strategies for improving quality of life and symptom burden (eg, sparing normal tissue, critical white-matter tracts). These studies that are currently recruiting are discussed below.

NCT03075072 is a phase III trial comparing SRS (1–5 fractions) with WBRT (HA when possible; 30 Gy in 10 fractions) in radiation-naïve patients with 5 to 20 brain metastases. The primary outcome measure is quality of life utilizing the MD Anderson Symptom Inventory–Brain Tumor. Secondary measures are OS, neurologic survival, recurrence patterns, rates of radiation necrosis, incidence and time to neurocognitive decline, and performance status.

NCT05013892 is a phase II randomized trial evaluating the safety and efficacy of normal brain tissue sparing (NTS) WBRT plus SIB with HA-WBRT. Both treatment arms will be prescribed memantine. Primary outcomes are patient reported quality of life and patient reported symptom burden (both assessed using the Functional Assessment of Cancer Therapy–Brain). Secondary outcomes are local control rates; intracranial PFS; OS; neurocognitive function, mood, fatigue, neuroendocrine function, hearing, and alopecia changes; and treatment-related toxicity.

NCT04804644 is a phase III trial comparing SRS to HA-WBRT plus memantine in patients with pathologically proven diagnosis of small cell lung cancer. The primary outcome measure is time to neurocognitive failure with secondary outcomes measuring neurocognitive function, symptom burden, OS, and adverse events. Inclusion criteria include 10 or fewer brain metastases with a 3 cm or less diameter.

NCT04343157 is a phase II trial utilizing a novel imaging technique that uses diffusion tensor imaging and volumetric imaging to identify critical white-matter tracts and the hippocampus. The investigators will prospectively enroll 60 patients with 1 to 3 brain metastases who are eligible for SRS and use segmentation imaging studies for cognitive-sparing SRS planning. Primary outcomes include measuring changes in verbal memory, executive function, attention/processing speed, and language function from baseline 3 months after SRS.

Preoperative versus Postoperative Stereotactic Radiosurgery

Currently, there are several phase II and III trials (recruiting) comparing preoperative versus postoperative SRS outcomes. NCT04474925 is a phase III study comparing preoperative and postoperative SRS outcomes in radiation-naïve patients with brain metastases. The primary outcome is local control (assessed at 12 months) and

Table 1
Ongoing trials studying various radiation treatment strategies for brain metastases

Category	Trial	Phase	Sponsor	Intervention	Outcome Measures
WBRT	NCT03075072	III	Dana-Farber Cancer Institute	Comparing SRS with WBRT in patients with 5–20 brain metastases	Primary measure is quality of life (MD Anderson Symptom Inventory - Brain Tumor); secondary measures are OS, neurologic survival, recurrence patterns, rates of radiation necrosis, neurocognitive outcomes, and performance status
	NCT05013892	II	Massachusetts General Hospital	Comparing NTS WBRT plus SIB with HA-WBRT (both arms with memantine)	Primary outcomes are quality of life and patient-reported symptom burden; secondary outcomes are local control rates, intracranial PFS, survival outcomes, and treatment-related toxicities
	NCT04804644	III	NRG Oncology	Comparing SRS to HA-WBRT plus memantine	Primary outcome measure is time to neurocognitive failure; secondary outcomes are neurocognitive outcomes, symptom burden, survival outcomes, and adverse events
	NCT04343157	II	University of California, San Diego	Novel imaging technique using diffusion tensor for cognitive-sparing SRS planning imaging and volumetric imaging	Primary outcomes are changes in verbal memory, executive function, attention/ processing speed, language function

(continued on next page)

Table 1
(continued)

Category	Trial	Phase	Sponsor	Intervention	Outcome Measures
Preoperative vs postoperative SRS	NCT04474925	III	AHS Cancer Control Alberta	Comparing preoperative and postoperative SRS outcomes	Primary outcome is local control; secondary outcomes are distant control, MD, and cognitive outcomes
	NCT03741673	III	MD Anderson Cancer Center	Comparing preoperative and postoperative SRS outcomes	Primary outcome is leptomeningeal disease-free rates; secondary objectives are local control rates and survival outcomes
	NCT03750227	III	Mayo Clinic	Comparing preoperative and postoperative SRS outcomes in patients with 10 or fewer brain metastases	Primary outcome is time to first CNS event; secondary outcomes are OS, adverse events, quality of life, PFS, time to salvage treatment, and rate of neurosurgical morbidity
	NCT04503772 (STEP)	II	Center Jean Perrin	Preoperative SRS for patients with 4 or fewer brain metastases	Primary outcome is 6-mo local control; secondary outcome measures are radionecrosis, OS, toxicities, leptomeningeal relapse, cognitive function outcomes, and quality of life
Single-fractionated vs multifractionated SRS	NCT04114981 (Alliance A071801)	III	Alliance for Clinical Trials in Oncology	Comparing adjuvant single-fractionated vs multifractionated SRS	Primary outcome is surgical bed recurrence-free survival; secondary outcomes include quality of life, performance status, OS, adverse events, and radiation necrosis
	NCT05222620 (FRACTIONATE)	II	Mayo Clinic	Comparing single-fractionated vs multifractionated SRS for intact brain metastases	Primary outcome is time to treatment failure (either local recurrence or radionecrosis); secondary objectives are OS, adverse events, patterns of failure, and quality of life

secondary outcomes are local control (assessed at 6 and 24 months), distant brain recurrence, leptomeningeal recurrence, and cognitive function (Hopkins Verbal Learning Test, Controlled Oral Word Association, and Trial Making Test).

NCT03741673 is a phase III trial where the primary objective is assessing MD-free rates. Secondary objectives investigate local and distant control rates and OS. Symptom burden, neurocognitive function, and health outcomes will also be measured. Fractionated treatments are eligible for inclusion. There is no limit to number of brain metastases but the primary lesion cannot have a maximum diameter of 4 cm for single-fraction or 7 cm for multifraction therapy.

NCT03750227 is a phase III trial comparing preoperative and postoperative SRS in patients with 10 or fewer brain metastases with the primary outcome measuring the time from study randomization to first CNS event (up to 5 years). Secondary outcomes include OS, adverse events, patient reported quality of life, PFS, time to subsequent treatment, and rate of neurosurgical morbidity. Exclusion criteria include brain metastases greater than 5 cm in size.

NCT04503772 is a phase II trial assessing 6-month local control after preoperative SRS for patients with 4 or fewer brain metastases. Secondary outcome measures include local control rate after 1 year, radionecrosis, OS, acute and delayed toxicities, leptomeningeal relapse, cognitive function (Mini-Mental State Examination), and quality of life (European Organization for Research and Treatment of Cancer Quality of Life Questionnaire–Core 30).

Single-fractionated versus Multifractionated Stereotactic Radiosurgery

The Alliance A071801 Trial (NCT04114981) is a phase III study comparing single-fractionated with multifractionated SRS in patients with resected brain metastases. The primary outcome measured is surgical bed recurrence-free survival from time of randomization (up to 2 years postradiation). Secondary outcomes include quality of life changes, performance status, OS, adverse events, and radiation necrosis.

The FRACTIONATE trial (NCT05222620) is a phase II study comparing single-fraction to multifraction SRS for the treatment of intact brain metastases. The primary objective is assessing if the composite endpoint of cumulative treatment failure (local failure or radionecrosis of the largest lesion) is increased with fractionated versus single-fraction SRS. Secondary objectives include measuring OS, treatment-related adverse events, patterns of failure, and quality of life outcomes.

The ongoing clinical trials discussed above are summarized in **Table 1**.

SUMMARY

Radiotherapy techniques for the treatment of brain metastases are rapidly evolving. Historically, WBRT has been associated with increased morbidity, but researchers are actively seeking ways to mitigate quality of life and cognitive function decline by sparing critical structures such as the hippocampus. SRS has become increasingly utilized as a precise and effect treatment alternative that preserves cognition without decreasing OS. Over the past decade, more attention has been devoted to preoperative SRS; recent studies have suggested preoperative SRS may be associated with lower rates of radiation necrosis and leptomeningeal disease, and numerous ongoing clinical trials are being conducted in this space. Single-fractionated and multifractionated SRS have also been compared, and studies have found multifraction SRS results in lower rates of local recurrence and radiation necrosis. Further prospective evaluation of these treatment techniques is warranted.

DECLARATION OF INTERESTS

All authors deny conflicts of interest related to this article.

REFERENCES

1. Ostrom QT, Wright CH, Barnholtz-Sloan JS. Chapter 2 - Brain metastases: epidemiology. In: *Handbook of clinical neurology*, 149. Cambridge, MA: Elsevier; 2018. p. 27–42.
2. Chao JH, Phillips R, Nickson JJ. Roentgen-ray therapy of cerebral metastases. Cancer 1954;7(4):682–9.
3. Wilke C, Grosshans D, Duman J, et al. Radiation-induced cognitive toxicity: pathophysiology and interventions to reduce toxicity in adults. Neuro Oncol 2018;20(5):597–607.
4. Patchell RA, Tibbs PA, Walsh JW, et al. A Randomized Trial of Surgery in the Treatment of Single Metastases to the Brain. N Engl J Med 1990;322(8): 494–500.
5. Patchell RA, Tibbs PA, Regine WF, et al. Postoperative Radiotherapy in the Treatment of Single Metastases to the BrainA Randomized Trial. JAMA 1998;280(17): 1485–9.
6. Mulvenna P, Nankivell M, Barton R, et al. Dexamethasone and supportive care with or without whole brain radiotherapy in treating patients with non-small cell lung cancer with brain metastases unsuitable for resection or stereotactic radiotherapy (QUARTZ): results from a phase 3, non-inferiority, randomised trial. Lancet 2016;388(10055):2004–14.
7. Gondi V, Tomé WA, Mehta MP. Why avoid the hippocampus? A comprehensive review. Radiother Oncol 2010;97(3):370–6.
8. Eriksson PS, Perfilieva E, Björk-Eriksson T, et al. Neurogenesis in the adult human hippocampus. Nat Med 1998;4(11):1313–7.
9. Regine WF, Schmitt FA, Scott CB, et al. Feasibility of neurocognitive outcome evaluations in patients with brain metastases in a multi-institutional cooperative group setting: results of Radiation Therapy Oncology Group trial BR-0018. Int J Radiat Oncol Biol Phys 2004;58(5):1346–52.
10. Marsh JC, Herskovic AM, Gielda BT, et al. Intracranial Metastatic Disease Spares the Limbic Circuit: A Review of 697 Metastatic Lesions in 107 Patients. Int J Radiat Oncol Biol Phys 2010;76(2):504–12.
11. Gondi V, Pugh SL, Tome WA, et al. Preservation of Memory With Conformal Avoidance of the Hippocampal Neural Stem-Cell Compartment During Whole-Brain Radiotherapy for Brain Metastases (RTOG 0933): A Phase II Multi-Institutional Trial. J Clin Orthod 2014;32(34):3810–6.
12. Duman JG, Dinh J, Zhou W, et al. Memantine prevents acute radiation-induced toxicities at hippocampal excitatory synapses. Neuro Oncol 2018;20(5):655–65.
13. Chen H, Pellegrini J, Aggarwal S, et al. Open-channel block of N-methyl-D-aspartate (NMDA) responses by memantine: therapeutic advantage against NMDA receptor-mediated neurotoxicity. J Neurosci 1992;12(11):4427.
14. Chen HS, Lipton SA. Mechanism of memantine block of NMDA-activated channels in rat retinal ganglion cells: uncompetitive antagonism. J Physiol 1997; 499(1):27–46.
15. Brown PD, Pugh S, Laack NN, et al. Memantine for the prevention of cognitive dysfunction in patients receiving whole-brain radiotherapy: a randomized, double-blind, placebo-controlled trial. Neuro Oncol 2013;15(10):1429–37.

16. Gondi V, Deshmukh S, Brown PD, et al. Preservation of Neurocognitive Function (NCF) with Conformal Avoidance of the Hippocampus during Whole-Brain Radiotherapy (HA-WBRT) for Brain Metastases: Preliminary Results of Phase III Trial NRG Oncology CC001. Int J Radiat Oncol Biol Phys 2018;102(5):1607.
17. Rodríguez de Dios N, Couñago F, Murcia-Mejía M, et al. Randomized Phase III Trial of Prophylactic Cranial Irradiation With or Without Hippocampal Avoidance for Small-Cell Lung Cancer (PREMER): A GICOR-GOECP-SEOR Study. J Clin Orthod 2021;39(28):3118–27.
18. Kim JJ, Tannock IF. Repopulation of cancer cells during therapy: an important cause of treatment failure. Nat Rev Cancer 2005;5(7):516–25.
19. Wilson GA, Raiche AP, Sugeng F. 2.5D inversion of airborne electromagnetic data. null 2006;37(4):363–71.
20. Andrews DW, Scott CB, Sperduto PW, et al. Whole brain radiation therapy with or without stereotactic radiosurgery boost for patients with one to three brain metastases: phase III results of the RTOG 9508 randomised trial. Lancet 2004;363(9422):1665–72.
21. Westover KD, Mendel JT, Dan T, et al. Phase II trial of hippocampal-sparing whole brain irradiation with simultaneous integrated boost for metastatic cancer. Neuro Oncol 2020;22(12):1831–9.
22. Popp I, Rau S, Hintz M, et al. Hippocampus-avoidance whole-brain radiation therapy with a simultaneous integrated boost for multiple brain metastases. Cancer 2020;126(11):2694–703.
23. Grosu AL, Frings L, Bentsalo I, et al. Whole-brain irradiation with hippocampal sparing and dose escalation on metastases: neurocognitive testing and biological imaging (HIPPORAD) – a phase II prospective randomized multicenter trial (NOA-14, ARO 2015-3, DKTK-ROG). BMC Cancer 2020;20(1):532.
24. Palmer JD, Trifiletti DM, Gondi V, et al. Multidisciplinary patient-centered management of brain metastases and future directions. Neuro-Oncology Advances 2020;2(1):vdaa034.
25. Rolls ET. Limbic systems for emotion and for memory, but no single limbic system. Cortex 2015;62:119–57.
26. Connor M, Karunamuni R, McDonald C, et al. Regional susceptibility to dose-dependent white matter damage after brain radiotherapy. Radiother Oncol 2017;123(2):209–17.
27. Perlow H, Khaled D, Liu K, et al. Whole-Brain Radiation Therapy Versus Stereotactic Radiosurgery for Cerebral Metastases. Neurosurg Clin 2020;31(4):565–73.
28. Sahgal A, Aoyama H, Kocher M, et al. Phase 3 Trials of Stereotactic Radiosurgery With or Without Whole-Brain Radiation Therapy for 1 to 4 Brain Metastases: Individual Patient Data Meta-Analysis. Int J Radiat Oncol Biol Phys 2015;91(4):710–7.
29. Aoyama H, Shirato H, Tago M, et al. Stereotactic Radiosurgery Plus Whole-Brain Radiation Therapy vs Stereotactic Radiosurgery Alone for Treatment of Brain MetastasesA Randomized Controlled Trial. JAMA 2006;295(21):2483–91.
30. Chang EL, Wefel JS, Hess KR, et al. Neurocognition in patients with brain metastases treated with radiosurgery or radiosurgery plus whole-brain irradiation: a randomised controlled trial. Lancet Oncol 2009;10(11):1037–44.
31. Brown PD, Jaeckle K, Ballman KV, et al. Effect of Radiosurgery Alone vs Radiosurgery With Whole Brain Radiation Therapy on Cognitive Function in Patients With 1 to 3 Brain Metastases: A Randomized Clinical Trial. JAMA 2016;316(4):401–9.

32. Hughes RT, Masters AH, McTyre ER, et al. Initial SRS for Patients With 5 to 15 Brain Metastases: Results of a Multi-Institutional Experience. Int J Radiat Oncol Biol Phys 2019;104(5):1091–8.

33. Gondi V, Bauman G, Bradfield L, et al. Radiation Therapy for Brain Metastases: An ASTRO Clinical Practice Guideline. Practical Radiation Oncology 2022;12(4): 265–82.

34. Brown PD, Asher AL, Farace E. Adjuvant Whole Brain Radiotherapy: Strong Emotions Decide But Rational Studies Are Needed. Int J Radiat Oncol Biol Phys 2008;70(5):1305–9.

35. Roberge D, Brown P, Mason W, et al. CMET-48. CE7 canadian clinical trials group/alliance for clinical trials in oncology. a phase iii trial of stereotactic radio-surgery compared with whole brain radiotherapy (wbrt) for 5–15 brain metasta-ses. Neuro Oncol 2017;19(suppl_6):vi49.

36. Sankey EW, Tsvankin V, Grabowski MM, et al. Operative and peri-operative con-siderations in the management of brain metastasis. Cancer Med 2019;8(16): 6809–31.

37. Ahn JH, Lee SH, Kim S, et al. Risk for leptomeningeal seeding after resection for brain metastases: implication of tumor location with mode of resection: Clinical article. Journal of Neurosurgery JNS 2012;116(5):984–93.

38. Soltys SG, Adler JR, Lipani JD, et al. Stereotactic Radiosurgery of the Postoper-ative Resection Cavity for Brain Metastases. Int J Radiat Oncol Biol Phys 2008; 70(1):187–93.

39. Hyun JW, Jeong IH, Joung A, et al. Leptomeningeal metastasis: Clinical expe-rience of 519 cases. European Journal of Cancer 2016;56:107–14.

40. Katipally R, Koffer PP, Rava PS, et al. Surgical Resection and Posterior Fossa Location Increase the Incidence of Leptomeningeal Disease in Patients Treated with Stereotactic Radiosurgery for Brain Metastases. Int J Radiat Oncol Biol Phys 2017;99(2, Supplement):S173.

41. Udovicich C, Phillips C, Kok DL, et al. Neoadjuvant Stereotactic Radiosurgery: a Further Evolution in the Management of Brain Metastases. Curr Oncol Rep 2019; 21(8):73.

42. Patel KR, Burri SH, Asher AL, et al. Comparing Preoperative With Postoperative Stereotactic Radiosurgery for Resectable Brain Metastases: A Multi-institutional Analysis. Neurosurgery 2016;79(2). Available at: https://journals.lww.com/neurosurgery/Fulltext/2016/08000/Comparing_Preoperative_With_Postoperative. 24.aspx.

43. Patel KR, Burri SH, Boselli D, et al. Comparing pre-operative stereotactic radio-surgery (SRS) to post-operative whole brain radiation therapy (WBRT) for resectable brain metastases: a multi-institutional analysis. J Neuro Oncol 2017;131(3):611–8.

44. Prabhu RS, Press RH, Patel KR, et al. Single-Fraction Stereotactic Radiosurgery (SRS) Alone Versus Surgical Resection and SRS for Large Brain Metastases: A Multi-institutional Analysis. Int J Radiat Oncol Biol Phys 2017;99(2):459–67.

45. Asher AL, Burri SH, Wiggins WF, et al. A New Treatment Paradigm: Neoadjuvant Radiosurgery Before Surgical Resection of Brain Metastases With Analysis of Local Tumor Recurrence. Int J Radiat Oncol Biol Phys 2014;88(4):899–906.

46. Patel AR, Nedzi L, Lau S, et al. Neoadjuvant Stereotactic Radiosurgery Before Surgical Resection of Cerebral Metastases. World Neurosurgery 2018;120: e480–7.

47. Prabhu RS, Dhakal R, Vaslow ZK, et al. Preoperative Radiosurgery for Resected Brain Metastases: The PROPS-BM Multicenter Cohort Study. Int J Radiat Oncol Biol Phys 2021;111(3):764–72.

48. Palmer JD, Perlow HK, Matsui JK, et al. Fractionated pre-operative stereotactic radiotherapy for patients with brain metastases: a multi-institutional analysis. J Neuro Oncol 2022. https://doi.org/10.1007/s11060-022-04073-w.

49. Mahajan A, Ahmed S, McAleer MF, et al. Post-operative stereotactic radiosurgery versus observation for completely resected brain metastases: a single-centre, randomised, controlled, phase 3 trial. Lancet Oncol 2017;18(8):1040–8.

50. Brown PD, Ballman KV, Cerhan JH, et al. Postoperative stereotactic radiosurgery compared with whole brain radiotherapy for resected metastatic brain disease (NCCTG N107C/CEC·3): a multicentre, randomised, controlled, phase 3 trial. Lancet Oncol 2017;18(8):1049–60.

51. Kayama T, Sato S, Sakurada K, et al. Effects of Surgery With Salvage Stereotactic Radiosurgery Versus Surgery With Whole-Brain Radiation Therapy in Patients With One to Four Brain Metastases (JCOG0504): A Phase III, Noninferiority, Randomized Controlled Trial. J Clin Orthod 2018;36(33):3282–9.

52. Perlow HK, Ho C, Matsui JK, et al. Comparing pre-operative versus post-operative single and multi-fraction stereotactic radiotherapy for patients with resectable brain metastases. Clinical and Translational Radiation Oncology 2023;38:117–22.

53. Aliabadi H, Nikpour AM, Yoo DS, et al. Pre-operative stereotactic radiosurgery treatment is preferred to post-operative treatment for smaller solitary brain metastases. Chinese Neurosurgical Journal 2017;3(1):29.

54. El Shafie RA, Tonndorf-Martini E, Schmitt D, et al. Pre-Operative Versus Post-Operative Radiosurgery of Brain Metastases—Volumetric and Dosimetric Impact of Treatment Sequence and Margin Concept. Cancers 2019;11(3). https://doi.org/10.3390/cancers11030294.

55. Beard BW, Rahimian J. A Dosimetric Comparison of Preoperative Versus Postoperative Stereotactic Radiosurgery for Brain Metastases. Int J Radiat Oncol Biol Phys 2019;105(1):E758.

56. Soliman H, Ruschin M, Angelov L, et al. Consensus Contouring Guidelines for Postoperative Completely Resected Cavity Stereotactic Radiosurgery for Brain Metastases. Int J Radiat Oncol Biol Phys 2018;100(2):436–42.

57. Schaue D, Kachikwu EL, McBride WH. Cytokines in Radiobiological Responses: A Review. Radiat Res 2012;178(6):505–23.

58. Derks SHAE, van der Veldt AAM, Smits M. Brain metastases: the role of clinical imaging. BJR (Br J Radiol) 2022;95(1130):20210944.

59. Prabhu RS, Miller KR, Asher AL, et al. Preoperative stereotactic radiosurgery before planned resection of brain metastases: updated analysis of efficacy and toxicity of a novel treatment paradigm. Journal of Neurosurgery JNS 2019;131(5):1387–94.

60. Itshayek E, Cohen JE, Yamada Y, et al. Timing of stereotactic radiosurgery and surgery and wound healing in patients with spinal tumors: a systematic review and expert opinions. null 2014;36(6):510–23.

61. Williams BJ, Suki D, Fox BD, et al. Stereotactic radiosurgery for metastatic brain tumors: a comprehensive review of complications: Clinical article. Journal of Neurosurgery JNS 2009;111(3):439–48.

62. Blonigen BJ, Steinmetz RD, Levin L, et al. Irradiated Volume as a Predictor of Brain Radionecrosis After Linear Accelerator Stereotactic Radiosurgery. Int J Radiat Oncol Biol Phys 2010;77(4):996–1001.

63. Minniti G, Clarke E, Lanzetta G, et al. Stereotactic radiosurgery for brain metastases: analysis of outcome and risk of brain radionecrosis. Radiat Oncol 2011; 6(1):48.
64. Nedzi LA, Kooy H, Alexander E, et al. Variables associated with the development of complications from radiosurgery of intracranial tumors. Int J Radiat Oncol Biol Phys 1991;21(3):591–9.
65. Minniti G, Scaringi C, Paolini S, et al. Single-Fraction Versus Multifraction (3 × 9 Gy) Stereotactic Radiosurgery for Large (>2 cm) Brain Metastases: A Comparative Analysis of Local Control and Risk of Radiation-Induced Brain Necrosis. Int J Radiat Oncol Biol Phys 2016;95(4):1142–8.
66. Milano MT, Grimm J, Niemierko A, et al. Single- and Multifraction Stereotactic Radiosurgery Dose/Volume Tolerances of the Brain. Int J Radiat Oncol Biol Phys 2021;110(1):68–86.
67. Ernst-Stecken A, Ganslandt O, Lambrecht U, et al. Phase II trial of hypofractionated stereotactic radiotherapy for brain metastases: Results and toxicity. Radiother Oncol 2006;81(1):18–24.
68. Noordijk EM, Vecht CJ, Haaxma-Reiche H, et al. The choice of treatment of single brain metastasis should be based on extracranial tumor activity and age. Int J Radiat Oncol Biol Phys 1994;29(4):711–7.
69. Mintz AH, Kestle J, Rathbone MP, et al. A randomized trial to assess the efficacy of surgery in addition to radiotherapy in patients with a single cerebral metastasis. Cancer 1996;78(7):1470–6.
70. Sneed PK, Suh JH, Goetsch SJ, et al. A multi-institutional review of radiosurgery alone vs. radiosurgery with whole brain radiotherapy as the initial management of brain metastases. Int J Radiat Oncol Biol Phys 2002;53(3):519–26.
71. Sanghavi SN, Miranpuri SS, Chappell R, et al. Radiosurgery for patients with brain metastases: a multi-institutional analysis, stratified by the RTOG recursive partitioning analysis method. Int J Radiat Oncol Biol Phys 2001;51(2):426–34.
72. Kondziolka D, Patel A, Lunsford LD, et al. Stereotactic radiosurgery plus whole brain radiotherapy versus radiotherapy alone for patients with multiple brain metastases. Int J Radiat Oncol Biol Phys 1999;45(2):427–34.
73. Minniti G, D'Angelillo RM, Scaringi C, et al. Fractionated stereotactic radiosurgery for patients with brain metastases. J Neuro Oncol 2014;117(2):295–301.
74. Lehrer EJ, Peterson JL, Zaorsky NG, et al. Single versus Multifraction Stereotactic Radiosurgery for Large Brain Metastases: An International Meta-analysis of 24 Trials. Int J Radiat Oncol Biol Phys 2019;103(3):618–30.
75. Minniti G, Esposito V, Clarke E, et al. Multidose Stereotactic Radiosurgery (9 Gy × 3) of the Postoperative Resection Cavity for Treatment of Large Brain Metastases. Int J Radiat Oncol Biol Phys 2013;86(4):623–9.
76. Han JH, Kim DG, Chung HT, et al. Radiosurgery for Large Brain Metastases. Int J Radiat Oncol Biol Phys 2012;83(1):113–20.
77. Kotsarini C, Griffiths PD, Wilkinson ID, et al. A Systematic Review of the Literature on the Effects of Dexamethasone on the Brain From In Vivo Human-Based Studies: Implications for Physiological Brain Imaging of Patients With Intracranial Tumors. Neurosurgery 2010;67(6). Available at: https://journals.lww.com/neurosurgery/Fulltext/2010/12000/A_Systematic_Review_of_the_Literature_on_the.46.aspx.
78. McPherson CM, Warnick RE. Results of Contemporary Surgical Management of Radiation Necrosis using Frameless Stereotaxis and Intraoperative Magnetic Resonance Imaging. J Neuro Oncol 2004;68(1):41–7.

79. Srinivasan ES, Grabowski MM, Nahed BV, et al. Laser interstitial thermal therapy for brain metastases. Neuro-Oncology Advances 2021;3(Supplement_5): v16–25.
80. Ahluwalia M, Barnett GH, Deng D, et al. Laser ablation after stereotactic radiosurgery: a multicenter prospective study in patients with metastatic brain tumors and radiation necrosis. Journal of Neurosurgery JNS 2019;130(3):804–11.
81. Moussaieff A, Mechoulam R. Boswellia resin: from religious ceremonies to medical uses; a review of in-vitro, in-vivo and clinical trials. J Pharm Pharmacol 2009; 61(10):1281–93.
82. Kirste S, Treier M, Wehrle SJ, et al. Boswellia serrata acts on cerebral edema in patients irradiated for brain tumors. Cancer 2011;117(16):3788–95.
83. Tsao MN, Li YQ, Lu G, et al. Upregulation of Vascular Endothelial Growth Factor Is Associated with Radiation-Induced Blood-Spinal Cord Barrier Breakdown. J Neuropathol Exp Neurol 1999;58(10):1051–60.
84. Kim JH, Chung YG, Kim CY, et al. Upregulation of VEGF and FGF2 in Normal Rat Brain after Experimental Intraoperative Radiation Therapy. J Korean Med Sci 2004;19(6):879–86.
85. Gridley D, Loredo L, Slater J, et al. Pilot evaluation of cytokine levels in patients undergoing radiotherapy for brain tumor. Cancer Detect Prev 1998;22(1):20–9.
86. Levin VA, Bidaut L, Hou P, et al. Randomized Double-Blind Placebo-Controlled Trial of Bevacizumab Therapy for Radiation Necrosis of the Central Nervous System. Int J Radiat Oncol Biol Phys 2011;79(5):1487–95.
87. Pareek P, Sharma A, Thipparampalli Jr, et al. Pentoxifylline and vitamin E alone or in combination for preventing and treating side effects of radiation therapy and concomitant chemoradiotherapy. Cochrane Database Syst Rev 2016;3. https://doi.org/10.1002/14651858.CD012117.
88. Dion MW, Hussey DH, Osborne JW. The effect of pentoxifylline on early and late radiation injury following fractionated irradiation in C3H mice. Int J Radiat Oncol Biol Phys 1989;17(1):101–7.
89. Koh WJ, Stelzer KJ, Peterson LM, et al. Effect of pentoxifylline on radiation-induced lung and skin toxicity in rats. Int J Radiat Oncol Biol Phys 1995; 31(1):71–7.
90. Lefaix JL, Delanian S, Vozenin MC, et al. Striking regression of subcutaneous fibrosis induced by high doses of gamma rays using a combination of pentoxifylline and α-tocopherol: an experimental study. Int J Radiat Oncol Biol Phys 1999;43(4):839–47.
91. Jacobson G, Bhatia S, Smith BJ, et al. Randomized Trial of Pentoxifylline and Vitamin E vs Standard Follow-up After Breast Irradiation to Prevent Breast Fibrosis, Evaluated by Tissue Compliance Meter. Int J Radiat Oncol Biol Phys 2013;85(3):604–8.
92. Sudmeier L, Switchenko J, Eaton B, et al. RTHP-01. Pentoxifylline and vitamin e for the treatment of radiation necrosis after stereotactic radiosurgery. Neuro Oncol 2019;21(Supplement_6):vi210.
93. Chuang MT, Liu YS, Tsai YS, et al. Differentiating Radiation-Induced Necrosis from Recurrent Brain Tumor Using MR Perfusion and Spectroscopy: A Meta-Analysis. PLoS One 2016;11(1):e0141438.
94. Galldiks N, Law I, Pope WB, et al. The use of amino acid PET and conventional MRI for monitoring of brain tumor therapy. Neuroimage: Clinical 2017;13: 386–94.
95. Sasajima T, Ono T, Shimada N, et al. Trans-1-amino-3-18F-fluorocyclobutanecarboxylic acid (anti-18F-FACBC) is a feasible alternative to 11C-methyl-L-

methionine and magnetic resonance imaging for monitoring treatment response in gliomas. Nucl Med Biol 2013;40(6):808–15.

96. Parent EE, Benayoun M, Ibeanu I, et al. [18F]Fluciclovine PET discrimination between high- and low-grade gliomas. EJNMMI Res 2018;8(1):67.

97. Parent EE, Patel D, Nye JA, et al. [18F]-Fluciclovine PET discrimination of recurrent intracranial metastatic disease from radiation necrosis. EJNMMI Res 2020; 10(1):148.

98. Cao Y, Tsien CI, Nagesh V, et al. Clinical investigation survival prediction in high-grade gliomas by MRI perfusion before and during early stage of RT. Int J Radiat Oncol Biol Phys 2006;64(3):876–85.

99. Cha S, Johnson G, Wadghiri YZ, et al. Dynamic, contrast-enhanced perfusion MRI in mouse gliomas: Correlation with histopathology. Magn Reson Med 2003;49(5):848–55.

100. Cha S, Tihan T, Crawford F, et al. Differentiation of Low-Grade Oligodendrogliomas from Low-Grade Astrocytomas by Using Quantitative Blood-Volume Measurements Derived from Dynamic Susceptibility Contrast-Enhanced MR Imaging. Am J Neuroradiol 2005;26(2):266.

101. Law M, Yang S, Babb JS, et al. Comparison of Cerebral Blood Volume and Vascular Permeability from Dynamic Susceptibility Contrast-Enhanced Perfusion MR Imaging with Glioma Grade. Am J Neuroradiol 2004;25(5):746.

102. Hoefnagels FWA, Lagerwaard FJ, Sanchez E, et al. Radiological progression of cerebral metastases after radiosurgery: assessment of perfusion MRI for differentiating between necrosis and recurrence. J Neurol 2009;256(6):878–87.

103. Mitsuya K, Nakasu Y, Horiguchi S, et al. Perfusion weighted magnetic resonance imaging to distinguish the recurrence of metastatic brain tumors from radiation necrosis after stereotactic radiosurgery. J Neuro Oncol 2010;99(1):81–8.

Advances in Proton Therapy for the Management of Head and Neck Tumors

Jacob Trotter, MD, Alexander Lin, MD*

KEYWORDS

- Proton therapy • intensity-modulated radiotherapy • Head and neck tumors

KEY POINTS

- Radiation therapy is a standard and commonlyu used modality to treat cancers of the head and neck.
- Radiation therapy can cause significant side effects, negatively impacting quality of life.
- Proton therapy, through better sparing of normal tissues, may cause fewer side effects.
- Proton therapy is now being used to treat head and neck cancers, with increasing evidence supporting its use.

INTRODUCTION

The idea of using protons as a form of radiation therapy in the treatment of cancer was first proposed by the physicist Robert R Wilson in 1946 at the Harvard Cyclotron Laboratory who recognized that these charged particles deposited dose in a much more localized manner relative to photons given their qualities of having charge and mass.[1] Less than a decade later the first patient was treated using protons at the Lawrence Berkeley National Laboratory in 1954.[2] Since that initial patient, there have been many advances in proton beam radiotherapy (PBRT). Today, PBRT technologies such as pencil-beam scanning, intensity-modulated proton therapy (IMPT), and commercially available robust optimization algorithms offer the ability to deliver highly conformal radiation treatment plans with dosimetric superiority over conventional, photon-based (x-ray) intensity-modulated radiation therapy (IMRT).

With radiotherapy being a mainstay in the treatment of head and neck cancer in the definitive and adjuvant (postoperative) settings, and patients increasingly having geographic access to PBRT centers, practicing oncologists would benefit from a general understanding of this treatment modality and the evidence behind its use. In this article, the following will be discussed: the unique physical characteristics of proton

Department of Radiation Oncology, Perelman School of Medicine, University of Pennsylvania, 3400 Civic Center Boulevard, Philadelphia, PA 19104, USA
* Corresponding author.
E-mail address: Alexander.Lin2@pennmedicine.upenn.edu

Surg Oncol Clin N Am 32 (2023) 587–598
https://doi.org/10.1016/j.soc.2023.03.003
1055-3207/23/© 2023 Elsevier Inc. All rights reserved.

beam radiotherapy, its potential therapeutic clinical advantages and limitations, and possible future applications.

PROTON THERAPY

Limitations of Photon-Based Therapy

The fundamental aim in developing new radiation therapy technologies is to improve the therapeutic ratio. This involves delivering a therapeutic dose of radiation to control areas of tumor while minimizing dose to normal tissues to limit treatment-related toxicity. Over the past decade, there has been an increasing interest in the use of proton beam radiotherapy (PBRT) to further improve the therapeutic ratio in the treatment of patients with cancer. Protons are charged particles with unique physical properties compared with standard photon-based external beam radiotherapy (EBRT) that potentially allows for greater sparing of adjacent organs at risk. To understand the promise of PBRT, it is helpful to understand the limitations of traditional photon therapy techniques.

With standard photon-based EBRT, dose is deposited essentially at a steadily decreasing amount along the entire beam path from entrance into the patient until it exits the opposite side of the patient (**Fig. 1**). Thus, for a single beam of photons, the dose along the entrance path (entrance dose) is always higher than the dose to the target itself, and additional dose has to be deposited to the nontarget tissues distal to the target along the exit path (exit dose). Consequently, most of the radiation dose is actually deposited in nontarget tissues.

Many advanced photon-based techniques (three-dimensional conformal radiation therapy, tomotherapy, IMRT, and volumetric-modulated arc therapy) have been developed to offset this photon dose distribution problem by using multiple beams which conform high doses to tumor while distributing significantly lower doses to

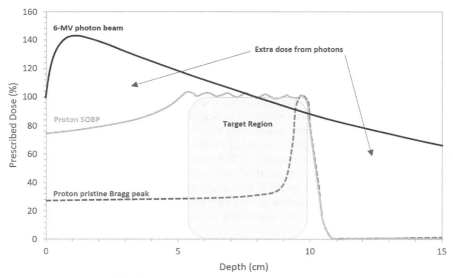

Fig. 1. Depth dose profiles for a 6-megavoltage (MV) photon beam (*purple*), a monoenergetic proton beam with a pristine Bragg peak (*blue*), and a polyenergetic proton beam with a spread-out Bragg peak (SOBP, *green*). Note the area under the 6-MV curve is significantly higher than for a proton SOBP leading to a higher integral dose for photon based beam (see *arrows* pointing out extra dose from photons).

the surrounding tissues. With these techniques, however, radiation to non-tumor tissues is merely redistributed rather than reduced. The end result is that more normal tissue is exposed to radiation, albeit at lower doses. This is because these complex beam arrangements concentrate high dose onto the tumor but in the process produce low exit dose in many areas of the normal tissues surrounding the tumor.

As the total dose to a tissue is a primary factor leading to toxicity, many toxicities can be reduced when using these advanced photon techniques. However, for some toxicities, the total volume of tissue irradiated is important, and even low doses increase the risk of certain toxicities when large volumes are treated and enough time has elapsed (eg, second malignancies and risk of pathologic fractures). This is especially problematic in patients who are expected to live a long enough time to experience distant late side effects and/or had a large volume of tissue irradiated. One such example is the pediatric population, for whom required radiation fields are large (such as craniospinal irradiation for select central nervous system malignancies), causing high rates of severe long-term toxicity interfering with independent living,[3] and where proton therapy offers significant gains in acute toxicity compared with photons.[4] In such cases, eliminating integral radiation exposure may be preferred to simply redistributing the dose, and gains in acute toxicity can translate to improvements in long-term toxicity rates and quality of life.

The Promise of Proton Therapy

Unlike photon-based techniques which simply redistribute dose, PBRT actually reduces the integral dose delivered. This is because protons have a different dose distribution pattern compared with photons. Although photons deliver dose continually along their path from entrance to exit, protons deliver their dose over a finite range. The characteristic dose deposition pattern of protons is known as the Bragg peak. In this pattern, a small nearly constant rate of dose is deposited along the entrance path followed by a sharp increase in dose deposition given over a very short range as the proton comes to a stop (see **Fig. 1**). No dose is deposited distally after the proton has stopped. This equates to a low entrance dose and a lack of an exit dose for a monoenergetic proton beam, as opposed to a high entrance dose and the presence of exit dose for a photon. Another way to understand this is that for a proton, most of its dose is delivered within the target, whereas for a photon, most of its dose is delivered outside the target as entrance and exit doses.

The distance a proton travels before stopping depends on its initial energy. Protons are generated from hydrogen gas and then are accelerated to treatment energies by either a cyclotron or synchrotron. Current technology allows acceleration of proton to energies high enough to treat tumors to depths of 35 cm within a patient. To make protons clinically useful, they are delivered over a range of energies, thus layering Bragg peaks together to create a spread-out Bragg peak (SOBP) that conforms dose to the shape of the target (see **Fig. 1**). The creation of an SOBP comes at the expense of increasing entrance dose, relative to a pristine monoenergetic beam, with the entrance dosing increasing proportional to the width of the target region. Given this, the principle dosimetric advantage of PBRT is the lack of exit dose compared with photon-based techniques.

POTENTIAL INDICATIONS OF PROTON THERAPY IN THE TREATMENT OF HEAD AND NECK CANCER

With the unique dosimetric advantages of protons and the advanced technologies now available, it is clear that protons therapy holds great promise in the treatment of cancer. However, given the advanced photon-based techniques that exist and their relative cheaper cost, it is important for clinicians and researchers to understand which situations are most likely to benefit from this type of therapy.

Radiotherapy is a standard and well-established treatment modality for cancers of the head and neck. It is indicated and used as a sole modality of therapy for early-stage disease,[5,6] postoperatively for improvement of locoregional control and overall survival,[7–10] or definitively with concurrent chemotherapy for organ preservation of advanced locoregional disease.[11–13] Its use, however, can lead to significant treatment-related morbidity[14–20] negatively impacting patient quality of life.[16] Therefore, approaches for toxicity mitigation are critically important, especially given the increasing incidence[21,22] and excellent long-term disease outcomes[23,24] seen in patients treated for human papillomavirus (HPV)-associated oropharyngeal squamous cell carcinoma (OPSCC).

The Particle Therapy Co-Operative Group (PTCOG) Head and Neck Subcommittee recently published consensus guidelines, based on promising results for the use of proton therapy in the treatment of cancers of the nasopharynx, sinonasal region, and oropharynx as well as in the postoperative and reirradiation settings.[25]

For nasopharynx cancer, these guidelines cite nonrandomized, comparative data in which patients who received treatment with proton therapy (as compared with IMRT) were found to have greater normal tissue sparing leading to less requirement for opioid pan medication at the end of treatment.[26] In a matched case-control study of patients treated with definitive chemoradiation for nasopharynx cancer, patients receiving proton beam radiotherapy, when compared with IMRT, had significantly lower doses delivered to the oral cavity and lower rates of requiring feeding tube during treatment (20 vs 65%).[27] While awaiting completion and results from randomized studies of proton versus photon radiation,[28] proton therapy can be considered in the treatment of nasopharynx cancers as a means to better spare normal tissue and decrease treatment morbidity.

For sinonasal cancers, recent single-institution, retrospective series have reported high long-term locoregional control rates of 80% or greater.[29,30] A systematic review and meta-analysis of 41 observational studies showed a significant improvement of 5-year disease-free survival and long-term locoregional control with proton therapy (vs IMRT) in the treatment of cancers of the paranasal sinuses and nasal cavity but with a greater risk of neurotoxicity.[31] Given the heterogeneity of tumor histologies, locations with the sinonasal region, and treatment indications (definitive vs postoperative), it is unlikely that large-scale, randomized trials of proton versus photon therapy will be conducted for this disease site. In the meantime, proton therapy can be considered a viable radiotherapy option to obtain high rates of disease control. Given concerns about treatment toxicity, all efforts should be made to use the most advanced forms of proton therapy (IMPT), coupled with daily anatomic imaging for quality assurance. Continued reports of comparative data for disease control and patient outcomes, using the most advanced forms of proton (IMPT) and photon (IMRT) will help inform the most proper use of radiotherapy in the future.

Oropharynx cancer, as mentioned above, with expected high rates of long-term patient survival, may represent the most compelling population for which proton therapy may be beneficial and for which data supporting the use of proton therapy have been the most robust comparative studies of proton RT versus IMRT for the treatment of oropharyngeal cancers in the definitive[32] and postoperative[33] settings have shown excellent disease outcomes, but with significant improvement in toxicity and quality of life in patients receiving proton therapy. These gains are likely due to the improved sparing and reduction of radiation dose to critical normal structures (**Fig. 2**), which may then translate to improvements in observed toxicity and patient-reported outcomes. There are two randomized phase III studies of proton therapy versus IMRT for

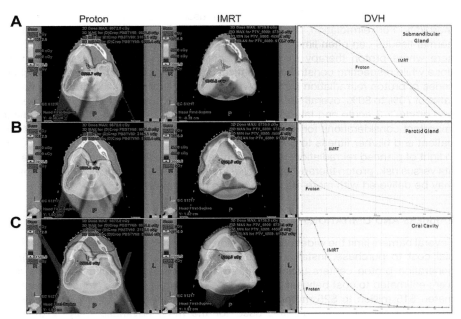

Fig. 2. Comparison of an IMRT plan and an intensity-modulated proton plan using a pencil beam scanning technique for a patient with T1N2b (AJCC v7) HPV + squamous cell carcinoma of the right tonsil requiring bilateral neck radiation. The figure illustrates the relative sparing of structures such as the submandibular gland (*A*), parotid gland (*B*), and the oral cavity (*C*) that can be achieved using modern proton techniques. On the left are the dose color washes for the proton plans. In the center are the similar dose color washes for the IMRT plan. On the right are the dose volume histograms for the organ of interest at that level. (*A*) The relative sparing of the contralateral submandibular gland circled in yellow. The mean dose to the left submandibular gland was 40 Gy with IMRT and 33 Gy with protons. (*B*) The relative sparing of the contralateral parotid gland circled in pink. The mean dose to the left parotid gland was 18 Gy with IMRT and 9 Gy with protons. (*C*) The relative sparing of the oral cavity circled in blue/purple. The mean dose to the oral cavity was 13.5 Gy with IMRT and 1.3 Gy with protons. DVH, dose volume histogram.

definitive, organ-preservation treatment of oropharynx cancer: a completed, multicenter study in the United States[34] (NCT01893307), for which results are pending, and a currently accruing trial in the United Kingdom (TORPEdO) being conducted by the National Health Service.[35] The PTCOG guidelines therefore recommend participation in clinical trial whenever possible, and otherwise strongly encourage consideration of proton therapy in the postoperative or definitive settings, given the existing data suggestive of clinical benefit.[25]

In the postoperative setting, consideration can be given for treating with proton therapy. Patients who have received postoperative proton therapy for oropharynx cancer seem to have better posttreatment salivary function and taste when compared with a comparable cohort of patients receiving IMRT.[33] Even in situations where the radiation field is less extensive, such as that seen for postoperative salivary gland and unilateral neck radiation, proton therapy may result in less severe toxicity with respect to mucositis, nausea, and taste changes.[36]

Reirradiation of recurrent or new primary head and neck cancer represents a particularly difficult therapeutic challenge, where curative options (salvage surgery or chemo-reirradiation) are limited, and often associated with significant potential morbidity. For reirradiation, the proximity of disease to previously irradiated critical normal tissues can often limit the ability to give a meaningful dose of radiation. It is here where proton therapy may be a viable option to both deliver a tumoricidal dose while respecting constraints on critical organs at risk. Several recent published series of proton reirradiation have shown promising results, with locoregional control rates of 70% to 80%, overall survival of 65% to 80% at 12 months and 35% at 2 years, and grade $\geq$ 3 acute and late toxicity rates of 12% to 30%.[37–39] Although the most important considerations for reirradiation remain, such as thorough evaluation of the patient and his/her fitness to undergo treatment, review of the prior radiation course in light of planned reirradiation, and a careful and detailed discussion weighing benefits versus risk, proton therapy can be considered as one option for which reirradiation may be delivered with more efficacy and less risk of severe toxicity.

BARRIERS AND LIMITATIONS

Several barriers limit the widespread adoption of proton therapy. One is the high financial cost to purchase, install, operate, and maintain a proton center.[40] The first-generation proton centers usually consisted of three to five treatment rooms and were estimated to cost between $100 and $200 million US dollars along with an estimated $15 million to $25 million in annual operating costs.[41,42] For comparison, a state-of-the-art linear accelerator, used for the most advanced delivery of non-proton therapeutic radiation, typically costs less than $5 million. Recently, advances in proton therapy technologies has allowed for more compact designs and the development of single-room proton centers. These newer centers are substantially cheaper, but with estimated startup costs of $30 to 40 million US dollars, and are still not without significant financial risk.[43] In order to cover these significant costs and maintain viability, proton centers must sustain a substantial clinical volume.[44]

For patients, access is the largest barrier to PBRT, with several contributing factors. First, there is simply much less access to proton therapy as compared with traditional photon-based radiation. At the time of this writing, there are only 40 operating proton centers in the United States, mostly confined to metropolitan areas. Second, many health care providers may not know indications for considering proton therapy and therefore may not understand when a proton referral is warranted. Even when referral is offered, many patients are unwilling or unable to travel significant distances for treatments or cannot afford the additional transportation and housing costs as well as potential wage loss during their time away for a course of treatment that often spans several weeks.

Affordable access can also be an issue given challenges with insurance coverage, especially given the higher treatment cost and reimbursement associated with proton therapy. A significant number of patients deemed to be medically appropriate for proton therapy were denied coverage by major US insurance companies, pointing to a lack of definitive evidence that PBRT is clinically superior to the most advanced, non-proton radiation techniques.[45] Currently, most payers in the United States still do not reimburse for proton beam radiotherapy,[46] with insurance approval representing one of the most significant barriers to patient access[47] and resultant increased resource utilization for appeals[47] and significant delays in initiating cancer therapy.[47,48]

Finally, although there is a body of published literature documenting clinical and cost-effective gains with proton beam radiotherapy,[49,50] we still await similar results via prospective randomized controlled trials. Accrual to some proton therapy trials in other disease sites (non-head and neck) has been affected by issues such as insurance denials for those randomized to protons as well as an unwillingness of many patient and/or providers to enroll given a perceived lack of equipoise.[46] However, for patients receiving definitive chemoradiation for the treatment of oropharynx cancer, there exist two prospective, randomized controlled trials comparing IMPT with IMRT, as mentioned above: a multicenter trial in the United States (NCT01893307)[34] and one being run by the National Health System in the United Kingdom.[35] In the absence of level 1 evidence, alternative methods to evaluate PBRT benefit have been developed such as the model-based approach used in the Netherlands which uses individual treatment plans and biological models of complications to predict who would benefit most from PBRT.[51,52] These models have been used with some success but the probabilities predicted by these models maintain some level of uncertainty.[53]

CURRENT AND FUTURE DIRECTIONS

Despite the limitations that exist around PBRT implementation, the technology as a whole continues to evolve and advance. Currently, there are efforts in implementing a number of technological advances in PBRT including but not limited to proton arc therapy, in vivo range verification techniques, online adaptive therapy, and beam control based on patient's respiratory cycle.[54–56] All of these offer improvement on current delivery techniques with possibility to further improve the therapeutic ratio.

One of the most intriguing research focuses on PBRT in recent years involves implementation of ultra-high dose rate FLASH radiotherapy (FLASH-RT). FLASH-RT is defined as delivery of radiation at dose rates greater than 40 Gy/s (~400–1000x conventional dose rates). FLASH-RT has been demonstrated in a number of preliminary in vivo studies using electrons, x-rays, or protons to substantially spare normal tissues while maintaining equivalent tumor control as compared with traditional EBRT at conventional dose rates, and most effectively given at high doses per fraction, over just several fractions[57–61] (which can be given over a short course, as opposed to a multiple month course of conventional RT). The physical and biological mechanisms that lead to these stunning results are currently being investigated and may represent a paradigm shift in radiation therapy if further validated. There is strong interest in proton FLASH-RT, as it combines the novel aspect of toxicity mitigation via delivery of RT dose at ultra-high dose rates, but also dosimetrically, with proton's ability to treat deep-seated tumors (a limitation of electrons, which can only treat superficial lesions) and better spare normal tissue (via the Bragg Peak) as compared with photon x-rays. Delivery of proton FLASH beams is feasible with modifications of existing clinical proton systems[62–64] and has demonstrated decreased late gut fibrosis after abdominal radiation.[62] However, challenges remain in clinical implementation with dosimetry, the ability to modulate the beam at such an ultra-high dose rate, and determining whether FLASH-RT need to be delivered in the fewest number of beams possible to harness the benefit of the technology (and thus potentially reducing the benefits of FLASH-RT compared with IMPT or IMRT approaches). Although this technology is still in its preliminary stages with further studies needed, its potential to significantly reduce toxicity and total treatment duration may greatly benefit patients in terms of quality of life as well as convenience.

SUMMARY

Proton therapy is a safe and established radiation treatment modality with many dosimetric advantages over standard photon-based techniques. Cost and insurance coverage remain significant barriers to its uptake and further efforts are needed to address these limitations. Potential indications for PBRT include situations where standard EBRT techniques produce long-term control at the expense of significant acute, late, or long-term toxicities or when local control is suboptimal with standard EBRT due to the inability to safely deliver a therapeutic dose. Enrollment in clinical trials, particularly phase III randomized trials comparing PBRT with IMRT, is strongly encouraged to better determine the optimal role of PBRT in cancer treatments. The future applications of proton beam radiotherapy, such as with FLASH-RT, have the potential to positively and significantly impact patient outcomes and quality of life.

CLINICS CARE POINTS

- Retrospective data suggests that proton therapy may be beneficial in decreasing treatment-related toxicity and improving patient-reported outcomes, as well as improving disease outcomes in the treatment of head and neck cancers.

- Randomized, prospective trials comparing proton therapy to non-proton therapy are currently ongoing, the results of which will further define and inform the proper indications and usage of proton therapy.

DISCLOSURES

The authors have no relevant disclosures to report.

REFERENCES

1. Wilson RR. Radiological use of fast protons. Radiology 1946;47:487–91.
2. Lawrence JH, Tobias CA, Born JL, et al. Pituitary irradiation with high-energy proton beams: a preliminary report. Cancer Res 1958;18:121–34.
3. Christopherson KM, Rotondo RL, Bradley JA, et al. Late toxicity following craniospinal radiation for early-stage medulloblastoma. Acta Oncol 2014;53:471–80.
4. Liu KX, Ioakeim-Ioannidou M, Susko MS, et al. A Multi-institutional Comparative Analysis of Proton and Photon Therapy-Induced Hematologic Toxicity in Patients With Medulloblastoma. Int J Radiat Oncol Biol Phys 2021;109:726–35.
5. O'Sullivan B, Warde P, Grice B, et al. The benefits and pitfalls of ipsilateral radiotherapy in carcinoma of the tonsillar region. Int J Radiat Oncol Biol Phys 2001;51:332–43.
6. Yamazaki H, Nishiyama K, Tanaka E, et al. Radiotherapy for early glottic carcinoma (T1N0M0): results of prospective randomized study of radiation fraction size and overall treatment time. Int J Radiat Oncol Biol Phys 2006;64:77–82.
7. Bernier J, Domenge C, Ozsahin M, et al. Postoperative irradiation with or without concomitant chemotherapy for locally advanced head and neck cancer. N Engl J Med 2004;350:1945–52.
8. Cooper JS, Pajak TF, Forastiere AA, et al. Postoperative concurrent radiotherapy and chemotherapy for high-risk squamous-cell carcinoma of the head and neck. N Engl J Med 2004;350:1937–44.
9. Bernier J, Cooper JS, Pajak TF, et al. Defining risk levels in locally advanced head and neck cancers: a comparative analysis of concurrent postoperative radiation plus chemotherapy trials of the EORTC (#22931) and RTOG (# 9501). Head Neck 2005;27:843–50.

10. Lundahl RE, Foote RL, Bonner JA, et al. Combined neck dissection and postoperative radiation therapy in the management of the high-risk neck: a matched-pair analysis. Int J Radiat Oncol Biol Phys 1998;40:529–34.

11. Forastiere AA, Goepfert H, Maor M, et al. Concurrent chemotherapy and radiotherapy for organ preservation in advanced laryngeal cancer. N Engl J Med 2003;349:2091–8.

12. Wolf GT, Fisher SG, Hong WK, et al. Induction chemotherapy plus radiation compared with surgery plus radiation in patients with advanced laryngeal cancer. N Engl J Med 1991;324:1685–90.

13. Al-Sarraf M, LeBlanc M, Giri PG, et al. Chemoradiotherapy versus radiotherapy in patients with advanced nasopharyngeal cancer: phase III randomized Intergroup study 0099. J Clin Oncol 1998;16:1310–7.

14. Dorresteijn LD, Kappelle AC, Boogerd W, et al. Increased risk of ischemic stroke after radiotherapy on the neck in patients younger than 60 years. J Clin Oncol 2002;20:282–8.

15. Eisbruch A, Lyden T, Bradford CR, et al. Objective assessment of swallowing dysfunction and aspiration after radiation concurrent with chemotherapy for head-and-neck cancer. Int J Radiat Oncol Biol Phys 2002;53:23–8.

16. Lin A, Kim HM, Terrell JE, et al. Quality of life after parotid-sparing IMRT for head-and-neck cancer: a prospective longitudinal study. Int J Radiat Oncol Biol Phys 2003;57:61–70.

17. Smith GL, Smith BD, Buchholz TA, et al. Cerebrovascular disease risk in older head and neck cancer patients after radiotherapy. J Clin Oncol 2008;26:5119–25.

18. Smith GL, Smith BD, Garden AS, et al. Hypothyroidism in older patients with head and neck cancer after treatment with radiation: a population-based study. Head Neck 2009;31:1031–8.

19. Tsai CJ, Hofstede TM, Sturgis EM, et al. Osteoradionecrosis and radiation dose to the mandible in patients with oropharyngeal cancer. Int J Radiat Oncol Biol Phys 2013;85:415–20.

20. Swisher-McClure S, Mitra N, Lin A, et al. Risk of fatal cerebrovascular accidents after external beam radiation therapy for early-stage glottic laryngeal cancer. Head Neck 2014;36:611–6.

21. Gillison ML, Chaturvedi AK, Anderson WF, et al. Epidemiology of Human Papillomavirus-Positive Head and Neck Squamous Cell Carcinoma. J Clin Oncol 2015;33:3235–42.

22. Chaturvedi AK, Engels EA, Pfeiffer RM, et al. Human papillomavirus and rising oropharyngeal cancer incidence in the United States. J Clin Oncol 2011;29:4294–301.

23. Ang KK, Harris J, Wheeler R, et al. Human papillomavirus and survival of patients with oropharyngeal cancer. N Engl J Med 2010;363:24–35.

24. O'Sullivan B, Huang SH, Siu LL, et al. Deintensification candidate subgroups in human papillomavirus-related oropharyngeal cancer according to minimal risk of distant metastasis. J Clin Oncol 2013;31:543–50.

25. Lin A, Chang JHC, Grover RS, et al. PTCOG Head and Neck Subcommittee Consensus Guidelines on Particle Therapy for the Management of Head and Neck Tumors. Int J Part Ther 2021;8:84–94.

26. McDonald MW, Liu Y, Moore MG, et al. Acute toxicity in comprehensive head and neck radiation for nasopharynx and paranasal sinus cancers: cohort comparison of 3D conformal proton therapy and intensity modulated radiation therapy. Radiat Oncol 2016;11:32.

27. Holliday EB, Garden AS, Rosenthal DI, et al. Proton Therapy Reduces Treatment-Related Toxicities for Patients with Nasopharyngeal Cancer: A Case-Match Control Study of Intensity-Modulated Proton Therapy and Intensity-Modulated Photon Therapy. International Journal of Particle Therapy 2015;2(1):19–28.
28. Shanghai Proton and Heavy Ion Center. Proton versus photon radiotherapy for nasopharyngeal carcinoma. ClinicalTrials.gov Identifier: NCT04528394. Available at: https://clinicaltrials.gov/ct2/show/NCT04528394. Accessed February 14, 2023.
29. Dagan R, Bryant C, Li Z, et al. Outcomes of Sinonasal Cancer Treated With Proton Therapy. Int J Radiat Oncol Biol Phys 2016;95:377–85.
30. Russo AL, Adams JA, Weyman EA, et al. Long-Term Outcomes After Proton Beam Therapy for Sinonasal Squamous Cell Carcinoma. Int J Radiat Oncol Biol Phys 2016;95:368–76.
31. Patel SH, Wang Z, Wong WW, et al. Charged particle therapy versus photon therapy for paranasal sinus and nasal cavity malignant diseases: a systematic review and meta-analysis. Lancet Oncol 2014;15:1027–38.
32. Blanchard P, Garden AS, Gunn GB, et al. Intensity-modulated proton beam therapy (IMPT) versus intensity-modulated photon therapy (IMRT) for patients with oropharynx cancer - A case matched analysis. Radiother Oncol 2016;120:48–55.
33. Sharma S, Zhou O, Thompson R, et al. Quality of Life of Postoperative Photon versus Proton Radiation Therapy for Oropharynx Cancer. Int J Part Ther 2018;5:11–7.
34. MD Anderson Cancer Center. Randomized trial of intensity-modulated proton beam therapy (IMPT) versus intensitymodulated photon therapy (IMRT) for the treatment of oropharyngeal cancer of the head and neck. ClinicalTrials.gov Identifier: NCT01893307. Available at: https://clinicaltrials.gov/ct2/show/NCT01893307. Accessed February 14, 2023.
35. Thomson DJ, Cruickshank C, Baines H, et al. TORPEdO: A phase III trial of intensity-modulated proton beam therapy versus intensity-modulated radiotherapy for multi-toxicity reduction in oropharyngeal cancer. Clin Transl Radiat Oncol 2023;38:147–54.
36. Romesser PB, Cahlon O, Scher E, et al. Proton beam radiation therapy results in significantly reduced toxicity compared with intensity-modulated radiation therapy for head and neck tumors that require ipsilateral radiation. Radiother Oncol 2016;118:286–92.
37. Phan J, Sio TT, Nguyen TP, et al. Reirradiation of Head and Neck Cancers With Proton Therapy: Outcomes and Analyses. Int J Radiat Oncol Biol Phys 2016;96:30–41.
38. McDonald MW, Zolali-Meybodi O, Lehnert SJ, et al. Reirradiation of Recurrent and Second Primary Head and Neck Cancer With Proton Therapy. Int J Radiat Oncol Biol Phys 2016;96:808–19.
39. Romesser PB, Cahlon O, Scher ED, et al. Proton Beam Reirradiation for Recurrent Head and Neck Cancer: Multi-institutional Report on Feasibility and Early Outcomes. Int J Radiat Oncol Biol Phys 2016;95:386–95.
40. Elnahal SM, Kerstiens J, Helsper RS, et al. Proton beam therapy and accountable care: the challenges ahead. Int J Radiat Oncol Biol Phys 2013;85:e165–72.
41. Hug EB, Loredo LN, Slater JD, et al. Proton radiation therapy for chordomas and chondrosarcomas of the skull base. J Neurosurg 1999;91:432–9.
42. Kim DJ, Wells C, Khangura S, et al. Budget impact analysis. Canadian Agency for Drugs and Technologies in Health; 2017. Available at: https://www.ncbi.nlm.nih.gov/books/NBK531700/. Accessed September 28, 2022.

43. Kerstiens J, Johnstone GP, Johnstone PAS. Proton Facility Economics: Single-Room Centers. J Am Coll Radiol 2018;15:1704–8.
44. Johnstone PA, Kerstiens J, Richard H. Proton facility economics: the importance of "simple" treatments. J Am Coll Radiol 2012;9:560–3.
45. Shah A, Ricci KI, Efstathiou JA. Beyond a moonshot: insurance coverage for proton therapy. Lancet Oncol 2016;17:559–61.
46. Bekelman JE, Denicoff A, Buchsbaum J. Randomized Trials of Proton Therapy: Why They Are at Risk, Proposed Solutions, and Implications for Evaluating Advanced Technologies to Diagnose and Treat Cancer. J Clin Oncol 2018;36: 2461–4.
47. Ning MS, Gomez DR, Shah AK, et al. The Insurance Approval Process for Proton Radiation Therapy: A Significant Barrier to Patient Care. Int J Radiat Oncol Biol Phys 2019;104:724–33.
48. Gupta A, Khan AJ, Goyal S, et al. Insurance Approval for Proton Beam Therapy and its Impact on Delays in Treatment. Int J Radiat Oncol Biol Phys 2019;104: 714–23.
49. Verma V, Mishra MV, Mehta MP. A systematic review of the cost and cost-effectiveness studies of proton radiotherapy. Cancer 2016;122:1483–501.
50. Sher DJ, Tishler RB, Pham NL, et al. Cost-Effectiveness Analysis of Intensity Modulated Radiation Therapy Versus Proton Therapy for Oropharyngeal Squamous Cell Carcinoma. Int J Radiat Oncol Biol Phys 2018;101:875–82.
51. Langendijk JA, Lambin P, De Ruysscher D, et al. Selection of patients for radiotherapy with protons aiming at reduction of side effects: the model-based approach. Radiother Oncol 2013;107:267–73.
52. Widder J, van der Schaaf A, Lambin P, et al. The Quest for Evidence for Proton Therapy: Model-Based Approach and Precision Medicine. Int J Radiat Oncol Biol Phys 2016;95:30–6.
53. Rwigema JM, Langendijk JA, Paul van der Laan H, et al. A Model-Based Approach to Predict Short-Term Toxicity Benefits With Proton Therapy for Oropharyngeal Cancer. Int J Radiat Oncol Biol Phys 2019;104:553–62.
54. Ding X, Li X, Zhang JM, et al. Spot-Scanning Proton Arc (SPArc) Therapy: The First Robust and Delivery-Efficient Spot-Scanning Proton Arc Therapy. Int J Radiat Oncol Biol Phys 2016;96:1107–16.
55. Parodi K, Polf JC. In vivo range verification in particle therapy. Med Phys 2018;45: e1036–50.
56. Schreuder AN, Shamblin J. Proton therapy delivery: what is needed in the next ten years? Br J Radiol 2020;93:20190359.
57. Zlobinskaya O, Siebenwirth C, Greubel C, et al. The effects of ultra-high dose rate proton irradiation on growth delay in the treatment of human tumor xenografts in nude mice. Radiat Res 2014;181:177–83.
58. Favaudon V, Caplier L, Monceau V, et al. Ultrahigh dose-rate FLASH irradiation increases the differential response between normal and tumor tissue in mice. Sci Transl Med 2014;6:245ra93.
59. Schüler E, Trovati S, King G, et al. Experimental Platform for Ultra-high Dose Rate FLASH Irradiation of Small Animals Using a Clinical Linear Accelerator. Int J Radiat Oncol Biol Phys 2017;97:195–203.
60. Vozenin MC, De Fornel P, Petersson K, et al. The Advantage of FLASH Radiotherapy Confirmed in Mini-pig and Cat-cancer Patients. Clin Cancer Res 2019; 25:35–42.
61. Bourhis J, Montay-Gruel P, Gonçalves Jorge P, et al. Clinical translation of FLASH radiotherapy: Why and how? Radiother Oncol 2019;139:11–7.

62. Diffenderfer ES, Verginadis II, Kim MM, et al. Design, Implementation, and in Vivo Validation of a Novel Proton FLASH Radiation Therapy System. Int J Radiat Oncol Biol Phys 2020;106:440–8.
63. Patriarca A, Fouillade C, Auger M, et al. Experimental Set-up for FLASH Proton Irradiation of Small Animals Using a Clinical System. Int J Radiat Oncol Biol Phys 2018;102:619–26.
64. Beyreuther E, Brand M, Hans S, et al. Feasibility of proton FLASH effect tested by zebrafish embryo irradiation. Radiother Oncol 2019;139:46–50.

Advances in MRI-Guided Radiation Therapy

Michael D. Chuong, MD[a],*, Russell F. Palm, MD[b], Michael C. Tjong, MD, MPH[c], Daniel E. Hyer, PhD[d], Amar U. Kishan, MD[e]

KEYWORDS

- MRI • Radiation therapy • Image guidance

KEY POINTS

- MRI-guided radiation therapy offers superior soft tissue contrast compared to CT guidance, intrafraction imaging, and online adaptive replanning.
- MRI-guided radiation therapy facilitates tumor dose escalation, normal organ sparing, and shorter fractionation compared to CT-guided radiation therapy.
- MRI-guided radiation therapy is more costly and resource-intense than CT-guided radiation therapy, especially when performing online adaptive replanning and clinical data are needed to clarify for which situations MRI guidance is medically necessary.

INTRODUCTION

MRI-guided radiotherapy (MRgRT) is a novel approach that was developed to overcome key challenges of conventional radiotherapy (RT).[1] Modern MRgRT systems represent the current state of the art regarding image guidance for soft tissue targets and couple an MRI scanner with a linear accelerator (LINAC), enabling clinicians to visualize internal anatomy with excellent soft tissue contrast directly before treatment delivery (**Fig. 1**).[2] MRgRT systems uniquely provide continuous imaging of the internal anatomy, called cine imaging, throughout treatment that is not possible on traditional LINACs that use x-ray-based imaging. This is due to the fact that MRI is nonionizing and can be used during treatment delivery without additional radiation exposure to the patient. This continuous feed of cine images during treatment enables even further technical developments, such as automated respiratory gating[3] or multi-leaf

[a] Department of Radiation Oncology, Miami Cancer Institute, 8900 North Kendall Drive, Miami, FL 33176, USA; [b] Department of Radiation Oncology, Moffitt Cancer Center, 12902 USF Magnolia Drive, Tampa, FL 33612, USA; [c] Department of Radiation Oncology, Dana-Farber Cancer Institute, 450 Brookline Avenue, Boston, MA 02215, USA; [d] Department of Radiation Oncology, University of Iowa, 200 Hawkins Dr, Iowa City, IA 52242, USA; [e] Department of Radiation Oncology, University of California Los Angeles, 1338 S Hope Street, Los Angeles, CA 90015, USA
* Corresponding author.
E-mail address: michaelchu@baptisthealth.net

Surg Oncol Clin N Am 32 (2023) 599–615
https://doi.org/10.1016/j.soc.2023.02.008
1055-3207/23/© 2023 Elsevier Inc. All rights reserved.

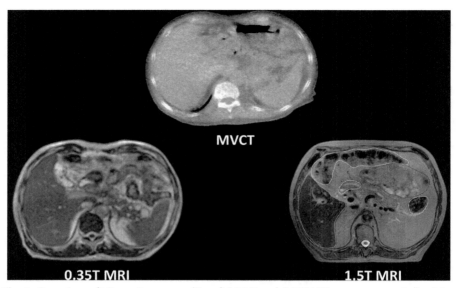

Fig. 1. Superior soft tissue image quality of 0.35 T and 1.5 T MRI versus computerized to-mography (CT). All scans were acquired without administering oral or intravenous contrast.

collimator tumor tracking,[4] both of which may reduce the volume of normal tissue irradiated during treatment by restricting the delivery of dose to a fraction of the entire motion envelope. In addition, the direct visualization of the target via cine-MRI substantially reduces the uncertainty of treating moving targets in comparison with traditional approaches that typically rely on an external surrogate or implanted fiducial marker.[5]

The typical RT planning paradigm includes acquiring simulation images of the patient in the treatment position at least several days to over 1 week before treatment delivery. The planning time accounts for delineation of target volumes and optimization of a treatment plan that aims to deliver the prescribed dose to the target while minimizing dose to uninvolved organs. A fundamental assumption in this paradigm is that the patient's anatomy is essentially unchanged across each delivered fraction. Unfortunately, this assumption rarely holds true. To account for the uncertainty of these anatomic changes, margins of at least 5 to 10 mm are commonly used, which contributes to organ-at-risk (OAR) dose and therefore the probability of adverse effects. If anatomic changes are consistently large enough, then the radiation oncologist may opt to have a new treatment plan created using an offline adaptive planning process that is usually done over several days.[6] MRgRT enables online adaptive replanning during which the treatment plan is modified immediately before treatment delivery, whereas the patient remains in the treatment position.[6] Online adaptive replanning is especially beneficial to satisfy OAR constraints despite anatomic changes that occur from 1 day of treatment to the next (interfraction) and can also be used to optimize target volume coverage if there is a favorable shift of OARs further from the target. **Fig. 2** illustrate a prostate patient undergoing MRgRT in which the original contours from the simulation imaging, particularly the rectum and seminal vesicles, did not match the shape of the organs seen on the daily imaging. In this situation, the contours are edited to reflect the anatomy on the treatment day and the treatment plan is then reoptimized over several minutes, whereas the patient remains on the

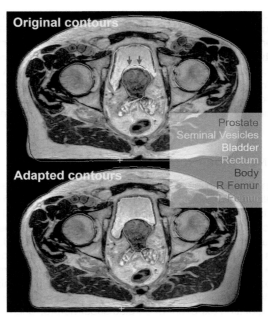

Fig. 2. Original contours derived from the simulation anatomy overlaid on the MRI of the day. The arrows in the top panel indicate the changes that were needed to the bladder and seminal vesicle contours.

treatment table. Although a margin around the target is still necessary to account for changes during the treatment delivery (intrafraction), this margin is frequently reduced to 3 to 5 mm.

MRgRT systems offer the unique ability to provide more than just anatomic information regarding the tumor. For example, diffusion-weight imaging (DWI) can provide quantitative information about the tumor known as the apparent diffusion coefficient (ADC). Recent literature suggests that an increase in the ADC may be correlated with pathologic findings and predict tumor response.[7] Ultimately, imaging biomarkers such as ADC may be used to perform dose painting to areas of the tumor that are more resistant to radiation or screen for patients that may not be responding well to their treatment and perform individual dose escalation.

At the time of this publication, three FDA-approved MR-LINACs are commercially available in the United States. These systems all combine a single-energy LINAC (6–7 MV) with an MRI scanner. Although all of these systems provide improved soft tissue contrast compared with those that use x-ray or cone-beam computerized tomography for image guidance, their designs differ significantly in the strength of the magnetic field which is 0.35 Tesla (T), 0.5 T, and 1.5 T for the ViewRay MRIdian,[8] MagnetTx Aurora-RT,[9] and Elekta Unity,[10] respectively. In general, as the magnetic field strength is increased, the signal-to-noise ratio also increases. With regard to dosimetry, a magnetic field oriented perpendicular to the beam, as is the case with MRIdian or Unity, will result in an electron return effect (ERE). The ERE refers to the process in which the electrons liberated through photon interactions follow a curved path due to the Lorentz force. For clinical cases, the ERE is modeled in the treatment planning system and the impact is reduced when multiple fields are used for treatment. The Aurora-

RT takes a different approach by orienting the magnetic field parallel to the radiation beam and placing the MRI and LINAC on the same rotating gantry. With the magnetic field configuration parallel to the radiation axis, the Lorentz force is significantly reduced, eliminating the ERE while generating greater beam collimation.

Emerging clinical outcomes of MRgRT demonstrate that this novel technology can reduce toxicity, improve local control (LC), potentially prolong overall survival (OS), and reduce fractionation for tumors in various anatomic locations.[11] In the following sections, the authors review MRgRT outcomes for thoracic, gastrointestinal, and genitourinary cancers.

CLINICAL OUTCOMES: THORACIC

There has been an increasing interest in using MRI guidance for thoracic cancers, especially related to delivering stereotactic body radiation therapy (SBRT) for central and ultracentral lung targets.[12] With its superior soft tissue contrast MRI can improve target and OAR delineation over CT especially for tumors invading adjacent mediastinal and hilar structures.[13] The ability to hold treatment (automatically or manually depending on which MRgRT system is used) based on the position of the target allows for an internal target volume (ITV) to be potentially avoided.[14] This can reduce the margin required to account for cardiorespiratory motions, thus minimizing OAR dose while maintaining adequate target coverage. With emerging data on increased risk of adverse cardiac events and worse OS due to radiation exposure of cardiac substructures such as the coronary arteries, MRgRT can achieve significant dose sparing of these substructures.[15] The phase II HILUS trial demonstrated a narrow therapeutic window of CT-guided ultracentral lung SBRT, with 34% grade 3 or higher toxicities and 15% treatment-related deaths.[16,17] MRgRT may widen this therapeutic window by enabling safe delivery of SBRT in high-risk locations such as ultracentral lung and mediastinum and permit safe dose escalation for radioresistant histologies such as colorectal metastases. A prospective study of MRgRT for ultracentral lung tumors demonstrated a reduction of planning objective violations from 94% to 17% by using online adaptive replanning.[18]

Published MRgRT outcomes for thoracic tumors are limited to phase I data and retrospective series. Henke and colleagues published a phase I trial of stereotactic MRI-guided adaptive radiation therapy (SMART) for five ultracentral lung tumor patients (one primary, four oligometastasis) prescribed 50 Gy in 5 fractions and treated on MRIdian.[19] Ten of 25 fractions were adapted, 70% to avoid predicted OAR violations and 30% to improve target volume coverage. No local failures or grade ≥3 toxicities were reported at 6 months. Finazzi and colleagues published the largest retrospective series to date of SMART on MRIdian for high-risk lung tumors that included 50 patients (54 tumors: 30 central, 17 after prior radiation, and 7 with interstitial lung disease).[20] SMART was delivered during breath-hold with sagittal cine tumor tracking and automatic beam gating. With median follow-up of 21.7 months, 12-month LC of 95.6% was achieved with grade 3 toxicity of 8% and no grade 4 or 5 toxicity. Another study from this group of single-fraction lung SBRT delivered on MRIdian prescribed to 34 Gy identified challenges with long treatment times (median 2 hours) and unreliable tracking for small tumors.[21] A case report from the Miami Cancer Institute of single-fraction lung SBRT in breath-hold on MRIdian described treatment time of only 17 minutes[22]; a prospective trial of single-fraction SBRT (25–40 Gy) is ongoing for primary or secondary cancers in the lung, liver, pancreas, adrenal gland, kidney, and abdominal/pelvic lymph nodes(NCT04939246). With mounting evidence supporting SBRT for oligometastases, MRI guidance may be clinically beneficial especially for treating such lesions in high-risk thoracic locations to decrease toxicity and improve LC.[23,24]

Additional ongoing trials are investigating MRgRT for thoracic tumors. MAGELLAN (NCT04925583) is a phase I dose-escalation trial exploring the maximum tolerated dose for ultracentral lung tumors and will enroll ~38 patients. The phase II LUNG STAAR trial (NCT04917224) is recruiting 60 patients with central (50 Gy/5 fractions) and ultracentral (60 Gy/8 fractions) lung tumors. Another phase II single-arm trial (NCT03916419) is investigating MR-guided adaptive hypofractionated (60 Gy/15 fractions) concurrent chemoradiation (CRT) followed by consolidation durvalumab for stage IIB-IIIC non-small cell lung cancer (NSCLC) patients. Nano SMART (NCT04789486) is a seamless phase I/II trial investigating SMART in conjunction with AGuIX, a gadolinium-based radiosensitizing nanoparticle aiming to recruit 100 patients with central lung tumors and pancreatic cancers. The emerging combinations of SMART with theranostics such as AGuIX have the potential to further widen the therapeutic window of MRgRT. Last, Dana-Farber Cancer Institute has a master prospective phase I-II trial (NCT04115254) investigating SMART for multitude of cancers with sub-protocols for early-stage NSCLC, mesothelioma, nodal metastases, and postoperative lung cancers. For each sub-protocol, the phase I study will assess feasibility and safety of SMART, whereas the phase II component will evaluate SMART efficacy in tumor control and patient-reported outcomes improvements. Despite the exciting early results of MRgRT, future comparative safety and efficacy data for SMART versus CT-guided SBRT in high-risk thoracic tumors will be required.

Aside from thoracic malignancies, MRgRT has been explored for treating refractory and sustained ventricular tachycardia (VT), which is an emerging indication for SBRT.[25] In a 71-year-old man with sustained VT refractory to antiarrhythmic medications and two endocardial radiofrequency ablations, Mayinger and colleagues performed the first human application of MR-guided SBRT (25 Gy in 1 fraction) using gating and respiratory motion management with cine-tracking of the heart motion. Alongside CT and invasive 3D-electroanatomical mapping of the clinical VT during electrophysiological studies, MRI was also used to delineate anatomic scarring and critical substrate to build the target volume. The treatment was successful, with cessation of sustained VT requiring implantable cardioverter-defibrillator shocks in the 3 months following SBRT.[26] With the ongoing refinement of cardiorespiratory motion management, there may be an increasing role of MRgRT for cardiac radioablation of refractory, sustained VT.[27]

CLINICAL OUTCOMES: GASTROINTESTINAL
Esophagus

Neoadjuvant CRT has long been a standard of care for locally advanced esophageal cancer, and definitive CRT is routinely offered to patients who refuse surgery or are medically inoperable.[28] However, 5-year OS remains poor in modern series particularly for inoperable patients, and it has been demonstrated that late radiation-related cardiopulmonary toxicity can contribute to death after CRT for esophageal cancer.[29,30]

MRgRT could improve outcomes by reducing unintended dose to the heart and lungs, especially for patients with distal esophageal and gastroesophageal cancers that are subject to potentially substantial respiratory motion.[31] MRgRT delivery systems provide excellent soft tissue imaging of the upper abdomen and uniquely provide continuous intrafraction cine-MRI that facilitates the use of smaller margins.[32] MRgRT systems that have automatic beam gating allow for an ITV to not be used thereby further reducing the volume of tissue that is intentionally irradiated.[33] Investigators from the University of Wisconsin demonstrated significant sparing of all evaluated cardiac substructures with respiratory-gated plans delivered with the MRIdian system versus free-breathing on a traditional LINAC.[33] Online adaptive replanning also may benefit some patients with esophageal cancer. Initial clinical investigations have demonstrated that daily adaptive treatments of esophageal cancer are associated with reductions in mean dose to both lungs and heart.[34] Although there are potential benefits of MRgRT for esophageal cancer, there is currently a lack of published clinical outcomes.

Areas of additional investigation include DWI-MRI that may be able to provide earlier response information during CRT and facilitate personalization of treatment.[35] Although dose escalation has not improved OS in randomized trials,[36] there is the potential for subsets of patients to benefit that could be made better tolerated using MRgRT through the use of smaller margins and online adaptive replanning.[37]

Liver

Liver RT was historically limited to low-dose palliation for metastases due to technical limitations in the ability to spare uninvolved liver parenchyma.[38] As the ability to deliver highly conformal treatment plans improved over the last several decades, the ability to safely dose escalate also improved. The safe delivery of ablative dose is typically limited to a subset of liver tumors that are relatively small and in favorable anatomic locations; emerging data demonstrate that the MRI guidance is poised to improve the therapeutic ratio of SBRT for primary or secondary liver cancer.[39]

Several single-institution retrospective studies have reported the feasibility of MRgRT for liver cancer without implanted fiducial markers, delivered with abdominal compression or respiratory gating.[40–42] Rosenberg and colleagues published a retrospective multi-institutional analysis of 26 patients (6 hepatocellular carcinoma [HCC], 2 cholangiocarcinoma, 18 metastatic) treated with MRIdian to a median dose of 50 Gy in 5 fractions without daily adaptive treatment planning.[43] The freedom from local progression for patients with HCC, colorectal metastasis, and all other lesions were 100%, 75%, and 83%, respectively. Grade 3 gastrointestinal toxicity was 7.7%, and there was no grade 4 or 5 toxicity.

Investigators from Washington University in St Louis completed a phase I trial that prescribed 50 Gy in 5 fractions in 20 patients for the treatment of primary malignancies of the abdomen, 10 who had liver tumors.[19] They found that 83.5% of fractions were adapted due to the initial plan violation of OAR constraints (61/97) or observed opportunity for target volume dose escalation (20/97). Plan adaptation increased planning target volume (PTV) coverage in 66% (64/97) of fractions. In the 10 patients with liver tumors, 66% (31/47) benefited from online adaptation, of which 14/47 was related to improved PTV coverage. In 3/10 liver patients, the location of OARs more than 2 cm from the target volume on day one permitted dose escalation such that the treatment course could be condensed to 4 fractions. Importantly, treatment was well tolerated and no grade ≥ 3 treatment-related toxicities were observed within 6 months.

The outcomes of a phase I trial completed at University of California Los Angeles (UCLA) of 20 patients with primary or metastatic liver cancer were recently published.[44] The median prescription dose was 54 Gy in 3 fractions. With median follow-up of nearly 19 months, the 1-and 2-year LC rates were 95% and 80%, respectively. One patient experienced grade 3 duodenal ulceration and grade 4 sepsis that thought to be secondary to a loop of bowel adjacent to the target receiving V35 Gy of 0.46 cc. No further toxicity was noted after a volumetric max constraint of V35 Gy less than 0.35 cc was mandated.

The MAESTRO randomized phase II trial (NCT05027711) is comparing MRgRT (MRIdian) and ITV-based SBRT for hepatic metastases ≤ 5 cm (or sum of 3 metastases $\leq$ 12 cm) with a primary endpoint is grade 3 or higher hepatobiliary or gastrointestinal toxicity.[45]

Future directions for liver MRgRT include personalizing therapy through MRI radiomics,[39,46] incorporation of functional MRI data, increasing utilization of single-fraction SBRT especially for multiple hepatic oligometastases,[47] and online adaptive planning to dose-escalate tumors adjacent to nonliver OARs such as bowel.[48]

Pancreas

Most patients diagnosed with pancreas cancer are not surgical candidates either due to local and/or distant metastatic disease. Although chemotherapy is the cornerstone of management for locally advanced pancreas cancer (LAPC), randomized data demonstrate that RT improves LC compared with chemotherapy alone.[49] Non-ablative radiation dose is routine for treating pancreas cancer primarily due to the proximity of luminal gastrointestinal OARs that are intolerant of high dose. There is growing evidence that radiation dose escalation beyond conventional doses may achieve more durable LC and improve OS, especially for LAPC patients.[50,51] Routine dose escalation has not been possible using CT guidance due to limitations in soft tissue resolution to identify OARs, lack of intrafraction imaging, and the inability to perform daily online adaptive replanning to account for variations in internal tumor and/or OAR anatomy. However, MR guidance addresses each of these challenges.[52]

Rudra and colleagues were among the first to demonstrate clinical benefits of dose escalation using MRgRT for patients with inoperable pancreas cancer.[51] They published outcomes from a multi-institutional retrospective analysis of 44 patients treated with various fractionation schedules on a MRIdian cobalt unit.[51] Two-year OS was significantly higher among patients prescribed a biologically effective dose (BED$_{10}$) greater than 70 Gy versus $\leq$70 Gy (49% vs 30%, P = .03), and there was no grade 3 or higher toxicity in the higher dose cohort.

Subsequent single institution retrospective studies have demonstrated encouraging LC, OS, and toxicity outcomes. Investigators at Washington University in St Louis published the results of 44 patients with inoperable pancreas cancer prescribed 50 Gy in 5 fractions (BED$_{10}$ = 100 Gy) and treated with MRIdian.[53] Severe toxicity was uncommon (4.6%). Although 2-year OS (37.9%) was higher than historical expectations, the results likely were influenced by 26% having Eastern Cooperative Oncology Group (ECOG) performance status of 2 or 3. Chuong and colleagues from the Miami Cancer Institute published their initial outcomes of 35 inoperable patients treated on MRIdian in breath hold with a prescribed dose of 50 Gy in 5 fractions. With median follow-up 10.3 months from treatment, 1-year LC was 87.8% and 1-year OS was 58.9%. Acute and late grade 3 toxicity rates were 2.9% each. A more recent publication from the Miami Cancer Institute in 62 inoperable patients who received induction chemotherapy was recently published.[54] Most patients were treated with a clinical target volume to cover areas of potential microscopic disease.[55] With median follow-up of 18.6 months from diagnosis, the 2-year LC and OS were 87.7% and 45.5%, respectively, which are significantly higher than historical outcomes of non-ablative RT. Acute and late grade 3 or higher toxicity rates were 4.8% each. The feasibility of ablative MRgRT with abdominal compression on Unity has been reported,[42,56] although there are not yet published clinical outcomes.

The reason why OS may be positively impacted through radiation dose escalation is uncertain. It is well understood that patients with pancreas cancer frequently die from distant metastases, but up to one-third of deaths might be attributed to local progression.[57] Thus, it is plausible that radiation dose escalation might prevent or delay death due to local progression, thereby impacting OS.[58]

Prospective studies are needed to confirm that ablative MRgRT is both safe and more effective than non-ablative RT, as suggested by retrospective data. The only prospective evaluation of ablative MRgRT for inoperable pancreas cancer to date was published by Kim and colleagues who completed a phase I trial of concurrent gemcitabine/nab-paclitaxel and 15 to 25 fractions delivered on an MRIdian cobalt unit.[59] The investigators concluded that the highest radiation dose level (67.5 Gy in 15 fractions) was safe. A phase 2 multi-institutional trial (NCT03621644) of ablative MRIdian SMART (50 Gy in 5 fractions) for borderline resectable and LAPC completed accrual in late 2021; the primary endpoint was met since no patient had acute grade 3 or higher gastrointestinal toxicity definitely attributable to SMART.[60] The phase 3 multi-institutional LAP-ABLATE trial (NCT05585554) is currently enrolling LAPC patients who are randomized to chemotherapy ± ablative 5-fraction MRIdian SMART; the primary endpoint is 2-year OS.

Rectum

MRI provides advantages over CT for treatment planning, including lower interobserver contouring variability.[61] Because of the uncertainty on CT in distinguishing tumor from normal tissue, it is common that CT-based target volumes overestimate the true extent of disease, thus increasing normal tissue dose. Several studies demonstrate that MRI-based volumes can be significantly smaller than those delineated using CT, and that this difference may be largest for anorectal tumors.[62,63] As such, MRI-based volumes may result in a meaningful reduction in dose to normal tissues such as the anal sphincter and reduce the risk of morbidity.[64]

MRI can aid in the evaluation of posttreatment tumor response following neoadjuvant CRT.[65] MRI can also aid in the evaluation of residual tumor after neoadjuvant treatment or surgery. MRI-based radiomics may be useful for assessing treatment response.[66,67] Changes in ADC during CRT for rectal cancer correlate with tumor downstaging on pathology at the time of surgery following neoadjuvant therapy.[68-70] Pre- and post-CRT delta radiomics demonstrate statistically significant associations with clinical outcomes.[71] Palmisano and colleagues demonstrated a correlation between the percent volumetric changes of the tumor on MRI at week 3 of CRT with the probability of pathologic complete response.[72] Lambregts and colleagues prospectively demonstrated that the addition of DWI-MRI to standard MRI sequences increased the sensitivity of detecting pathologic complete response from 0% to 40% to 52% to 64%,[73] and these findings were later validated in a bi-institutional study.[74] The ability to acquire DWI-MRI on a daily basis likely will further improve our ability to identify treatment responders versus nonresponders and thus tailor treatment accordingly.

Chiloiro and colleagues have published the only clinical experience to date of MRgRT for rectal cancer.[75] All 22 patients were treated using the MRIdian cobalt system. A simultaneous integrated boost of 55 Gy in 25 fractions to gross disease and 45 Gy in 25 fractions to elective regions was delivered. A total of 19 patients went on to surgery with three having a pathologic complete response (15.8%). In total, 27% of patients achieved either a complete clinical or pathologic response to treatment. Acute grade 3 gastrointestinal toxicities occurred in 22.7%.

Online adaptive MRgRT has several potential benefits for rectal cancer.[76] First, rectal cancers can decrease substantially in volume over the 5 to 6 weeks of CRT and plan adaptation would decrease OAR dose.[77] Second, online adaptive replanning may facilitate safe dose escalation that could improve clinical outcomes for some patients including the probability of achieve complete clinical/pathologic complete response and negative margins.[78,79]

CLINICAL OUTCOMES: GENITOURINARY
Prostate: Definitive

MRgRT offers several theoretic advantages in the definitive treatment of prostate cancer.[80,81] These benefits include the ability to reduce the PTV margins that are used to ensure adequate target dosing.[82] Because the high-dose regions of the PTV often overlap portions of the bladder, rectum, and other nearby structures, a larger PTV margin is likely to be associated with increased toxicity.[83–86]

First, MRI-guided LINACs can substantially improve motion management in prostate RT. Historically, interfraction motion monitoring has relied on implanting fiducial markers into the prostate that serve as a surrogate for the prostate's position.[87,88] Intrafraction motion monitoring can be achieved in several ways, including leveraging a rapid treatment time or frequently (once every 30–60 seconds) obtaining orthogonal X-rays to triangulate the prostate based on the position of the fiducial markers. With MRgRT, the prostate can be directly visualized for alignment before treatment (entirely bypassing the need for fiducial markers). A cine-MRI in the sagittal plane can be obtained 4 to 8 times per second to track the prostate using MRIdian.[89] The physician can specify a "gating window" around the prostate; for instance, he or she could stipulate that if greater than 10% of the prostate volume moved outside a 3-mm gating boundary placed around the prostate on any given slice of the cine MRI, an automatic beam-hold will be initiated. As a result, the PTV margin needed for motion uncertainty can be reduced significantly.

Uncertainties related to contouring (which constitute a part of the PTV margin) can also be minimized in an MRgRT workflow. The prostate is best visualized with MRI, and thus when designing a radiation plan, diagnostic MRI images are often "fused" to the CT-based images that are obtained for planning. This cross-modality fusion introduces residual error, which necessitates a larger margin when formulating the treatment volumes. This error can be minimized with the direct utilization of MRI images for contouring; even if a diagnostic MRI were to be fused, this would be an MRI–MRI fusion with minimal uncertainty.[81,90] A corollary principle applies to urethral delineation. The urethra—which is best visualized on MRI—is considered to be an extremely critical OAR with respect to urinary toxicity after RT.[91] The urethra itself is not seen on traditional RT planning CT scans, and thus an MRI-CT fusion is always needed to delineate the urethra for the purposes of dose minimization. An MRgRT delivery system can minimize the uncertainties in urethral delineation.

The ability to leverage an MRgRT system to reduce PTV margins has been studied in the phase III randomized MIRAGE trial (NCT04384770), in which patients received SBRT to the prostate using CT guidance with a standard-of-care 4 mm margin, versus SBRT to the same dose using MRIdian with a standard-of-care 2 mm margin. The trial was closed early to accrual when clinically significant reductions in acute grade 2+ genitourinary toxicity (24.4% vs. 43.4%; $P = .01$) and acute grade 2+ gastrointestinal toxicity (0.0% vs. 10.5%; $P = .003$) were found favoring the MRIdian arm.[92] The post-SBRT decrement in patient-reported urinary and bowel quality of life metrics was also minimized with MRI guidance. This trial provides level 1 evidence that the enhanced image guidance offered by MRgRT can translate into meaningful benefits for patients. Future work will investigate whether further adjustments of dosing to the prostate, and the dominant intraprostatic lesion could optimize the therapeutic ratio.

Prostate: Postoperative

In the context of postoperative RT, a major challenge is that the target volume is "invisible" and is in fact a potential space that is delimited by the adjacent bladder and rectum, both of which are highly deformable and will vary in size and shape from day-to-day.[93,94] This variation has implications both for toxicity (potential overdosing of these adjacent organs) and efficacy (potentially underdosing the target volume). A solution is online adaptive RT, and dosimetric studies have shown this approach can improve target coverage and reduce doses to adjacent organs.[95] Because of the improved soft tissue contrast with MRI compared with CT, adaptive MRgRT is likely to be more accurate than CT-based adaptive therapy, and this may lead to improved outcomes.

Beyond adaptive RT, the advantages of an MRI-LINAC in the intact setting generally also apply to the postprostatectomy setting. For instance, management of intrafraction motion—which can be substantial and is not accounted for in most CT-based workflows—can be achieved by tracking the anterior rectal wall. Early results from the phase II SCIMITAR trial of SBRT to the prostate fossa (NCT03541850) found an improved side effect profile with MRgRT versus CT-guided RT in this context.[96] Specifically, MRgRT was associated with a 30.5% reduction in any grade acute gastrointestinal toxicity and with improved posttreatment bowel quality of life. Although nonrandomized comparisons should be taken with caution, this study provides prospective data supporting the benefit of MRgRT for post-prostatectomy radiation and builds on the principles of the MIRAGE trial in the intact prostate setting.

Bladder and Kidney

Although prostate cancer is the main genitourinary malignancy treated with RT, compelling data support RT for bladder and renal cell carcinomas as well.[97] In the context of bladder cancer, the enhanced visualization of soft tissue and the ability to perform online adaptive RT are the key features of MRI-LINACs that support their use in this context.[98,99] For renal cell carcinoma, emerging data suggest excellent LC and survival with SBRT.[100] As tumors in the upper abdomen are highly mobile and surrounding critical structures such as the duodenum and stomach are highly deformable, MRgRT seems uniquely poised to optimize the therapeutic ratio. Indeed, preliminary data suggest that this is well tolerated[101] and the results of the fully accrued MRI-MARK trial (NCT04580836) are highly anticipated.

CLINICS CARE POINTS

- MRI guidance for radiation therapy has recently become available, providing technological advantages over other forms of image guided radiation therapy.
- The majority of MRI guided radiation therapy outcomes have been published for the treatment of tumors in the thorax, abdomen, pelvis and demonstrate particular advantages for tumors that are subject to intrafraction motion and those that benefit from dose escalation.
- MRI guidance offers the potential to guide radiation therapy by incorporating novel imaging biomarkers.

DISCLOSURES

Dr M.D. Chuong reports honoraria, consulting fees, and research funding from View-Ray. Dr D.E. Hyer reports consulting fees and research funding from Elekta, Inc Dr A.U. Kishan reports consulting fees, research funding, stock ownership from View-Ray, United States.

REFERENCES

1. Hall WA, Paulson ES, van der Heide UA, et al. The transformation of radiation oncology using real-time magnetic resonance guidance: A review. Eur J Cancer 2019;122:42–52.
2. Noel CE, Parikh PJ, Spencer CR, et al. Comparison of onboard low-field magnetic resonance imaging versus onboard computed tomography for anatomy visualization in radiotherapy. Acta Oncol 2015;54(9):1474–82.
3. Charters JA, Abdulkadir Y, O'Connell D, et al. Dosimetric evaluation of respiratory gating on a 0.35-T magnetic resonance-guided radiotherapy linac. J Appl Clin Med Phys 2022;10:e13666.
4. Uijtewaal P, Borman PTS, Woodhead PL, et al. First experimental demonstration of VMAT combined with MLC tracking for single and multi fraction lung SBRT on an MR-linac. Radiother Oncol 2022;174:149–57.
5. Snyder JE, Flynn RT, Hyer DE. Implementation of respiratory-gated VMAT on a Versa HD linear accelerator. J Appl Clin Med Phys 2017;18(5):152–61.
6. Green OL, Henke LE, Hugo GD. Practical Clinical Workflows for Online and Offline Adaptive Radiation Therapy. Semin Radiat Oncol 2019;29(3):219–27.
7. Chin S, Eccles CL, McWilliam A, et al. Magnetic resonance-guided radiation therapy: A review. J Med Imaging Radiat Oncol 2020;64(1):163–77.
8. Kluter S. Technical design and concept of a 0.35 T MR-Linac. Clin Transl Radiat Oncol 2019;18:98–101.
9. Fallone BG. The rotating biplanar linac-magnetic resonance imaging system. Semin Radiat Oncol 2014;24(3):200–2.
10. Raaymakers BW, Lagendijk JJ, Overweg J, et al. Integrating a 1.5 T MRI scanner with a 6 MV accelerator: proof of concept. Phys Med Biol 2009;54(12): N229–37.
11. Keall PJ, Brighi C, Glide-Hurst C, et al. Integrated MRI-guided radiotherapy - opportunities and challenges. Nat Rev Clin Oncol 2022;19(7):458–70.
12. Henke LE, Olsen JR, Contreras JA, et al. Stereotactic MR-Guided Online Adaptive Radiation Therapy (SMART) for Ultracentral Thorax Malignancies: Results of a Phase 1 Trial. Adv Radiat Oncol 2019;4(1):201–9.
13. Crockett CB, Samson P, Chuter R, et al. Initial Clinical Experience of MR-Guided Radiotherapy for Non-Small Cell Lung Cancer. Front Oncol 2021;11:617681.
14. Finazzi T, Palacios MA, Haasbeek CJA, et al. Stereotactic MR-guided adaptive radiation therapy for peripheral lung tumors. Radiother Oncol 2020;144:46–52.
15. Tjong MC, Bitterman DS, Brantley K, et al. Major adverse cardiac event risk prediction model incorporating baseline Cardiac disease, Hypertension, and Logarithmic Left anterior descending coronary artery radiation dose in lung cancer (CHyLL). Radiother Oncol 2022;169:105–13.
16. Lindberg K, Grozman V, Karlsson K, et al. The HILUS-Trial-a Prospective Nordic Multicenter Phase 2 Study of Ultracentral Lung Tumors Treated With Stereotactic Body Radiotherapy. J Thorac Oncol 2021;16(7):1200–10.
17. Rosenberg SA, Mak R, Kotecha R, et al. The Nordic-HILUS Trial: Ultracentral Lung Stereotactic Ablative Radiotherapy and a Narrow Therapeutic Window. J Thorac Oncol 2021;16(10):e79–80.
18. Regnery S, Buchele C, Weykamp F, et al. Adaptive MR-Guided Stereotactic Radiotherapy is Beneficial for Ablative Treatment of Lung Tumors in High-Risk Locations. Front Oncol 2021;11:757031.
19. Henke L, Kashani R, Robinson C, et al. Phase I trial of stereotactic MR-guided online adaptive radiation therapy (SMART) for the treatment of oligometastatic

or unresectable primary malignancies of the abdomen. Radiother Oncol 2018; 126(3):519–26.

20. Finazzi T, Haasbeek CJA, Spoelstra FOB, et al. Clinical Outcomes of Stereotactic MR-Guided Adaptive Radiation Therapy for High-Risk Lung Tumors. Int J Radiat Oncol Biol Phys 2020;107(2):270–8.

21. Finazzi T, van Sornsen de Koste JR, Palacios MA, et al. Delivery of magnetic resonance-guided single-fraction stereotactic lung radiotherapy. Phys Imaging Radiat Oncol 2020;14:17–23.

22. Chuong MD, Kotecha R, Mehta MP, et al. Case report of visual biofeedback-driven, magnetic resonance-guided single-fraction SABR in breath hold for early stage non-small-cell lung cancer. Med Dosim. Autumn 2021;46(3):247–52.

23. Gomez DR, Tang C, Zhang J, et al. Local Consolidative Therapy Vs. Maintenance Therapy or Observation for Patients With Oligometastatic Non-Small-Cell Lung Cancer: Long-Term Results of a Multi-Institutional, Phase II, Randomized Study. J Clin Oncol 2019;37(18):1558–65.

24. Siva S, Bressel M, Mai T, et al. Single-Fraction vs Multifraction Stereotactic Ablative Body Radiotherapy for Pulmonary Oligometastases (SAFRON II): The Trans Tasman Radiation Oncology Group 13.01 Phase 2 Randomized Clinical Trial. JAMA Oncol 2021;7(10):1476–85.

25. Robinson CG, Samson PP, Moore KMS, et al. Phase I/II Trial of Electrophysiology-Guided Noninvasive Cardiac Radioablation for Ventricular Tachycardia. Circulation 2019;139(3):313–21.

26. Mayinger M, Kovacs B, Tanadini-Lang S, et al. First magnetic resonance imaging-guided cardiac radioablation of sustained ventricular tachycardia. Radiother Oncol 2020;152:203–7.

27. Akdag O, Borman PTS, Woodhead P, et al. First experimental exploration of real-time cardiorespiratory motion management for future stereotactic arrhythmia radioablation treatments on the MR-linac. Phys Med Biol 2022;67(6). https://doi. org/10.1088/1361-6560/ac5717.

28. Sjoquist KM, Burmeister BH, Smithers BM, et al. Survival after neoadjuvant chemotherapy or chemoradiotherapy for resectable oesophageal carcinoma: an updated meta-analysis. Lancet Oncol 2011;12(7):681–92.

29. Wang X, Palaskas NL, Yusuf SW, et al. Incidence and Onset of Severe Cardiac Events After Radiotherapy for Esophageal Cancer. J Thorac Oncol 2020;15(10): 1682–90.

30. Pao TH, Chang WL, Chiang NJ, et al. Cardiac radiation dose predicts survival in esophageal squamous cell carcinoma treated by definitive concurrent chemotherapy and intensity modulated radiotherapy. Radiat Oncol 2020;15(1):221.

31. Lee SL, Bassetti M, Meijer GJ, et al. Review of MR-Guided Radiotherapy for Esophageal Cancer. Front Oncol 2021;11:628009.

32. Lips I, Lever F, Reerink O, et al. SU-E-J-57: MRI-Linac (MRL) Guided Treatment for Esophageal Cancer. Med Phys 2012;39(6Part6):3665.

33. Lee SL, Mahler P, Olson S, et al. Reduction of cardiac dose using respiratory-gated MR-linac plans for gastro-esophageal junction cancer. Med Dosim. Summer 2021;46(2):152–6.

34. Boekhoff MR, Bouwmans R, Doornaert PAH, et al. Clinical implementation and feasibility of long-course fractionated MR-guided chemoradiotherapy for patients with esophageal cancer: An R-IDEAL stage 1b/2a evaluation of technical innovation. Clin Transl Radiat Oncol 2022;34:82–9.

35. van Rossum PS, van Lier AL, van Vulpen M, et al. Diffusion-weighted magnetic resonance imaging for the prediction of pathologic response to neoadjuvant

chemoradiotherapy in esophageal cancer. Radiother Oncol 2015;115(2): 163–70.

36. Hulshof M, Geijsen ED, Rozema T, et al. Randomized Study on Dose Escalation in Definitive Chemoradiation for Patients With Locally Advanced Esophageal Cancer (ARTDECO Study). J Clin Oncol 2021;39(25):2816–24.

37. Zhang W, Luo Y, Wang X, et al. Dose-escalated radiotherapy improved survival for esophageal cancer patients with a clinical complete response after standard-dose radiotherapy with concurrent chemotherapy. Cancer Manag Res 2018;10:2675–82.

38. Hoyer M, Swaminath A, Bydder S, et al. Radiotherapy for liver metastases: a review of evidence. Int J Radiat Oncol Biol Phys 2012;82(3):1047–57.

39. Witt JS, Rosenberg SA, Bassetti MF. MRI-guided adaptive radiotherapy for liver tumours: visualising the future. Lancet Oncol 2020;21(2):e74–82.

40. Feldman AM, Modh A, Glide-Hurst C, et al. Real-time Magnetic Resonance-guided Liver Stereotactic Body Radiation Therapy: An Institutional Report Using a Magnetic Resonance-Linac System. Cureus 2019;11(9):e5774.

41. Boldrini L, Romano A, Mariani S, et al. MRI-guided stereotactic radiation therapy for hepatocellular carcinoma: a feasible and safe innovative treatment approach. J Cancer Res Clin Oncol 2021;147(7):2057–68.

42. Stanescu T, Shessel A, Carpino-Rocca C, et al. MRI-Guided Online Adaptive Stereotactic Body Radiation Therapy of Liver and Pancreas Tumors on an MR-Linac System. Cancers 2022;14(3). https://doi.org/10.3390/cancers1403071.

43. Rosenberg SA, Henke LE, Shaverdian N, et al. A Multi-Institutional Experience of MR-Guided Liver Stereotactic Body Radiation Therapy. Adv Radiat Oncol 2019; 4(1):142–9.

44. van Dams R, Wu TC, Kishan AU, et al. Ablative radiotherapy for liver tumors using stereotactic MRI-guidance: A prospective phase I trial. Radiother Oncol 2022;170:14–20.

45. Hoegen P, Zhang KS, Tonndorf-Martini E, et al. MR-guided adaptive versus ITV-based stereotactic body radiotherapy for hepatic metastases (MAESTRO): a randomized controlled phase II trial. Radiat Oncol 2022;17(1):59.

46. Dreher C, Linde P, Boda-Heggemann J, et al. Radiomics for liver tumours. Strahlenther Onkol 2020;196(10):888–99.

47. Folkert MR, Meyer JJ, Aguilera TA, et al. Long-Term Results of a Phase 1 Dose-Escalation Trial and Subsequent Institutional Experience of Single-Fraction Stereotactic Ablative Radiation Therapy for Liver Metastases. Int J Radiat Oncol Biol Phys 2021;109(5):1387–95.

48. Mayinger M, Ludwig R, Christ SM, et al. Benefit of replanning in MR-guided online adaptive radiation therapy in the treatment of liver metastasis. Radiat Oncol 2021;16(1):84.

49. Hammel P, Huguet F, van Laethem JL, et al. Effect of Chemoradiotherapy vs Chemotherapy on Survival in Patients With Locally Advanced Pancreatic Cancer Controlled After 4 Months of Gemcitabine With or Without Erlotinib: The LAP07 Randomized Clinical Trial. JAMA 2016;315(17):1844–53.

50. Krishnan S, Chadha AS, Suh Y, et al. Focal Radiation Therapy Dose Escalation Improves Overall Survival in Locally Advanced Pancreatic Cancer Patients Receiving Induction Chemotherapy and Consolidative Chemoradiation. Int J Radiat Oncol Biol Phys 2016;94(4):755–65.

51. Rudra S, Jiang N, Rosenberg SA, et al. Using adaptive magnetic resonance image-guided radiation therapy for treatment of inoperable pancreatic cancer. Cancer Med 2019;8(5):2123–32.

52. Hall WA, Small C, Paulson E, et al. Magnetic Resonance Guided Radiation Therapy for Pancreatic Adenocarcinoma, Advantages, Challenges, Current Approaches, and Future Directions. Front Oncol 2021;11:628155.

53. Hassanzadeh C, Rudra S, Bommireddy A, et al. Ablative Five-Fraction Stereotactic Body Radiation Therapy for Inoperable Pancreatic Cancer Using Online MR-Guided Adaptation. Advances in Radiation Oncology 2020;6(1):100506.

54. Chuong MD, Herrera R, Kaiser A, et al. Induction Chemotherapy and Ablative Stereotactic Magnetic Resonance Image-Guided Adaptive Radiation Therapy for Inoperable Pancreas Cancer. Front Oncol 2022;12:888462.

55. Chuong MD, Kharofa J, Sanford NN. Elective Target Coverage for Pancreatic Cancer: When Less Does Not Clearly Achieve More. Int J Radiat Oncol Biol Phys 2022;112(1):143–5.

56. Tyagi N, Liang J, Burleson S, et al. Feasibility of ablative stereotactic body radiation therapy of pancreas cancer patients on a 1.5 Tesla magnetic resonance-linac system using abdominal compression. Phys Imaging Radiat Oncol 2021; 19:53–9.

57. Iacobuzio-Donahue CA, Fu B, Yachida S, et al. DPC4 gene status of the primary carcinoma correlates with patterns of failure in patients with pancreatic cancer. J Clin Oncol 2009;27(11):1806–13.

58. Chuong MD, Herrera R, Ucar A, et al. Causes of death among initially inoperable pancreas cancer patients after induction chemotherapy and ablative 5-fraction stereotactic magnetic resonance image-guided adaptive radiation therapy. Advances in Radiation Oncology 2022;8(1):101084.

59. Kim H, Olsen JR, Green OL, et al. MR-Guided Radiation Therapy With Concurrent Gemcitabine/Nab-Paclitaxel Chemotherapy in Inoperable Pancreatic Cancer: A TITE-CRM Phase I Trial. Int J Radiat Oncol Biol Phys 2022;115(1):214–23.

60. Parikh PJ, Lee P, Low D, et al. Stereotactic MR-Guided On-Table Adaptive Radiation Therapy (SMART) for Patients with Borderline or Locally Advanced Pancreatic Cancer: Primary Endpoint Outcomes of a Prospective Phase II Multi-Center International Trial. Int J Radiat Oncol Biol Phys 2022;114(5):1062–3.

61. Burbach JP, Kleijnen JP, Reerink O, et al. Inter-observer agreement of MRI-based tumor delineation for preoperative radiotherapy boost in locally advanced rectal cancer. Radiother Oncol 2016;118(2):399–407.

62. O'Neill BD, Salerno G, Thomas K, et al. MR vs CT imaging: low rectal cancer tumour delineation for three-dimensional conformal radiotherapy. Br J Radiol 2009;82(978):509–13.

63. Tan J, Lim Joon D, Fitt G, et al. The utility of multimodality imaging with CT and MRI in defining rectal tumour volumes for radiotherapy treatment planning: a pilot study. J Med Imaging Radiat Oncol 2010;54(6):562–8.

64. Arias F, Eito C, Asin G, et al. Fecal incontinence and radiation dose on anal sphincter in patients with locally advanced rectal cancer (LARC) treated with preoperative chemoradiotherapy: a retrospective, single-institutional study. Clin Transl Oncol 2017;19(8):969–75.

65. Kalisz KR, Enzerra MD, Paspulati RM. MRI Evaluation of the Response of Rectal Cancer to Neoadjuvant Chemoradiation Therapy. Radiographics 2019;39(2): 538–56.

66. Kim SH, Lee JY, Lee JM, et al. Apparent diffusion coefficient for evaluating tumour response to neoadjuvant chemoradiation therapy for locally advanced rectal cancer. Eur Radiol 2011;21(5):987–95.

67. Horvat N, Veeraraghavan H, Khan M, et al. MR Imaging of Rectal Cancer: Radiomics Analysis to Assess Treatment Response after Neoadjuvant Therapy. Radiology 2018;287(3):833–43.
68. Sun YS, Zhang XP, Tang L, et al. Locally advanced rectal carcinoma treated with preoperative chemotherapy and radiation therapy: preliminary analysis of diffusion-weighted MR imaging for early detection of tumor histopathologic downstaging. Radiology 2010;254(1):170–8.
69. Shaverdian N, Yang Y, Hu P, et al. Feasibility evaluation of diffusion-weighted imaging using an integrated MRI-radiotherapy system for response assessment to neoadjuvant therapy in rectal cancer. The Br J Radiol 2017;90(1071):20160739.
70. Nougaret S, Vargas HA, Lakhman Y, et al. Intravoxel Incoherent Motion-derived Histogram Metrics for Assessment of Response after Combined Chemotherapy and Radiation Therapy in Rectal Cancer: Initial Experience and Comparison between Single-Section and Volumetric Analyses. Radiology 2016;280(2):446–54.
71. Jeon SH, Song C, Chie EK, et al. Delta-radiomics signature predicts treatment outcomes after preoperative chemoradiotherapy and surgery in rectal cancer. Radiat Oncol 2019;14(1):43.
72. Palmisano A, Esposito A, Rancoita PMV, et al. Could perfusion heterogeneity at dynamic contrast-enhanced MRI be used to predict rectal cancer sensitivity to chemoradiotherapy? Clin Radiol 2018;73(10):911 e1–e911 e7.
73. Lambregts DM, Vandecaveye V, Barbaro B, et al. Diffusion-weighted MRI for selection of complete responders after chemoradiation for locally advanced rectal cancer: a multicenter study. Ann Surg Oncol 2011;18(8):2224–31.
74. Lambregts DM, Rao SX, Sassen S, et al. MRI and Diffusion-weighted MRI Volumetry for Identification of Complete Tumor Responders After Preoperative Chemoradiotherapy in Patients With Rectal Cancer: A Bi-institutional Validation Study. Ann Surg 2015;262(6):1034–9.
75. Chiloiro G, Boldrini L, Meldolesi E, et al. MR-guided radiotherapy in rectal cancer: First clinical experience of an innovative technology. Clin Transl Radiat Oncol 2019;18:80–6.
76. Boldrini L, Intven M, Bassetti M, et al. MR-Guided Radiotherapy for Rectal Cancer: Current Perspective on Organ Preservation. Front Oncol 2021;11:619852.
77. Van den Begin R, Kleijnen JP, Engels B, et al. Tumor volume regression during preoperative chemoradiotherapy for rectal cancer: a prospective observational study with weekly MRI. Acta Oncol 2018;57(6):723–7.
78. Bonomo P, Lo Russo M, Nachbar M, et al. 1.5 T MR-linac planning study to compare two different strategies of rectal boost irradiation. Clin Transl Radiat Oncol 2021;26:86–91.
79. Passoni P, Fiorino C, Slim N, et al. Feasibility of an adaptive strategy in preoperative radiochemotherapy for rectal cancer with image-guided tomotherapy: boosting the dose to the shrinking tumor. Int J Radiat Oncol Biol Phys 2013;87(1):67–72.
80. Hall WA, Paulson E, Li XA, et al. Magnetic resonance linear accelerator technology and adaptive radiation therapy: An overview for clinicians. CA Cancer J Clin 2022;72(1):34–56.
81. Pathmanathan AU, van As NJ, Kerkmeijer LGW, et al. Magnetic Resonance Imaging-Guided Adaptive Radiation Therapy: A "Game Changer" for Prostate Treatment? Int J Radiat Oncol Biol Phys 2018;100(2):361–73.
82. Antolak JA, Rosen II. Planning target volumes for radiotherapy: how much margin is needed? Int J Radiat Oncol Biol Phys 1999;44(5):1165–70.

83. Willigenburg T, van der Velden JM, Zachiu C, et al. Accumulated bladder wall dose is correlated with patient-reported acute urinary toxicity in prostate cancer patients treated with stereotactic, daily adaptive MR-guided radiotherapy. Radiother Oncol 2022;171:182–8.

84. Mylona E, Acosta O, Lizee T, et al. Voxel-Based Analysis for Identification of Urethrovesical Subregions Predicting Urinary Toxicity After Prostate Cancer Radiation Therapy. Int J Radiat Oncol Biol Phys 2019;104(2):343–54.

85. Alayed Y, Davidson M, Quon H, et al. Dosimetric predictors of toxicity and quality of life following prostate stereotactic ablative radiotherapy. Radiother Oncol 2020;144:135–40.

86. Spratt DE, Lee JY, Dess RT, et al. Vessel-sparing Radiotherapy for Localized Prostate Cancer to Preserve Erectile Function: A Single-arm Phase 2 Trial. Eur Urol 2017;72(4):617–24.

87. Dang A, Kupelian PA, Cao M, et al. Image-guided radiotherapy for prostate cancer. Transl Androl Urol 2018;7(3):308–20.

88. O'Neill AG, Jain S, Hounsell AR, et al. Fiducial marker guided prostate radiotherapy: a review. Br J Radiol 2016;89(1068):20160296.

89. Green OL, Rankine LJ, Cai B, et al. First clinical implementation of real-time, real anatomy tracking and radiation beam control. Med Phys 2018. https://doi.org/10.1002/mp.13002.

90. Pathmanathan AU, Schmidt MA, Brand DH, et al. Improving fiducial and prostate capsule visualization for radiotherapy planning using MRI. J Appl Clin Med Phys 2019;20(3):27–36.

91. Leeman JE, Chen YH, Catalano P, et al. Radiation Dose to the Intraprostatic Urethra Correlates Strongly With Urinary Toxicity After Prostate Stereotactic Body Radiation Therapy: A Combined Analysis of 23 Prospective Clinical Trials. Int J Radiat Oncol Biol Phys 2022;112(1):75–82.

92. Kishan AU, Ma TM, Lamb JM, et al. Magnetic Resonance Imaging-Guided vs Computed Tomography-Guided Stereotactic Body Radiotherapy for Prostate Cancer: The MIRAGE Randomized Clinical Trial. JAMA Oncol 2023. https://doi.org/10.1001/jamaoncol.2022.6558.

93. Yoon S, Cao M, Aghdam N, et al. Prostate bed and organ-at-risk deformation: Prospective volumetric and dosimetric data from a phase II trial of stereotactic body radiotherapy after radical prostatectomy. Radiother Oncol 2020;148:44–50.

94. Ost P, De Meerleer G, De Gersem W, et al. Analysis of prostate bed motion using daily cone-beam computed tomography during postprostatectomy radiotherapy. Int J Radiat Oncol Biol Phys 2011;79(1):188–94.

95. Cao M, Gao Y, Yoon SM, et al. Interfractional Geometric Variations and Dosimetric Benefits of Stereotactic MRI Guided Online Adaptive Radiotherapy (SMART) of Prostate Bed after Radical Prostatectomy: Post-Hoc Analysis of a Phase II Trial. Cancers 2021;13(11). https://doi.org/10.3390/cancers13112802.

96. Ma TM, Ballas LK, Wilhalme H, et al. Quality-of-Life Outcomes and Toxicity Profile Among Patients with Localized Prostate Cancer After Radical Prostatectomy Treated With Stereotactic Body Radiation: The SCIMITAR Multi-Center Phase 2 Trial. Int J Radiat Oncol Biol Phys 2022. https://doi.org/10.1016/j.ijrobp.2022.08.041.

97. Kerkmeijer LGW, Kishan AU, Tree AC. Magnetic Resonance Imaging-guided Adaptive Radiotherapy for Urological Cancers: What Urologists Should Know. Eur Urol 2022;82(2):149–51.

98. Hunt A, Hanson I, Dunlop A, et al. Feasibility of magnetic resonance guided radiotherapy for the treatment of bladder cancer. Clin Transl Radiat Oncol 2020;25:46–51.

99. Hijab A, Tocco B, Hanson I, et al. MR-Guided Adaptive Radiotherapy for Bladder Cancer. Front Oncol 2021;11:637591.

100. Siva S, Louie AV, Warner A, et al. Pooled analysis of stereotactic ablative radiotherapy for primary renal cell carcinoma: A report from the International Radiosurgery Oncology Consortium for Kidney (IROCK). Cancer 2018;124(5):934–42.

101. Tetar SU, Bohoudi O, Senan S, et al. The Role of Daily Adaptive Stereotactic MR-Guided Radiotherapy for Renal Cell Cancer. Cancers 2020;12(10). https://doi.org/10.3390/cancers12102763.

Advances in Radiotherapy Immune Modulation

From Bench-to-Bedside and Back Again

Charles X. Wang, MD, PhD[1], Jared Hunt[1], Shera Feinstein, MD[1], Soo Kyoung Kim, MD, Arta M. Monjazeb, MD, PhD*

KEYWORDS

- Radiotherapy • Immunotherapy • Immune checkpoint inhibitor • Immuno-oncology

KEY POINTS

- Pre-clinical and clinical data clearly demonstrate the immune modulatory effects of radiotherapy (RT).
- Most clinical trials investigating the benefit of combining RT + immunotherapy have been equivocal.
- Improved understanding of radiation immune modulation and how parameters of RT delivery (site and number of lesions, dose, fractionation, timing) influence immune modulation are needed.
- Many investigations focus on combining RT with immune checkpoint inhibitors but partnering RT with other immunotherapy strategies may also be fruitful.

INTRODUCTION

Metastatic cancer accounts for nearly 90% of cancer deaths and thus is critically important, but clinically challenging to manage.[1] Historically, chemotherapy and targeted therapies were the mainstays of clinical management, but many patients with systemic disease also received radiotherapy (RT) with palliative intent. The advent of immune checkpoint inhibitor (ICI) immunotherapy has made tremendous strides in improving the outcomes of patients with metastatic disease, and is now being moved into the management of patients with localized disease. There is considerable interest in combining RT with immunotherapy based on evidence suggesting that RT can act as an "in-situ" vaccination and induce inflammation which can support an anti-tumor immune response.[2] This in-situ vaccine effect was first proposed by reports of

UC Davis Health, Department of Radiation Oncology, 4501 X-Street, Sacramento, CA 95817, USA

[1] Co-first authors, these authors contributed equally to this work.

* Corresponding author. Laboratory of Cancer Immunology, UC Davis Comprehensive Cancer Center, 4501 X-Street, Suite G-120, Sacramento, CA 95817.

E-mail address: ammonjazeb@ucdavis.edu

Surg Oncol Clin N Am 32 (2023) 617–629
https://doi.org/10.1016/j.soc.2023.02.009
1055-3207/23/© 2023 Elsevier Inc. All rights reserved.

surgonc.theclinics.com

radiation triggering out-of-field responses to metastatic disease (termed an "abscopal effect"). Reports of an abscopal effect of RT date back to as early as the 1950s to 1970s.[3–6] After widespread speculations of the underlying mechanism, data supporting an immune-mediated mechanism came from seminal studies in mouse models where immune-deficient mice could not produce an abscopal response.[7] A pivotal report of a RT-induced abscopal response that induced ICI sensitivity in a resistant patient opened the floodgates of interest in the abscopal effect and in combining RT and immunotherapy.[8] It appeared that we had cracked the formula to inducing abscopal responses, and we rapidly moved from bench-to-bedside. In the excitement of the immunotherapy revolution, the number of randomized clinical trials combining immunotherapy and RT rapidly multiplied.[9] However, now a decade on, despite a body of strongly supportive pre-clinical and correlative clinical data, there remains limited clinical evidence from these randomized clinical trials to support the clinical synergy of RT and ICI.[10–15] Despite these missteps, we believe the exploration of combining RT and immunotherapy is only beginning. Radiation therapy has had a long, rich history in cancer treatment spanning over a century, and the immune modulatory effects of RT are firmly established.[2] Reflection on what we have learned and what gaps in knowledge remain, on our successes and failures, will allow us to take a more rational and data-driven approach to advance the field. We can thereby determine how best to exploit the immune modulatory effects of RT and more effectively partner with immunotherapy. We must return to the bench to effectively approach the bedside. In this review, we aim to succinctly summarize the known interactions of radiation and the immune system, explore current strategies of combining RT with immunotherapy, and postulate on future directions for the field.

DISCUSSION
The Tumor Microenvironment

The tumor microenvironment (TME) comprises numerous different cell types with various functions, including tumor-infiltrating immune cells. From an immunologic standpoint, the TME can be viewed as a continuum of archetypes that promote or suppress anti-tumor immunity.[16] Through alterations in DNA, RNA, and protein-misfolding, tumor cells can express novel antigens (neoantigens) that the immune system can recognize as non-self.[17] Concurrently, damage-associated molecular patterns (DAMPs) in the TME can induce the production and release of cytokines such as interferons, which are critical to anti-tumor immunity.[18] For example, DAMPs such as inappropriately exposed DNA and RNA localization into the cellular cytoplasm compartment or release of high mobility group box 1 (HMGB1) into the extracellular matrix can activate pattern recognition receptors such as Cyclic GMP–AMP synthase\Stimulator of interferon genes (cGAS/STING),[19–22] mitochondrial antiviral-signaling protein/etinoic acid-inducible gene I (MAVS/RIG-1),[23–25] and toll-like receptor (TLR) 4[26] respectively, to trigger interferon (IFN) and nuclear factor kappa-light-chain-enhancer of activated B cells (NF-κB) signaling. This signaling recruits immune cells into the TME and activates dendritic cells (DCs), both of which are critical for anti-tumor immunity.[18] DCs, such as CD103+ DCs can migrate from the TME to their respective lymph nodes (LNs) and present tumor neoantigens through major histocompatibility complex (MHC) class I receptors (cross-presentation) to cytotoxic T lymphocytes (CTLs).[27] These CTLs then migrate from the LNs and infiltrate into the TME. These activated CD103+ DCs support CTLs in the TME by producing cytokines such as IL-12.[28] Several studies also suggest that Tim3 signaling and natural killer cells are essential in activating the anti-tumor effects of CD103+ DCs.[27,29,30] Furthermore,

CD103+ DCs may also be necessary to prime T-cells in anti-tumor immunity.[31] Even if the above components are in the right place at the right time, tumors can limit the generation of immune responses. Moreover, various factors in the TME, such as physical (desmoplastic reaction), chemical (pH, nutritional desert), and biological (Treg, myeloid-derived suppressor cells) factors, can limit the efficacy of the generated immune response.[32] For example, a lack of DAMP-induced cytokine production will inhibit the generation of an effective anti-tumor immune response.[18,22] Furthermore, hypoxic regions in the TME can promote T-cell dysfunction and an exhausted T-cell phenotype limiting the efficacy of generated anti-tumor responses.[33] In an ideal situation, all the partners and signals work in concert leading to the eradication of tumor cells by CTLs via cytotoxic degranulation or induction of tumor cell apoptosis.[34] These components are visually summarized in **Fig. 1** left panel. This process may eradicate transformed cells before they become clinically detectable malignancies but generally cannot eliminate established clinically detectable tumors.

The Irradiated Tumor Microenvironment

RT can have pleomorphic effects on the immune compartment of the TME, which can evolve and have been previously reviewed in detail.[35] Initially, radiation therapy can shift multiple aspects of the TME in favor of an immune response (**Fig. 1**). Radiation increases cell stress and immunogenic cell death, causing the release of the DAMPs, resulting in the upregulation of interferons and activation of the inflammatory cascade.[26,36,37] This RT-induced inflammation can increase cytokines and chemokines[38] and alter TME structure[39] to improve homing and diapedesis of immune cells into the TME. This results in a surge of infiltrating immune cells, including the cross-priming dendritic cells[18] and various lymphocytes.[35] RT augments type 1 IFN signaling,[36] TLR expression,[40] and MHCI receptor count and the diversity of peptides presented.[41,42] This acute inflammation is sometimes observed on imaging within days to weeks of radiation administration as slight increases in the size of the irradiated lesion. This pseudoprogression has been best described in intracranial tumors[43] and has recently been used as a marker for response to ICI.[44]

RT may also influence immunity at a subcellular level beyond the induction of DAMPs and cytokines. Cancer cell-intrinsic DNA repair defects, primarily the error-

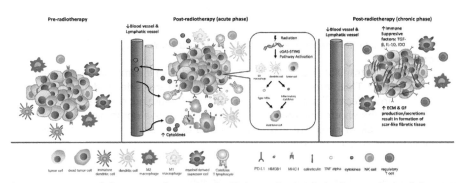

Fig. 1. Overview of the TME. Schematic of cellular and subcellular interactions of the TME demonstrating: a suppressive TME at baseline (pre-RT, left panel); an influx of inflammatory cells and cytokines resulting from stress response to DNA damage (acute post-RT, middle panel); and eventual upregulation of suppressive factors, recruitment of suppressive cells, and fibrosis due to chronic inflammation and rebound immune suppression (chronic post-RT, right panel).

free homologous recombination pathway defects, may push radiation-induced DNA damage toward error-prone repair methods,[45] thereby causing the production of diverse neoantigens.[46,47] These may eventually translate to increased diversity of neo-antigen-specific T-cells and presumably a more effective anti-tumor immune response.[48,49] Indeed, some clinical trial data have suggested that a significant contribution of RT in combination with immunotherapy is to increase T-cell diversity,[50-52] mismatch repair,[53] and microsatellite instability/genomic instability[54] best exemplify these DNA repair defect-dependent reverberations on anti-tumor immune responses. This is visually summarized in **Fig. 1**, middle panel.

However, like many things in biology, RT-induced immune cell infiltration and inflammation can be a double-edged sword. Not all immune cells attracted to the TME after irradiation drive the TME toward tumor cell kill. As the initial burst of acute inflammation wears off and chronic inflammation sets in, spanning weeks to months, immunosuppressive networks may begin to dominate in a process termed "rebound immune suppression".[55,56] The influx of proinflammatory cells gives way to the infiltration of immune suppressive cells. Myeloid-derived suppressor cells, which inhibit T-cells through nutritional depletion[32] and other mechanisms, are seen to increase in the TME weeks after irradiation.[57] Heterogeneous populations of tumor-associated macrophages with M2 polarization can also be upregulated weeks after RT.[58] They can function to inhibit T-cells[59] and produce immunosuppressive cytokines such as vascular endothelial growth factor (VEGF), interleukin-10 (IL-10), and transforming growth factor beta (TGF-β).[60,61] Immune-suppressive regulatory T-cells (Tregs) infiltration can also infiltrate or persist in the TME after the radiation.[55] Master regulators orchestrating immune suppression following RT may involve the upregulation of molecules such as PD-L1[62] and indolamine-2,3,-dioxygenase (IDO).[55,56] Paradoxically, sustained cytokine signaling cascades such as interferon is immune suppressive.[63] These sustained inflammatory pathways leading to chronic inflammation and deleterious effects have also been described after RT.[64,65] Tissue remodeling of the TME also occurs, leading to fibrosis and decreased lymphatic/blood vessels[66] which can limit immune access to the TME. Thus, the duration of inflammatory cascades may be critical, as a burst of interferon is proinflammatory, whereas chronic inflammatory cascades promote immune tolerance.[67] This is reflected in patients with preexisting conditions that trigger chronic inflammatory states like obesity leading to chronic immune suppression.[68] This is visually summarized in **Fig. 1**, right panel.

Consideration of immune modulatory effects based on timing, dose, and fractionation

As we attempt to translate our fundamental knowledge of the immunological response of the irradiated TME into clinical practice, we must consider radiation's practical application and effects. Thus, here we will consider the timing, dose, and fractionation of RT. Among the shortcomings of our initial clinical forays combining RT and immunotherapy, a lack of sufficient investigation and consideration of these variables is arguably the most conspicuous.

Timing. Several studies have reported meaningful abscopal responses when combining immunotherapy and RT. Pre-clinical studies have shown that the timing of immunotherapy can impact efficacy.[69] In one study, tumor-bearing mice were treated with 20 Gy combined with either an anti-cytotoxic T-lymphocyte associated protein 4 (CTLA4) antibody or anti-OX40 (CD134) agonist antibody at a single time point around the delivery of radiation.[70] They found that the ideal timing depended on the mechanism of action of the immunotherapy agent, with anti-CTLA4 being most effective when given before RT due to depletion of regulatory T-cells and anti-OX40 agonist antibody being most effective when given 1 day following RT during the period of increased antigen presentation. Meanwhile, another study found that anti-PD-L1 antibodies have higher efficacy when delivered concurrently with RT.[71] Ongoing clinical studies use regimens that start immunotherapy before, after, and concurrent with RT treatment generally without a strong rationale for the timing. More pre-clinical and clinical trials evaluating how the timing of therapies can influence the synergy of RT in combination with various immunotherapy agents will clarify the ideal timing. It is also possible that this will depend to an extent on the tumor type, the type of immunotherapy, and the status of the TME.

Dose and fractionation. Similarly, there is no established consensus on the optimal dose and fractionation of RT in combination with immunotherapy to maximize efficacy and generate an abscopal effect. Different RT regimens are likely to produce distinct immune modulatory effects.[69] One frequently cited study compared three regimens on mouse breast tumors, specifically 20 Gy in a single fraction, 8 Gy x 3 fractions, and 6 Gy x 5 fractions. Their findings suggested that hypofractionated RT was better at stimulating anti-tumor immune responses in combination with anti-CTLA4, with the 8 Gy x 3 being the most effective.[72] Alternatively, single ablative doses of RT (>20 Gy) have been shown to substantially increase T-cell priming, CD8+ T-cell infiltration, and tumor regression in breast, lung, and melanoma mouse models.[73] High-dose RT is hypothesized to be required for an efficient immune response by showering the immune system with antigens. However, there is pre-clinical evidence that doses above 10 Gy may reduce immune response via induction of DNA exonuclease TREX1.[37] Conversely, it has been posited that ablative stereotactic body radiotherapy (SBRT) doses promote more immunogenic changes in the TME[74] due to the promotion of cell death by necrosis and senescence, which is considered a more immunogenic form of cell death compared with apoptosis.[26] It has been shown that conventional fractionation might reduce tumor-infiltrating CD8+ T-cells during treatment due to radiation-induced cell death of tumor-infiltrating, immune-effector cells.[74] Finally, a recent meta-analysis of pre-clinical studies suggests that the higher biologically effective dose (BED) (greater than 60) are most effective at inducing the abscopal effects of RT.[75] Ultimately, the complexity of radiation dose, fractionation, type, and volume does not support a "one-size-fits-all" approach. Emerging data suggest that dose and fractionation may need to be tailored to tumor characteristics and the type of immunotherapy used.[69]

Future study. Future studies should further optimize RT delivery to maximize the immunomodulatory benefit. Further pre-clinical and clinical studies evaluating the influence of these variables on RT-induced immune modulation and the effects of combined radio-immunotherapy are needed. Efforts should also evaluate methods to avoid lymphopenia commonly observed during and following clinical RT, which can negate RT-induced pro-immunogenic effects.[76] One option is to prevent elective nodal radiation in cases where it is not clinically indicated. In addition, FLASH RT (FLASH-RT) delivers radiation treatment at an ultra-high-dose rate. Although computational modeling supports the case for FLASH-RT sparing effect on circulating immune cells, there are limited biological studies investigating the impact of FLASH-RT on circulating immune cells and the TME.[77] Studies further evaluating a combination of FLASH-RT and immunotherapeutic agents in pre-clinical tumor models are needed. In addition to FLASH-RT, future studies should work on identifying the ideal metastatic site (or sites) to treat, the number of sites to treat, and the effects of intentional partial tumor radiation (lattice therapy) to optimize immune system activation and synergy with immunotherapy.[78]

Clinical Studies

Combination immunotherapy and radiotherapy for locally advanced malignancies

There have been increasing efforts to incorporate immunotherapy into the standard of care for locally advanced malignancies, where RT is already part of the treatment paradigm. The PACIFIC trial presented the most significant results to date. The double-blinded phase III trial demonstrated the impact of durvalumab when delivered sequentially after chemoradiotherapy (CRT) for stage III non-small cell lunng cancer (NSCLC). The 18-month progression-free survival (PFS) increased from 27.0% to 44.2%, and the overall survival (OS) was significantly prolonged with a hazard ratio of 0.68.[79] In support of the above data regarding the importance of timing, the analysis of timing demonstrated patients with delayed initiation of ICI derived less benefit. The addition of immunotherapy to CRT is now the standard of care in the management of unresectable stage III NSCLC. Another practice-changing trial in locally advanced esophageal or gastroesophageal junction cancer was Keynote 577[80] which demonstrated that the addition of nivolumab to trimodality therapy in patients with residual viable disease on pathology doubled the disease free survival (DFS) from 11 months (95% CI: 8.3, 14.3) to 22.4 months (95% CI: 16.6, 34.0; HR 0.69; 95% CI: 0.56, 0.85; $P = 0.0003$).

Despite these gains, there have been many failures. For example, locally advanced rectal cancer has also been the subject of multiple combination immunotherapy–RT trials, given the proven benefit of neoadjuvant RT. In NRG Oncology GI002, Rahma and colleagues[81] randomized 185 patients with locally advanced rectal cancer to total neoadjuvant therapy (including chemoradiation) with or without pembrolizumab and found that whereas this combination was suggested to be safe, the neoadjuvant rectal score difference (a measure of response to neoadjuvant therapy) did not support further study. Other trials in this space also failed to conclusively demonstrate the benefit of the addition of ICI.[82] Results of studies investigating the combination of immunotherapy and RT in the curative intent treatment of other locally advanced malignancies have also been equivocal.

Combination of immunotherapy and radiotherapy for metastatic disease

Numerous studies have evaluated the combination immunotherapy + RT in treating metastatic disease and a comprehensive review of all of these is beyond the scope of this discussion. Studies in melanoma and lung cancer have been at the forefront and an examination of these may provide some insights. In metastatic melanoma, a systematic review of 451 patients from 16 studies evaluating the incidence of the abscopal effect in patients treated with RT and ipilimumab (ipi) found that the median abscopal response rate and OS were 26.5% and 19 months, and the median survival for patients with abscopal responses was significantly longer at 22.4 months compared with 8.3 months in patients without abscopal responses. The authors concluded that combining ipilimumab and RT may improve survival in patients with metastatic melanoma.[83] Further, a retrospective analysis of 101 patients with metastatic melanoma who received ipilimumab showed that median OS was significantly increased in those treated with concurrent RT compared with those treated with ipi alone (19 vs 10 months, $P = 0.01$). Rates of complete response were also significantly higher in the ipi-RT group at 25.7% versus 6.5% in the ipi alone group ($P = 0.04$).[84] In the setting of metastatic NSCLC treated with ICI targeting PD-1/PD-L1 results have been equivocal. PEMBRO-RT is a phase II trial that randomized 92 patients with metastatic NSCLC to pembrolizumab alone or pembrolizumab after 8 Gy x 3 to a single tumor site which found a trend toward improved overall response rate (ORR) at 12 weeks from 18% in the control arm to 36% in the experimental arm ($P = 0.07$).

Median PFS was significantly longer after the addition of RT from 1.9 months to 6.6 months ($P = 0.019$) and OS from 7.6 months to 15.9 months.[15] The PD-L1-negative subgroup largely influenced these results, and this trial failed to meet its primary endpoint. However, the results from the PD-L1-negative subgroup have led to a larger randomized phase II/III trial combining SBRT with immunotherapy or chemoimmunotherapy in this PD-L1-negative patient population (Alliance A082002). Furthermore, a combined analysis of 148 NSCLC patients treated with pembrolizumab versus pembrolizumab and RT, pooled from the PEMBRO-RT trial and the MD Anderson Cancer Center (MDACC) trial, demonstrated a significant increase in abscopal responses (19·7% vs 41·7%, odds ratio [OR] 2·96, 95% CI 1·42–6·20; $P = 0·0039$), and median overall survival (8·7 months vs 19·2 months; $P = 0·0004$) with the addition of RT (PMID: 33096027).

A phase 2 multicenter study for patients with NSCLC with progression during the previous PD(L)-1 therapy randomized patients 1:1:1 to durvalumab plus tremelimumab alone or with low-dose RT (0.5 Gy delivered twice daily repeated 2 days during each of the first four cycles of therapy) or with hypofractionated RT (8 Gy x 3 fractions during the first cycle only) 1 week after initial durvalumab–tremelimumab administration. Although the treatments were able to induce a response in patients previously resistant to single-agent ICI, there were no differences in overall response rates among all three arms, demonstrating no benefit of RT in addition to dual ICI.[11] It is unclear if the differences among the above-quoted studies are to be attributed to the difference in melanoma versus NSCLC or differences in targeting CTLA-4 versus PD-1/PD-L1. Given the differences in mechanism, with CTLA-4 inhibitors targeting regulatory T-cells and the priming phase of the T-cell response versus PD-1/PD-L1 inhibitors targeting the effector phase, a better understanding of how RT partners with each of these ICI strategies individually, and as dual ICI, is needed.

(Not so) Novel approaches

The immunotherapy revolution is not limited to ICI, although our attempts at combining immunotherapy + RT largely have been in the setting of combinations with ICI. It is possible that ICI is not the most synergistic immunotherapy partner for RT, and additional pre-clinical and clinical evaluations of novel combinations are needed. RT alone rarely induces abscopal responses indicating that its immunomodulatory effects may not be strong enough to induce a vaccine effect. It is therefore possible, that as opposed to ICI which aims at reversing immune suppression, RT will better partner with immuno-stimulatory therapies. Agonists of stimulatory T-cell co-receptors, vaccine approaches, and cellular therapies are also promising partners for RT. The use of cytokines and bacterial products to stimulate an inflammatory anti-tumor response are among the oldest immunotherapy approaches. The pre-clinical and clinical data combining RT with these type of approaches have been very encouraging and represent some of the most promising clinical results combining RT + immunotherapy.[55,85,86]

SUMMARY

The focus of this review has been to highlight a few key areas where improved attempts at combining RT + immunotherapy are needed.

- First, although pre-clinical and clinical data clearly demonstrate the immune modulatory effects of RT, much of the clinical data to date is equivocal in terms of a clinical benefit to combining RT + immunotherapy. A majority of the clinical data is limited to phase I/II trials that lack proper control arms and in-depth correlative assays, restricting our ability to differentiate between the systemic effects of immunotherapy and RT out-of-field effects.

- Second, we do not fully understand how practical parameters of RT delivery (site and number of lesions, dose, fractionation, timing) influence its immune modulatory effects, and therefore, how it should optimally be combined with immunotherapy.
- Third, much of our effort has been focused on combining RT with anti-PD-1/PD-L1 ICI but it is possible that other ICIs or other immunotherapy strategies may better partner with RT.

Other topics not discussed in this review also need to be considered. The incongruity between the pre-clinical studies and the clinical reality of combining radiation therapy and immunotherapy may also be explained by a mismatch between our pre-clinical models and clinical patients. For instance, most animal models employ adolescent mice implanted with syngeneic tumor cells or young genetically engineered mice which do not reflect the cellular evolution of clinical malignancy and the complexity of human cancer patients. The next wave of advances in combining RT and immunotherapy will require a bedside back-to-the-bench approach where more clinically-relevant pre-clinical models and evaluation of correlative samples from current clinical studies address the gaps in knowledge and provide rational design for the next generation of RT + immunotherapy clinical trials. Eventually, combining RT + immunotherapy is likely to be most efficacious after several iterations of a "bench-to-bedside and back again" approach which will allow us to take a precision medicine approach where the RT dose, timing, irradiated site(s), and immunotherapy partner are tailored to the TME, genetic, metabolic, and immune characteristics of each patient.

FUNDING SOURCE

A.M. Monjazeb was supported by R01CA240751.

DISCLOSURE

A.M. Monjazeb research support: Merck, BMS, Transgene, Incyte, Trisalus, Genentech. *A.M. Monjazeb Consulting fees:* Zosano. *A.M. Monjazeb Advisory boards:* BMS, AstraZeneca, Incyte, Dynavax. *AMM Stock options:* MultiplexThera.

REFERENCES

1. Dillekås H, Rogers MS, Straume O. Are 90% of deaths from cancer caused by metastases? Cancer Med 2019;8(12):5574–6.
2. Weichselbaum RR, Liang H, Deng L, et al. Radiotherapy and immunotherapy: a beneficial liaison? Nat Rev Clin Oncol 2017;14(6):365–79.
3. Mole RH. Whole body irradiation; radiobiology or medicine? Br J Radiol 1953; 26(305):234–41.
4. Nobler MP. The abscopal effect in malignant lymphoma and its relationship to lymphocyte circulation. Radiology 1969;93(2):410–2.
5. Ehlers G, Fridman M. Abscopal effect of radiation in papillary adenocarcinoma. Br J Radiol 1973;46(543):220–2.
6. Kingsley DP. An interesting case of possible abscopal effect in malignant melanoma. Br J Radiol 1975;48(574):863–6.
7. Demaria S., Ng B., Devitt M.L., et al., Ionizing radiation inhibition of distant untreated tumors (abscopal effect) is immune mediated, Int J Radiat Oncol Biol Phys, 58 (3), 2004, 862–870.

8. Postow M.A., Callahan M.K., Barker C.A., et al., Immunologic correlates of the ab-scopal effect in a patient with melanoma, N Engl J Med, 366 (10), 2012, 925–931.
9. Daly ME, Monjazeb AM, Kelly K. Clinical trials integrating immunotherapy and ra-diation for non-small-cell lung cancer. J Thorac Oncol 2015;10(12):1685–93.
10. McBride S., Sherman E., Tsai C.J., et al., Randomized phase II trial of nivolumab with stereotactic body radiotherapy versus nivolumab alone in metastatic head and neck squamous cell carcinoma, J Clin Oncol, 39 (1), 2021, 30–37.
11. Schoenfeld J.D., Giobbie-Hurder A., Ranasinghe S., et al., Durvalumab plus tremelimumab alone or in combination with low-dose or hypofractionated radio-therapy in metastatic non-small-cell lung cancer refractory to previous PD(L)-1 therapy: an open-label, multicentre, randomised, phase 2 trial, Lancet Oncol, 23 (2), 2022, 279–291.
12. Pakkala S., Higgins K., Chen Z., et al., Durvalumab and tremelimumab with or without stereotactic body radiation therapy in relapsed small cell lung cancer: a randomized phase II study,Immunother Cancer, 8 (2), 2020, e001302, doi:10.1136/jitc-2020-001302.
13. Welsh J, Menon H, Chen D, et al. Pembrolizumab with or without radiation therapy for metastatic non-small cell lung cancer: a randomized phase I/II trial. J Immun-other Cancer 2020;8(2):e001001. https://doi.org/10.1136/jitc-2020-001001.
14. Theelen W., Chen D., Verma V., et al., Pembrolizumab with or without radiotherapy for metastatic non-small-cell lung cancer: a pooled analysis of two randomised trials, Lancet Respir Med, 9 (5), 2021, 467–475.
15. Theelen W., Peulen H.M.U., Lalezari F., et al., effect of pembrolizumab after ste-reotactic body radiotherapy vs pembrolizumab alone on tumor response in pa-tients with advanced non-small cell lung cancer: results of the PEMBRO-RT Phase 2 randomized clinical trial, JAMA Oncol, 5 (9), 2019, 1276–1282.
16. Mujal AM, Krummel MF. Immunity as a continuum of archetypes. Science 2019; 364(6435):28–9.
17. Wells D.K., van Buuren MM., Dang K.K., et al., key parameters of tumor epitope immunogenicity revealed through a consortium approach improve neoantigen prediction, Cell, 183 (3), 2020, 818–834.e13.
18. Fuertes M.B., Kacha A.K., Kline J., et al., Host type I IFN signals are required for antitumor CD8+ T cell responses through CD8{alpha}+ dendritic cells, J Exp Med, 208 (10), 2011, 2005–2016.
19. Guillerme JB, Boisgerault N, Roulois D, et al. Measles virus vaccine-infected tu-mor cells induce tumor antigen cross-presentation by human plasmacytoid den-dritic cells. Clin Cancer Res 2013;19(5):1147–58.
20. Dunn GP, Bruce AT, Sheehan KCF, et al. A critical function for type I interferons in cancer immunoediting. Nat Immunol 2005;6(7):722–9.
21. Dighe AS, Richards E, Old LJ, et al. Enhanced in vivo growth and resistance to rejection of tumor cells expressing dominant negative IFNγ receptors. Immunity 1994;1(6):447–56.
22. Woo S.-R., Fuertes M.B., Corrales L., et al., STING-dependent cytosolic DNA sensing mediates innate immune recognition of immunogenic tumors, Immunity, 41 (5), 2014, 830–842.
23. Kim Y, Lee JH, Park JE, et al. PKR is activated by cellular dsRNAs during mitosis and acts as a mitotic regulator. Genes Dev 2014;28(12):1310–22.
24. Ahmad S., Mu X., Yang F., et al., Breaching self-tolerance to Alu Duplex RNA un-derlies MDA5-mediated inflammation, Cell, 172 (4), 2018, 797–810.e13.

25. Michallet M.C., Meylan E., Ermolaeva M.A., et al., TRADD protein is an essential component of the RIG-like helicase antiviral pathway, Immunity, 28 (5), 2008, 651–661.

26. Apetoh L., Ghiringhelli F., Tesniere A., et al., Toll-like receptor 4-dependent contribution of the immune system to anticancer chemotherapy and radiotherapy, Nat Med, 13 (9), 2007, 1050–1059.

27. de Mingo Pulido Á., Gardner A., Hiebler S., et al., TIM-3 regulates CD103(+) dendritic cell function and response to chemotherapy in breast cancer, Cancer Cell, 33 (1), 2018, 60–74.e6.

28. Sharma M.D., Rodriguez P.C., Koehn B.H., et al., Activation of p53 in immature myeloid precursor cells controls differentiation into Ly6c(+)CD103(+) monocytic antigen-presenting cells in tumors, Immunity, 48 (1), 2018, 91–106.e6.

29. Böttcher J.P., Bonavita E., Chakravarty P., et al., NK cells stimulate recruitment of cDC1 into the tumor microenvironment promoting cancer immune control, Cell, 172 (5), 2018, 1022–1037.e14.

30. Barry K.C., Hsu J., Broz M.L., et al., A natural killer–dendritic cell axis defines checkpoint therapy–responsive tumor microenvironments, Nat Med, 24 (8), 2018, 1178–1191.

31. Ferris S.T., Durai V., Wu R., et al., cDC1 prime and are licensed by CD4(+) T cells to induce anti-tumour immunity, Nature, 584 (7822), 2020, 624–629.

32. Gabrilovich DI, Nagaraj S. Myeloid-derived suppressor cells as regulators of the immune system. Nat Rev Immunol 2009;9(3):162–74.

33. Scharping N.E., Rivadeneira D.B., Menk A.V., et al., Mitochondrial stress induced by continuous stimulation under hypoxia rapidly drives T cell exhaustion, Nat Immunol, 22 (2), 2021, 205–215.

34. Martínez-Lostao L, Anel A, Pardo J. how do cytotoxic lymphocytes kill cancer cells? Clin Cancer Res 2015;21(22):5047–56.

35. Monjazeb A.M., Schalper K.A., Villarroel-Espindola F., et al., Effects of radiation on the tumor microenvironment, Semin Radiat Oncol, 30 (2), 2020, 145–157.

36. Burnette BC, Liang H, Lee Y, et al. The efficacy of radiotherapy relies upon induction of type i interferon-dependent innate and adaptive immunity. Cancer Res 2011;71(7):2488–96.

37. Vanpouille-Box C, Alard A, Aryankalayil MJ, et al. DNA exonuclease Trex1 regulates radiotherapy-induced tumour immunogenicity. Nat Commun 2017;8:15618.

38. Matsumura S, Wang B, Kawashima N, et al. Radiation-induced CXCL16 release by breast cancer cells attracts effector T cells. J Immunol 2008;181(5):3099–107.

39. Ganss R., Ryschich E., Klar E., et al., Combination of T-cell therapy and trigger of inflammation induces remodeling of the vasculature and tumor eradication, Cancer Res, 62 (5), 2002, 1462–1470.

40. Yoneyama M, Onomoto K, Jogi M, et al. Viral RNA detection by RIG-I-like receptors. Curr Opin Immunol 2015;32:48–53.

41. Sharma A, Bode B, Studer G, et al. Radiotherapy of human sarcoma promotes an intratumoral immune effector signature. Clin Cancer Res 2013;19(17):4843–53.

42. Reits E.A., Hodge J.M., Herberts C.A., et al., Radiation modulates the peptide repertoire, enhances MHC class I expression, and induces successful antitumor immunotherapy, J Exp Med, 203 (5), 2006, 1259–1271.

43. Thust SC, van den Bent MJ, Smits M. Pseudoprogression of brain tumors. J Magn Reson Imaging 2018;48(3):571–89.

44. Butner J.D., Elganainy D., Wang C.X., et al., Mathematical prediction of clinical outcomes in advanced cancer patients treated with checkpoint inhibitor immunotherapy, Sci Adv, 6 (18), 2020, eaay6298.

45. Chatterjee N, Walker GC. Mechanisms of DNA damage, repair, and mutagenesis. Environ Mol Mutagen 2017;58(5):235–63.
46. Chae Y.K., Anker J.F., Oh M.S., et al., Mutations in DNA repair genes are associated with increased neoantigen burden and a distinct immunophenotype in lung squamous cell carcinoma, Sci Rep, 9 (1), 2019, 3235.
47. Lippert TP, Greenberg RA. The abscopal effect: a sense of DNA damage is in the air. J Clin Invest 2021;131(9).
48. van Rooij N, van Buuren MM, Philips D, et al. Tumor exome analysis reveals neoantigen-specific T-cell reactivity in an ipilimumab-responsive melanoma. J Clin Oncol 2013;31(32):e439–42.
49. Matsushita H., Vesely M.D., Koboldt D.C., et al., Cancer exome analysis reveals a T-cell-dependent mechanism of cancer immunoediting, Nature, 482 (7385), 2012, 400–404.
50. Twyman-Saint Victor C., Rech A.J., Maity A., et al., Radiation and dual checkpoint blockade activate non-redundant immune mechanisms in cancer, Nature, 520 (7547), 2015, 373–377.
51. Monjazeb A.M., Giobbie-Hurder A., Lako A., et al., a randomized trial of combined PD-L1 and CTLA-4 inhibition with targeted low-dose or hypofractionated radiation for patients with metastatic colorectal cancer, Clin Cancer Res, 27 (9), 2021, 2470–2480.
52. Rudqvist N.P., Pilones K.A., Lhuillier C., et al., Radiotherapy and CTLA-4 blockade shape the TCR repertoire of tumor-infiltrating T cells, Cancer Immunol Res, 6 (2), 2018, 139–150.
53. Lu C., Guan J., Lu S., et al., DNA sensing in mismatch repair-deficient tumor cells is essential for anti-tumor immunity, Cancer Cell, 39 (1), 2021, 96–108.e6.
54. Roudko V., Bozkus C.C., Orfanelli T., et al., shared immunogenic poly-epitope frameshift mutations in microsatellite unstable tumors, Cell, 183 (6), 2020, 1634–1649.e17.
55. Monjazeb A.M., Michael S. Kent, Steven K. Grossenbacher, et al., Blocking indolamine-2,3-dioxygenase rebound immune suppression boosts antitumor effects of radio-immunotherapy in murine models and spontaneous canine malignancies, Clin Cancer Res, 22 (17), 2016, 4328–4340.
56. Li A., Barsoumian H.B., Schoenhals J.E., et al., ido1 inhibition overcomes radiation-induced "rebound immune suppression" by reducing numbers of IDO1-expressing myeloid-derived suppressor cells in the tumor microenvironment, Int J Radiat Oncol Biol Phys, 104 (4), 2019, 903–912.
57. Xu J, Escamilla J, Mok S, et al. CSF1R signaling blockade stanches tumor-infiltrating myeloid cells and improves the efficacy of radiotherapy in prostate cancer. Cancer Res 2013;73(9):2782–94.
58. Crittenden MR, Baird J, Friedman D, et al. Mertk on tumor macrophages is a therapeutic target to prevent tumor recurrence following radiation therapy. Oncotarget 2016;7(48):78653–66.
59. Mira E, Carmona-Rodríguez L, Tardáguila M, et al. A lovastatin-elicited genetic program inhibits M2 macrophage polarization and enhances T cell infiltration into spontaneous mouse mammary tumors. Oncotarget 2013;4(12):2288–301.
60. Fadok VA, Bratton DL, Konowal A, et al. Macrophages that have ingested apoptotic cells in vitro inhibit proinflammatory cytokine production through autocrine/paracrine mechanisms involving TGF-beta, PGE2, and PAF. J Clin Invest 1998;101(4):890–8.

61. Saccani A, Schioppa T, Porta C, et al. p50 nuclear factor-kappaB overexpression in tumor-associated macrophages inhibits M1 inflammatory responses and anti-tumor resistance. Cancer Res 2006;66(23):11432–40.
62. Deng L, Liang H, Burnette B, et al. Irradiation and anti-PD-L1 treatment synergistically promote antitumor immunity in mice. J Clin Invest 2014;124(2):687–95.
63. Benci J.L., Johnson L.R., Choa R., et al., opposing functions of interferon coordinate adaptive and innate immune responses to cancer immune checkpoint blockade, Cell, 178 (4), 2019, 933–948.e14.
64. Halle M, Gabrielsen A, Paulsson-Berne G, et al. Sustained inflammation due to nuclear factor-kappa B activation in irradiated human arteries. J Am Coll Cardiol 2010;55(12):1227–36.
65. Zhao W, Robbins ME. Inflammation and chronic oxidative stress in radiation-induced late normal tissue injury: therapeutic implications. Curr Med Chem 2009;16(2):130–43.
66. Avraham T, Yan A, Zampell JC, et al. Radiation therapy causes loss of dermal lymphatic vessels and interferes with lymphatic function by TGF-β1-mediated tissue fibrosis. Am J Physiol Cell Physiol 2010;299(3):C589–605.
67. Bakhoum S.F., Ngo B., Laughney A.M., et al., Chromosomal instability drives metastasis through a cytosolic DNA response, Nature, 553 (7689), 2018, 467–472.
68. Wang Z., Aguilar E.G., Luna J.I., et al., Paradoxical effects of obesity on T cell function during tumor progression and PD-1 checkpoint blockade, Nat Med, 25 (1), 2019, 141–151.
69. Demaria S., Guha C., Schoenfeld J., et al., Radiation dose and fraction in immunotherapy: one-size regimen does not fit all settings, so how does one choose?, J Immunother Cancer, 9 (4), 2021 Apr;9(4):e002038. doi: 10.1136/jitc-2020-002038.
70. Young K.H., Baird J.R., Savage T., et al., Optimizing timing of immunotherapy improves control of tumors by hypofractionated radiation therapy, PLoS One, 11 (6), 2016, e0157164.
71. Dovedi SJ, Adlard AL, Lipowska-Bhalla G, et al. Acquired resistance to fractionated radiotherapy can be overcome by concurrent PD-L1 blockade. Cancer Res 2014;74(19):5458–68.
72. Dewan MZ, Galloway AE, Kawashima N, et al. Fractionated but not single-dose radiotherapy induces an immune-mediated abscopal effect when combined with anti-CTLA-4 antibody. Clin Cancer Res 2009;15(17):5379–88.
73. Lee Y, Auh SL, Wang Y, et al. Therapeutic effects of ablative radiation on local tumor require CD8+ T cells: changing strategies for cancer treatment. Blood 2009; 114(3):589–95.
74. Filatenkov A, Baker J, Mueller AMS, et al. ablative tumor radiation can change the tumor immune cell microenvironment to induce durable complete remissions. Clin Cancer Res 2015;21(16):3727–39.
75. Marconi R., Strolin S., Bossi G., et al., A meta-analysis of the abscopal effect in preclinical models: is the biologically effective dose a relevant physical trigger?, PLoS One, 12 (2), 2017, e0171559.
76. Venkatesulu B.P., Mallick S., Lin S.H., et al., A systematic review of the influence of radiation-induced lymphopenia on survival outcomes in solid tumors, Crit Rev Oncol Hematol, 123, 2018, 42–51.
77. Jin J.Y., Gu A., Wang W., et al., Ultra-high dose rate effect on circulating immune cells: a potential mechanism for FLASH effect?, Radiother Oncol, 149, 2020, 55–62.

78. Aliru M.L., Schoenhals J.E., Venkatesulu B.P., et al., Radiation therapy and immunotherapy: what is the optimal timing or sequencing?, Immunotherapy, 10 (4), 2018, 299–316.
79. Antonia SJ, Villegas A, Daniel D, et al. Durvalumab after chemoradiotherapy in stage III non-small-cell lung cancer. N Engl J Med 2017;377(20):1919–29.
80. Kelly R.J., Ajani J.A., Kuzdzal J., et al., Adjuvant nivolumab in resected esophageal or gastroesophageal junction cancer, N Engl J Med, 384 (13), 2021, 1191–1203.
81. Rahma O.E., Yothers G., Hong T.S., et al., Use of Total neoadjuvant therapy for locally advanced rectal cancer: initial results from the pembrolizumab arm of a phase 2 randomized clinical trial, JAMA Oncol, 7 (8), 2021, 1225–1230.
82. Shamseddine A., Zeidan Y.H., El Husseini Z., et al., Efficacy and safety-in analysis of short-course radiation followed by mFOLFOX-6 plus avelumab for locally advanced rectal adenocarcinoma, Radiat Oncol, 15 (1), 2020, 233.
83. Chicas-Sett R., Morales-Orue I., Rodriguez-Abreu D., et al., Combining radiotherapy and ipilimumab induces clinically relevant radiation-induced abscopal effects in metastatic melanoma patients: a systematic review, Clin Transl Radiat Oncol, 9, 2018, 5–11.
84. Koller KM, Mackley HB, Liu J, et al. Improved survival and complete response rates in patients with advanced melanoma treated with concurrent ipilimumab and radiotherapy versus ipilimumab alone. Cancer Biol Ther 2017;18(1):36–42.
85. Brody JD, Ai WZ, Czerwinski DK, et al. In situ vaccination with a TLR9 agonist induces systemic lymphoma regression: a phase I/II study. J Clin Oncol 2010; 28(28):4324–32.
86. Curti B., Crittenden M., Seung S.K., et al., Randomized phase II study of stereotactic body radiotherapy and interleukin-2 versus interleukin-2 in patients with metastatic melanoma, J Immunother Cancer, 8 (1), 2020, 8(1):e000773. doi: 10.1136/jitc-2020-000773.